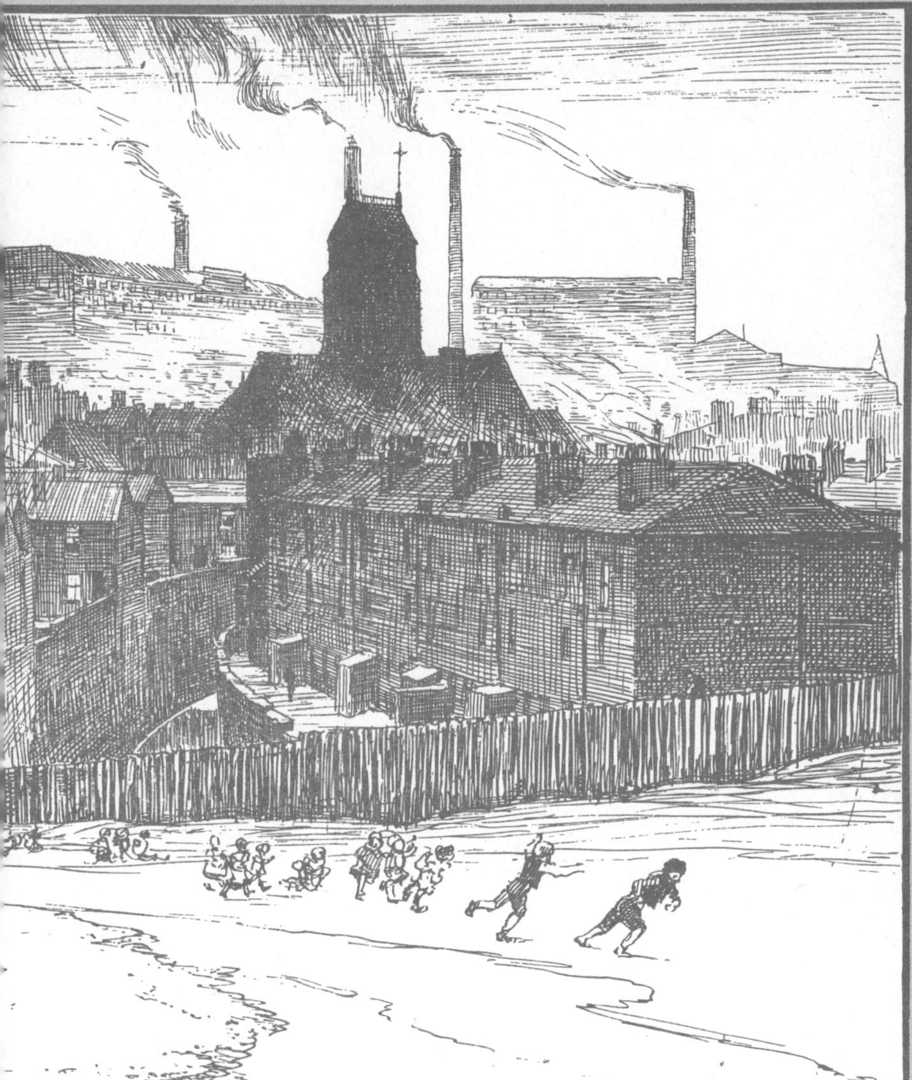

A DOCTOR'S LIFE

ALSO BY DAVID SELBOURNE

Plays

The Play of William Cooper and Edmund Dew-Nevett
The Two-Backed Beast
Dorabella
The Damned
Samson and Alison Mary Fagan

Non fiction

An Eye to India
An Eye to China
Through the Indian Looking-Glass
The Making of A Midsummer Night's Dream
Against Socialist Illusion: A Radical Argument
In Theory and in Practice: Essays on the Politics of
Jayaprakash Narayan (Ed.)
Left Behind: Journeys into British Politics

A DOCTOR'S LIFE

The Diaries of Hugh Selbourne M.D.
1960–63

Edited and with an Introduction by
DAVID SELBOURNE

JONATHAN CAPE
THIRTY-TWO BEDFORD SQUARE LONDON

First published 1989
© David Selbourne 1989
Jonathan Cape Ltd, 32 Bedford Square, London WC1B 3SG

A CIP catalogue record for this book
is available from the British Library

ISBN 0-224-02369-1

Printed in Great Britain by
Mackays of Chatham PLC

For Emilie Selbourne
(b. September 9th, 1965)
and Raphael Selbourne
(b. November 12th, 1968)

CONTENTS

PLATES

between pages 64 and 65

A child in Montmartre
At King's College, London
Dr Hugh Selbourne
Resident Medical Officer at Lewisham Hospital
Locum in London general practice

between pages 96 and 97

Engagement : Hugh and M.
In the Lake District, with Sunbeam Talbot
M. with David and Ruth as small children
Wartime general practitioner with M., at
Dukinfield

between pages 192 and 193

With Lancashire patient

The Family at Dukinfield
Works doctor at Arnfields, near Manchester
At Sherratt and Hughes, the Manchester bookseller

between pages 224 and 225

Worshipful Master of his Masonic Lodge
In Lindos, Rhodes
Dining out with M. in Manchester
Miss James, receptionist at St. John Street
David Selbourne, 1964
M., Judy and Hazel

The endpaper is from a lithograph by Frank L. Emanuel

There is a history in all men's lives . . .

William Shakespeare
Henry IV, Part 2, Act Three, Scene One

INTRODUCTION

As 1960 began, my father – a diarist from the 1930s to the 1970s – was fifty-three, and my mother ('M.') forty-four. He had by then been a doctor for thirty-two years, and a consultant physician since 1951. Though dogged by ill health, he was then at the height of his skills (especially as a diagnostician), securely established as one of 'Lowry-land's' leading doctors, and increasingly confiding to his diaries. I was twenty-two at the time and working in London; my elder sister, Ruth, was twenty and had herself married a doctor the previous June; my younger sister, Judy, was a fourteen-year-old Manchester schoolgirl.

My father wrote little for publication. In 1928, when he was twenty-two, he published a paper on ectopic gestation in the *British Medical Journal*; in 1936, short articles on congenital cysts of the lungs and Addison's disease. That is, essentially, all. Instead, and often late at night, including when he felt ill and exhausted, he made the day's entry in what he variously called his 'diary', his 'journal' and his 'ledger'. In the selection I have made from the years 1960–63, he reveals that he also destroyed 'old diaries', on the ground – so he tells his journal in September 1960 – that they were 'of no interest to others'. Twenty-two months later, in July 1962, he is regretting his earlier action, yet characteristically continuing with the destruction. At the same time, and very ambivalently, he has begun copying some of the interesting past items (from 1935) into the 1962 journal, on the grounds that 'the events are likely to be forgotten if the Diary is destroyed'. Three weeks later, in a turn of emotion typical of him, he resignedly declares that 'no one will read this Diary anyway'.

Yet the sense of personal obligation to his diary-keeping is very strong, and he confides in it increasingly as time passes through the 1960s. Did he really hope, then, that these journals, which he made no attempt to destroy, would one day be read and learned from, even published? Guardedly – for who knows for sure with the diarist? – the answer must be 'yes'. I think the diaries were too meticulously kept, year upon year, with their neat red underlinings, careful accounts, news comments, medical opinions and more-than-medical observations for it all to have been done without ulterior purpose, or at least aspiration.

At his death, and after his library had been taken away for safe-keeping, I found the diaries discarded in his room in a dusty tumble of letters and papers. His manuscript notes and reports on over a thousand of his patients lay abandoned in disorder in a wash-house, where they had been dumped for disposal. Over the next few years, at available moments, these latter papers – which supplement the diaries – I collated, identified and pieced together. Those which were dated, or could be accurately dated, were assembled in chronological order; and since my father each day kept careful note in his diaries of the names of many of the patients he had seen, especially of those who came to his rooms, it was possible to integrate the two sets of sources and thus to reconstitute the record of his daily work and passing observations.

This record provides a self-portrait, a medical portrait of a community, and one observant man's response to a time of flux in the early 1960s. Moreover, there is to be found in the circumstances which brought people down, and hence to my father's attentions, a complex part of the social history of our times, a part which is usually hidden. It was a period of cultural overlap, in which patients who could have stepped from the pages of Dickens, and who were 'bred by the conditions of the industrial revolution', rubbed shoulders with the first generation of post-war working class and welfare state teenagers.

My father was born in 1906 in Montmartre. At the outbreak of the First World War, he came with his parents, grandmother and elder brother to England, with a 'safe conduct' issued by the Military Government of Paris. The family settled in Mount Street, in the East End of London, and lived in humble circumstances. But the two sons of the family, 'driven' by their dressmaker mother, both became doctors, my father a month before his twenty-second birthday in 1928.

A student first at King's College, London, and then at St Bartholomew's Medical School, he went on to take his M.B., B.S. in 1929, gaining the only Distinction in Medicine to be awarded in his year. Even more distinguished were his M.D. (London) and his M.R.C.P., both of which he passed in 1931, and at the first attempt, when he was still only twenty-five. 'I have a very high opinion of his personal qualities and attainments, which I have observed since his student days', Lord Horder, physician-in-ordinary to the King, was to write later. 'He is well-trained, skilled, and scientific in his outlook.'

After a spell as a young assistant in general practice in Dowlais near Merthyr Tydfil, he became House Physician and then Resident Surgical Officer at St Bartholomew's Hospital, Rochester. From 1932 to 1935, he was Resident Medical officer, and unhappy, at Lewisham Hospital in South London, and at the same time Tutor in Medical Pathology at Bart's. At twenty-nine he moved to Southend General Hospital in the more senior post of Medical Registrar. It was at this time, in August 1936, that he married my mother, who had been brought up in a high rabbinical household in Belgium before becoming a student at the Institut Supérieur de Commerce in Antwerp. Nearly ten years her senior, my father at once abandoned his hospital work for general practice and took her north to the old mill-owner's red-brick house, overshadowed by Buckley's towering mill, in the main street of Dukinfield in Cheshire, where I was brought up until the age of fourteen. This was the unhealthy heart of 'Lowry-land', an area with death-rates uniformly above the national average. A fellow practitioner and a close colleague of my father's at the local Ashton Infirmary, Dr Alec Laing of Droylsden, was one of L. S. Lowry's first patrons. The painter died in the Woods Hospital in Glossop in February 1976, a hospital which is often mentioned in this volume.

The family stayed through and beyond the exhausting years of the war in the mill-owner's house amid the huddled terraces – an unlikely Parisian putting down roots in the world of Walter Greenwood's *Love on the Dole*. In summer, in our large house's dark shadows and recesses, I remember roses and garden flowers in cut glass vases, set upon flower stands and small tables. I recall my father among them, head in hands or smoking a cigarette. As for my elegant mother, lost in a grim mill-town and come to a point of no returning, her solitudes were deep beyond all fathoming. 'Your mother was called the "Quiet Lady", on the reserved side', one of my father's former patients told me.

In February 1948, my father became a consulting Honorary Physician to the Ashton Infirmary, a voluntary hospital founded in 1859 by philanthropic mill-owners. Yet, almost immediately after the introduction of the National Health Service in July of that year, what he called a 'bureaucratic stroke of the pen' demoted him, despite his qualifications, from his consultant's post. It led to a bitter three-year struggle for reinstatement, championed by the local Labour MP, the Revd Gordon Lang, in which the Minister of Health, Aneurin Bevan, had eventually to intervene on his behalf. He was restored to his post in November 1951, wearied by the battle and beginning to show the early symptoms of his long illness.

Nevertheless, from 1952 onwards, the pattern of his mature medical work and personal life, as it is reflected in this volume, quickly became settled. He was by then installed, as paterfamilias, in a large Edwardian house in a leafy south Manchester suburb, filled with the thousands of books he had collected. He was now a senior consultant physician to the Ashton, Hyde and Glossop group of hospitals, and also became visiting works' doctor at the Audenshaw engineering firm of Arnfield's. Day after day he was called out by local general practitioners (many of them friends) to give a consultant's judgment, a second opinion, under the system of 'domiciliary' or home visits funded by the Health Service. Besides these visits, which took him to every corner of the cotton district, he also had a considerable practice at his rooms in Manchester's St John Street (a Lancashire Harley Street) where he conducted life insurance examinations, carried on his medico-legal work and saw his private patients, many of whom were 'ordinary' working people.

In 1953, at the age of forty-seven, another pattern was set: he suffered a coronary thrombosis. 'What is this I hear about you, heart trouble?', wrote a former medical colleague, who had retired to London. 'You have been overdoing it for many years now, working night and day, giving yourself no rest and rushing about like a torpedo destroyer. To make matters worse, your pleasures have been as strenuous as your work.'

My recollection of him in the 1950s and early 1960s is somewhat different; a memory of a plump, but dapper, hurrying figure with thinning hair, who possessed a kind of Napoleonic gusto, by turns ebullient and in depression. At times he was jovial, amusing, debonair even, eyes twinkling; at other times inaccessible or despairing. He could be harsh in his judgments, but was always deeply caring and conscientious; conventional in some matters, aggressively rebellious and 'anti-Establishment' in others. He sought advancement for himself, but was often hostile to privilege and the abuse of privilege in others. A sociable man who did not easily share confidences, he could be coldly patriarchal and remotely proud in some private moods. In his work, he was a plain dealer, an entirely unsnobbish 'common man' – 'straight', 'down to earth', his patients called him.

Above all, he was dedicated to his patients and was loved for it. 'He was a friend to hundreds of people, he knew his customers, he was smashing', was one view; Lord Horder said of him that his 'human approach' to his patients was 'one of his chief assets'. But he was feared, too, for his sardonic impatience and angry swearing.

His intellectual interests, his enthusiasms and his reading, as the diaries reveal, were as wide-ranging as his prodigious library, and his friendships likewise. In particular, the news media of all kinds were a passion; he found time, most days, to make a record – however brief – of what he thought important in passing political events. Here, his judgment (a kind of diagnosis) is striking: his eye is for significant detail, whether in a patient's presenting symptoms or in the world's larger actions. Convulsively busy though he usually was, the diaries of the 1960s also show the importance to him of the information and stimulus he obtained from the BBC's

Panorama and *Tonight*, from the arts programme *Monitor*, from the *Face to Face* interviews conducted by John Freeman, and from the satirical television programme *That Was The Week That Was*.

Names like Alan Whicker, Robin Day, James Mossman recur frequently in his diaries. What they had to say about the changing world was important to him. If my father is a reliable example (who knows?) of the audience of the time which assiduously watched and learned from them, then their cultural impact must have been a large one; the kind of impact which has arguably much diminished now, a quarter of a century later. He was an avid reader above all of the *Manchester Guardian*, as it then was. It was as if he could not exist without it, just as he could not exist without broadcast classical music, the Hallé Orchestra and John Barbirolli. When the *Manchester Guardian* had been thrown out in error on one occasion, before his return home and before he had read it, the loss was serious.

In the editing of this volume, ''tis not the persons themselves, 'tis the example that is the thing aimed at' (as Daniel Defoe wrote in 1722, in one of the two books he wrote on the plague). Thus, I have been careful throughout to conceal the identities of all those – doctors, nurses, patients and hospital administrators – who had professional dealings with my father, giving them false initials randomly chosen. No other particular has been falsified. I have everywhere preferred omission to alteration, since it is important that this be a true record. Friends who did not have a professional relationship with him are mentioned sometimes by their first names followed by an initial, sometimes by their surnames; relatives by their first names only; public figures, employees and tradesmen – provided they were not also his patients – usually have their names given in full. As to the original documents, the diaries and papers, no one but me has been permitted to read them. Once my editorial work has been completed, they will be lodged in a secure place and sealed for twenty-five years from the date of publication of this volume.

Finally, I must acknowledge my principal debts. My first is to Graham C. Greene, for suggesting the form of this book to me and for his continuous encouragement of my work on it.

My second is to Tony Colwell and Judy Cooke, of Jonathan Cape, for their expert editorial advice and knowledge. My third, and greatest, is to my wife, for the constancy of her support, help and insight, as we reconsidered the past together. I would also like to record my gratitude to Dr B. S. Benedikz and Miss Christine Penney of the University of Birmingham for the help they gave me with bibliographical information and to Drs Sidney Agnew and Renwick Vickers for answering my medical queries, some of which arose from difficulties in deciphering my father's medical abbreviations. Mr S. F. Griffiths of Arnfield's was also helpful. Responsibility for all error is mine.

D. S.
April 1989

1960

Jan 14   Snow on the ground. Very cold. Anniversary of my father's death. Memorial light kindled. Ward round, 14, and to St. John St. Miss James [*receptionist and factotum*] nearly choked while gorging a large chunk of toast and being rude: eating and talking at the same time. Saw 5 cases.

2:15 p.m. [*Male, aged 20, single, bus conductor*] Riding his motor-cycle he collided with a car and lacerated his right knee three months ago. Eighteen stitches were inserted into the lacerations around the right knee-joint. He was off work for one month. On examination, he was a healthy young lad – who served in the RAF from 1956 to 1959 – but said that his knee 'still keeps aching after a day's work running up and down the stairs'. There was no swelling of the knee to be observed, and there was full range of movement. His scars were pigmented, but had healed soundly.

3:0 p.m. [*Male, aged 21, paper-mill worker*] He was a sallow young man, with some dilated venules on his cheeks, who lives with his parents. Eight months after 'signing up' in a Guards' regiment – 'for more experience' – he developed pains in his right ankle and in both shoulders. The pains became generalized in all his joints, he had severe pains in his chest, and his fingers and toes became stiff and painful. He was in bed for four months, suffering from acute rheumatic fever. On recovery, he was discharged from the Service, with a pension of 15/- a week for the next two years (followed by a final gratuity of £75), and a good character reference. He found a job fairly quickly at the Paper Mill. However, he had to work in steam and damp conditions, which caused him intermittent pain in the shoulders and ankles. He has therefore recently been transferred to another Department, but his pay has diminished from 5/- to 3/7d an hour.

[*Before decimalization there were 12 pence in one shilling and 20 shillings to the pound. Thus 5/- (five shillings) was equivalent to 25p today and 3/7d (three shillings and seven pence) to just under 18p.*]

Today, his hands were moist and clammy, creaking sounds could be obtained at both shoulder joints, and his left ankle was swollen. His pulse and blood pressure were normal, but over the apex of the heart there was a late diastolic murmur. His presenting symptoms are those of sub-acute rheumatism, but he has valvular disease of the heart, a consequence of his rheumatic fever. Although of mild degree at present, it is steadily progressive. In addition, one attack of rheumatic fever predisposes to another.

Jan 15　　Took Judy [*daughter*] to school, and thereafter to two domiciliaries: hypertension and congestive heart failure (aet [*aged*] 62, Hyde), and left pleural effusion (aet 37, Hyde, admitted). Ward round 15; lunch at 'The Organ', Hollingsworth, with Tony T. and George W. [*friends*]; and lengthy medical out-patients. Purchased fruit, 10/-.

Jan 17 [*Sunday*]　　To David [*son*] £10, before he returned to London. Rested, and read papers. [*£10 was generous; by some economists' calculations the equivalent in purchasing power of about £90 at late 1980s prices.*]

Jan 18　　Haircut, 3/-. Letters dictated, Ward Round, 7; 4 patients at St. John Street.

3:0 p.m. [*Male, aged 38, milk roundsman*] He was a thickset man of average height who said that until his accident he had worked 'seven days a week for four years' without a day off 'except for official holidays'. (He was invalided out of the army in 1947 with asthma but said he had had no attacks 'since 1950'.) Four months ago at the dairy while he was pulling a loaded milk 'truck' by its two shafts he fell backwards over a milk crate. He said that he tried to 'push the truck away' as he fell, but one of the steel shaft handles struck him on the inner side of the right thigh, causing a deep wound which required several stitches. 'It tore my trousers', he added.

A week after the accident he woke in the middle of the night intensely short of breath. He was off work thereafter for 10 weeks. On examination today, I heard diffuse wheezing in both lung fields with prolonged expiration. He said that he wakes up in the middle of the night 'coughing and wheezing'. He also had a scar on his right thigh just below the groin.

What happened was that his accident with the milk 'truck' precipitated his bronchospasm and rekindled his asthma; there is a direct relation between the events. That is, the emotional upset of the injury to his thigh disturbed the even tenor of his daily existence and provoked the renewed onset of asthmatic symptoms. How long he will continue wheezing like this is difficult to tell; he is unlikely to improve during these winter months. He told me that he now works '6 days a week only', and with 'a lad' to help him on his milk-round.

Watched TV, including 'Panorama' on Apartheid in South Africa. Note racialism in this wicked world.

Jan 19   Heavy rain. Received bottle of whisky from a patient, and gratitude from another, expressed verbally. Domiciliary visit in Openshaw: case of obstructive jaundice, admitted to hospital, aet 57.

Jan 20   Anginal attack of some severity this morning. It was the cold which precipitated it, and some annoyance caused by the simple-minded domestic, Rosina, who had run off all the hot water at 6.30 a.m. to wash a few dishes. To the County Court, to give medical evidence on behalf of a civil engineer, up for the fourth time for being drunk-in-charge. He was let off rather lightly with a £75 fine and 5 years suspension. Much jubilation [*on part of solicitors*]. Visited Bob Walmsley's Bookshop. He is a smug man, full of self-satisfaction and no particular friend of mine, I reckon. He seems to be eaten up by jealousy.

Jan 25   Domiciliary visit in Denton: a coronary(?), but patient, aet 57, refused admission [*to hospital*]. Home early. Watched interesting criticisms of Australian life by returning emigrants (zombies).

Jan 29   Ward Rounds; Saw C.D., case of coronary thrombosis, moribund. Dr. N. appears obsessed with stocks and shares. Interesting outpatients, including fascinating case of gout. Listened to General de Gaulle's speech on Algeria. A quiet evening of reading.

Jan 31 [*Sunday*]   Rose at 4.20 a.m. and wrote out in long-hand the first six pages of my lecture to the Optical Congress, and the gist of the subject matter in headings. It appears to be adequate, and I have ample hope of its success. Gave Geoffrey [*son-in-law, a physician*] Erasmus' *Roman History*, printed in Basle, 1517, and Foxe's *Book of Martyrs*, 3 vols, large copy; books worth anything from £20 to £50.

Feb 1   Ward rounds; letters dictated. No lunch; St. John St., 4 cases. Algiers – rebellion settled.

Feb 2   Domiciliary visit in Hadfield: angina of effort. Tumult and agitation by Dr. H. about hospital residents' accommodation.

Feb 3   Snack at lunch; appetite under better control.

Feb 5   11 a.m., lectured to the Nurses on disseminated sclerosis; D.E. from Glossop as subject for demonstration. Very lengthy out-patients. Fruit purchased, £2. 6s. od. Toffees, 10/-. Dr. Barbara Moore completes 1,000-mile walk, John O'Groats to Land's End. Phone-call, at 9 p.m., re M.R. [*private patient*], who has had another coronary thrombosis. Returned to the hospital, fog coming down. He died on my arrival.

Feb 8   Wakened at 2 a.m. by acid-regurgitation; relieved by milk and alkalis. Ward rounds. Purchased tooth paste, soap and powder in Hadfield, 14/9d. Very mean salesgirl; the last time I will purchase anything there. I am much more alert with no lunch today.

Feb 10   St. John Street, 6 cases.

3:0 p.m. [*Male, aged 32, light labourer*] He received an electric shock at work seven months ago, while insulating fridges, and fell on his back unconscious. At the hospital, he complained of severe pains in his neck and right shoulder but was not detained. He was given a collar made of cardboard to limit his movements – which he wore for 15 weeks – and was off work 18 weeks in all while he received physiotherapy.

Today, he said he no longer has 'dizzy-do's' but cant sleep 'much', although he could not say what keeps him awake. (He said that 'after a couple of hours in bed', he feels 'ready to get up'.) His main complaint today was of continuing pains in the back of his neck which 'come up' to the 'top' of his head. 'I cant bear the wireless on too loud', he added. He was a man of healthy appearance.

Feb 13 [*Saturday*]   Gave Geoffrey an early book on Radium. Will call a halt, for the time being, to the gift of books.

Feb 14   Valentine's Day. Tried to make the day as restful as possible by staying in bed late, but the process was hampered to a great extent by the presence of Mouli [*a widower-relative*], and his selfish and self-indulgent daughter Vivianne. She never gave up her seat to elders, never passed anything at the table, hurled herself into the most comfortable chairs, and snatched the newspapers without asking if anyone wished to have them. Intensely irritated by her conduct, but was unable to tell her without upsetting her father, for whom I feel sorry. Read the *British Medical Journal* – on head-lice, and on the use of hydro-cortisone in the shock of coronary thrombosis – book catalogues, and Ian Fleming on Honolulu. A day of generalized annoyance, [*due to a*] combination of factors. M. [*wife*] on the warpath, about reading in bed.

Feb 15   Judy's birthday, her 15th anniversary. Slush and snow, frost and cold. Took Mouli and his frightful daughter to Exchange Station. F.G., 65, Denton, admitted with coronary thrombosis; died shortly after. Dictated letters, and ordered items 36 and 320 from Guernsey book catalogue. Lunch at Masonic Temple. Gave Miss James [*receptionist*] 5/-. 'Panorama' on British Railways, and Communism in Trade Unions.

Feb 18   Slippery roads today; many accidents noticed on way to hospital. Ward Rounds, and 5 cases at St. John St., including car salesman with haemoptysis [*spitting blood*]. 7 p.m., to lecture at Manchester City Library on 'J. Ogilby and His Itineraries'. The speaker, Miss Wadsworth, had a pleasant, melodious voice.

Feb 19   Queen gives birth to a son at 4 p.m. Ramage on *Asthma* (1847) has arrived from Guernsey.

Feb 20 [*Saturday*]   The plate glass in the hall door was found broken tonight. Rosina [*the maid*] had slammed the door in anger, after quarrelling with her schizophrenic Albert.

Feb 22   The customary selfishness experienced today with these Masonic types. Full of gratitude when they need you, and the devil in them when they achieve their purpose. To bed early.

Feb 24   Ward Rounds, 12, 14, 15; H.I. thinks he is improving. False elation of poor man. At St. John Street. G.W., a humourless conveyancing clerk, with hypertension.

Feb 25   Cases of jaundice and dermatitis herpetiformis at St. John Street. Purchased 85 cigars, Upmann and Punch Havana, £23.13s.od. Mr. Aspinall called re book insurance. Showed him George Herbert's *The Temple*, 1633, Cambridge.

Feb 26   Rosina [*the maid*] leaves; paid her £3.10s.od. Informed the police of her departure. Lecture to the Nurses on Angina Pectoris. Ward round, 15. Dictated report on deceased patient.

[*Female, aged 54, housewife*] While walking in the street she was struck on the legs by a bale of cotton which fell from a passing lorry, and her left leg was fractured. It was in plaster for one month, and this immobilised her leg; it is quite probable that this set up a thrombosis in the deep veins of the calf muscles, and that an embolus became detached from it, which lodged itself in the pulmonary vessels. Three weeks after the removal of the plaster she died suddenly in her sleep, of a pulmonary embolism. There is an ever-present danger of such an event when the limb is immobile after an injury, especially where the lower limb veins are varicosed. An embolism also sometimes follows surgical operations on the hips and pelvis, when there is stasis, or stagnation, in the leg veins.

A striking example of such effects of stagnation, or immobilisation, was the increased number of deaths from pulmonary embolism among elderly people during the heavy air-raids on London. These elderly people sat for hours on deckchairs in the shelters, with a wooden cross-piece obstructing the circulation about the middle of the thighs. As soon as the sleeping bunks became more general, deaths from pulmonary embolism diminished. The only preventative measure, in the case of non-fractures, is to allow the limb to be moved about from time to time.

Toffees, 13/9. Engagement of Princess Margaret announced. Heavy rain.

Feb 28 [*Sunday*]　　My 54th anniversary. I am grateful to Almighty God for having survived to this middle-age, with my family intact and launched partly on their careers. May the Grace of God descend upon us, and may we be worthy of his everlasting care. Amen. Restful day. Gave Geoffrey [*son-in-law*] Martial's *Epigrams*, Mayence, 1527, and Jeremy Taylor's *Life of Christ*, with Faithorne illustrations, 1694. Fight between Ruth and Judy [*daughters*].

Feb 29　　Leap Year. Ward Rounds, 12 and 15; discussed some neurological cases with Dr A. To St. John Street, 4 cases. Purchased Simone de Beauvoir's *The Mandarins*. Watched

'Panorama' on: 1) the ignorance of modern children about recent history; 2) Eden's book *Full Circle* about Suez; 3) the question of golf-clubs and Jews. Dealt with inadequately.

March 1   St. John St.: physicist with one eye, and travel agent with alleged heart trouble. To bed at 9 p.m.

March 3   The thorough-going incompetence of Miss James [*receptionist*] increases with time. No silver lining.

March 4   Lecture to the Nurses on metabolic diseases. Talked to Dr. P. about one of his schizophrenics. Medical out-patients included chauffeur with postural scoliosis [*curvature of the spine*], and young girl with record of attempted suicide. Three domiciliary visits: pleural effusion (Audenshaw), congestive heart failure (Openshaw), and hypertension (Openshaw).

March 8   Freezing weather. Domiciliary visit in Denton: L.M., aet 69, cor pulmonale [*congestive heart failure*]. I explained the condition to [*the patient's*] husband and son, who have adopted a militant attitude towards their G.P. Saw H.I.; the poor man still thinks he is better. Watched Agadir earthquake pictures, and listened to Brahms' Piano Concerto.

March 11   Presented Walter S. [*friend*] with 1st edition of *Verses* (1868) by Cardinal Newman: light brown cloth, fine copy. Deposited My Last Will and Testament at Bank. Lecture to Nurses on Subarachnoid Haemorrhage and began Rheumatic Fever. Lunch at hospital, 3/-. Discussed 'sway-back' in sheep and multiple sclerosis in Man with Dr. A.

March 13 [*Sunday*]   Dr. M. calls for tea and stays too long. Chaos in my room.

March 16   Poor night worrying about tomorrow's lecture [*to Northern Optical Congress*]. Looked up Jacques Daniel's (1696–1742) treatment of cataract, and Dalton's account of colour blindness, 1794.

March 17   Southport. Long walk this morning. Icy winds. Gave Barker-Meadley Lecture, 'As a Physician Sees It'. In the course of the lecture, I said that there was a surfeit of small men who dub themselves medical scientists and a shortage of Doctors interested primarily in the art of living. The Hospital environment is an artificial environment, and hospital patients represent only a fraction of medical problems. We can say of clinical medicine what Simone de Beauvoir said of philosophy: 'It is in the street'. Life is not enclosed in a hospital ward . . .'

[*turning to the subject of the eye*] '. . . I have always laid great store by an understanding and careful examination of the human eye. The eye is an index of systemic disease. I was also taught by Foster Moore at Bart's that there is no such thing as eyestrain; that sewing, reading or other forms of near work do not cause myopia, cataract or glaucoma; and that no permanent ocular damage arises from wrongly prescribed glasses. The late Mr. Basil Lang used to tell of a man with 18 diopters of myopia in each eye who drove a taxicab for years in the crowded streets of Marseilles without wearing glasses. Such people can develop uncanny skill in the interpretation of blurred images, and if they take to spectacles suddenly in adult life may even find them intolerably confusing . . .'

[*on opticians*] '. . . You should regard your work as a Life Study, instead of being mere purveyors of spectacles in gaudier and more exotic frames; just as the job of a physician is not to hand out tranquillizers and euphoriants. You have a rigorous course of study and a difficult examination. I have seen some of the questions; Isaac Newton would have failed to answer them. But there are many doctors, and all sorts of graduates in the ancillary services, for whom a qualification means the end of long years of tiresome study. They are like Becky Sharp. When she left Miss Pinkerton's Academy she threw Johnson's *Dictionary* away, and leant back in the carriage, saying "Thank God, I'm out" . . .'

The lecture was well received. I felt much improved on seeing the enthusiastic reception.

March 18   Bitterly cold.

March 19 [*Saturday*]   H.I.'s condition deteriorating, sent home. Domiciliary visits: bronchogenic carcinoma (Clayton), and cancer of stomach, with secondaries in the liver (Hyde). Heard of lamented death of Herbert Smith, dentist at Hadfield. Tidied up one of my shelves: Titus Oates, anti-Popish tracts, Nehemiah Grew, and Sir Wm. Davenant's *Collected Works* (1673). Inspiring material.

March 20   Exhausted.

March 21   To M., £15.5.0d wages. After ward rounds, to town with Dr C. [*house physician*].

4:30 p.m. [*Female, aged 27, shorthand typist*] She was a thick-set, obese, florid girl, who was apprehensive and had a tremor of her outstretched hands. She is engaged to be married. She cannot sleep and feels 'all weak', is 'nervous and jumpy', and her 'mind is all worked up'. Five weeks ago she suffered trivial injuries in a car collision: she is having medicine for her nerves, and tablets for her back. She told me that she receives a great deal of sympathy from her fiancé: she probably enjoys her minor disability, and the sympathy it attracts from him.

Riots near Johannesburg. 56 Black people killed; trouble in Cape Town too.

March 22   Home early. Stupid-looking maid arrives, without baggage. Went out to dinner.

March 23   Maid had to be wakened at 8.0 a.m.; had orgy last night after we left. Promptly sacked this morning. Had taken radiator into her room, and left it on all night to dry some of her linen. A nymphomaniac. Immunized 60 to 70 cases against polio at Arnfield's. Left at noon. Lunch at Masonic, and proceeded to St. John St., 5 cases. In the evening, began John Bratby's *Breakdown*.

March 24   Serious reactions to shootings of 73 natives in South Africa.

March 26 [*Saturday*]   Siesta, then watched Grand National. Read *British Medical Journal* and *Lancet*. Passes for Africans are to be 'suspended' in South Africa, for the time being. Geoffrey and Ruth came this evening. Ruth expecting(?); God willing, so be it.

March 28   Collided with dog (mongrel) while driving in Rusholme. Reported dog accident to the police. Ward rounds, and 6 cases at St. John Street, including mathematician, aet 32, with glycosuria [*sugar in urine*].

March 29   St. John St, 3 cases.

3:45 p.m. [*Male, aged 31, bus driver*] He was driving his bus when he was involved last August in a minor accident with a female learner-driver. He says he was jerked violently in the cab and struck the right side of his chest on the door handle. He said he was 'a little shaken, but not much'. He carried on with his duties for the rest of the day, but was then off work for 10 weeks. I asked him why he had been off work for so long with such a trivial injury. He said it was because he could not sleep, and because the pain was acute at night, especially in hot weather. A few moments later he said the pain in his chest was worse in cold weather.

He smokes 20–30 cigarettes a day: his tongue was furred from cigarette smoking, and there was a smell of alcohol on his breath. He should not have been incapacitated for more than a fortnight; he stayed off work for 7 or 8 weeks too long. He says he is 'not all right' and has chest pains when 'pulling on heavy steering', but I thought he was a neurotic, and exaggerating.

April 1   Mrs K., ring [*for prolapse of uterus*] inserted, £1. Lecture to Nurses on acute pulmonary oedema. No cases to be demonstrated for a time, until general attention of class improves. Medical Out-patients finished early. Dr W. came round to the house this evening to apologise; he wishes me to stay as Fellow of Manchester Medical Society, and not resign. [*There had been some affront given by the Society, but it is not clear what this was*]. I showed him a few books, and deliberately 'gilded the lily'. Gave him a whisky. My reaction, after talking things over with M., is to leave resignation where it is, and to Hell with them! Very exhausted this evening.

April 2 [*Saturday*]   Bad night thinking about reply to Manchester Medical Society. Medical journals arrive; too much reading material to cope intelligently with it. Did not go to hospital. Oxford won Boat Race. Listened to Elgar's *Dream of Gerontius*. Sat up late collating books: J. Hunter on *The Blood, Inflammation and Gunshot Wounds* (1794) and John Browne's *Myographia Nova* (1698). To bed, 2 a.m.

April 3   Poor night's sleep. Chaos in the house, comings and goings. S. [*son of friend*] arrives with his mother for consultation. Provisional diagnosis: schizophrenia. Collated as perfect my presentation copy of Robert Hooke's *Lectiones Cutlerianae*, 1679, one of the rarest books in English scientific history. Also collated Charles White's *Treatise on the Management of Pregnant and Lying-in Women*, 1773; unbound and partly unopened, but browned and damp-stained. A great deal of work is required to get it into shape.

April 6   Dictated revised version of letter of resignation from Manchester Medical Society. Domiciliary visits; Wards, 12 and 15; St. John St., 4 cases. Ill-mannered drivers on the roads of England today. An evil spirit possesses uncouth working-class lorry drivers in particular. Some of them are militant, aggressive and villainous.

April 7   Purchased Fever Pamphlets by James Black, 1825 and 1826. Debit in Bank, £377.1s 1d. Visited Mrs. D. [*private patient*]; *in extremis*, with cerebral vascular lesion [*stroke*].

April 8   Lecture to the Nurses on cardiac arrhythmias; started diabetes mellitus. Bought fruit, 19/-. Ward rounds, 14, 15. Medical Out-patients: interviewed parents of boy of 22 with acute leukaemia. Box of Punch Havanas received from Albert J. [*a friend*] this evening.

April 9   Purchased Herman Wouk's *This is My God*,

Alec Waugh's *Fuel for the Flames*, and a *Life of Schumann*. Attempted assassination of Dr. Verwoerd, South African prime minister, in Johannesburg.

April 10 [*Sunday*]   Mrs. T. [*wife of private patient*] telephoned about her husband. The nature of her questioning showed a complete lack of realization of what her husband's condition is: cancer of the prostate, with secondary metastases [*migration of the cancer to another part of the body*]. Severish attack of vertigo in the afternoon, which lasted into the evening. Tidying up my library perhaps caused it. To bed early.

April 12   Passover. Blessed my children.

April 14   Visited Ante-Natal Ward: saw Mrs. W. of Dukinfield there. She has a large abdominal tumour. Domiciliary in Bradford, M/C 11: congestive heart failure. St. John Street, 8 cases; including cardiac ischaemia, with anxiety neurosis. 7/6 to Miss James. Very fatigued and tired out. Good Friday tomorrow.

April 16 [*Saturday*]   Read *Life of St. Francis of Assissi*.

April 17 [*Easter Day*]   Amazing treasures came to light, dusting shelves; wonderful books out of recesses and corners. Helped in the chores today. Saw TV film of Bali, made by Italians. Read article on apartheid by Rebecca West. Death of Mrs. D. at 10.15 p.m. [*see April 7*]. Visited the house at 11 p.m., and helped to lift the body. On return, tidied up further shelves, and unwrapped beautiful 16th century copy of Ovid's *Metamorphoses* [*Parma, 1505*].

April 18   Tinkering with books most of the day. Gave Geoffrey 1654 *Euclid*. Had a fresh look at Bright's *Diseases of the Kidneys* [*1827*].

April 19   Beautiful bright morning. Made breakfast for M. Interesting out-patients. Phoned Dr. C. re case of attempted suicide by coal-gas poisoning, aet 84. M. on the warpath when she got home from the Pictures; her nerves are very jaded.

April 20   Domiciliaries: broncho-pneumonia, and cor pulmonale. Ward Rounds. Talked to detective about attempted suicide case by delinquent patient, aet [*aged*] 27, with 8 convictions for larceny. Lunch at hospital, 3/-. St. John St., 3 cases. Changed into dinner jacket to go to Opera House for appalling play, *The Grass is Greener* by Hugh and Margaret Williams. Frightful tosh.

April 22   Lecture to Nurses. Threaded my way carefully through Treatment of Tape-worms with mepacrine, and distributed chart on Arthritides. Out-patients tedious.

April 25   Gloomy and miserable day. 10 bags of coal at 9/7d each. Haircut, 3/-. Full ward rounds.

April 26   Medical out-patients and Ward rounds at Glossop. St. John St., 5 cases.

4:25 p.m. [*Female, aged 56, housewife*] She has had pains in the chest for the past fortnight, and feels as if she is choking. She says that she has lost 10lbs in the last 4 months. She 'heaves', but does not vomit. She also has a 'musty smell in the nose' and is 'all of a tremble'. Her own doctor told her that it was 'due to the change of life' and 'worry', and gave her 'capsules for sleeping'. But this could be either Hashimoto's Disease or carcinoma of the pharynx. Admit, if no better.

To Lodge Meeting at 5.30 p.m.; home at 10.0 p.m. M. has been booked by police again for parking offence.

April 27   Domiciliaries: loss of weight and anaemia (Audenshaw), and narcolepsy (Ashton). Called on Dr. J. to return his copy of *Encounter*. St. John St., 2 cases. Watched 'Tonight' on Dr. Syngman Rhee(ruthless), and an undiscovered murder in Kent 50 years ago. Poor speeches by R.A. Butler and Lord Mountbatten from Royal Academy dinner.

April 30   Hospital board pay slip, £393.7s.2d. Resignation from Manchester Medical Society confirmed. M. back from London: the light of the household.

May 1 [*Sunday*]   Restful day, but not feeling well. Read extracts from the Bible in *This Year of Grace*, by Victor Gollancz.

May 2   Ward 15; St. John St., 5 cases. Caryl Chessman executed at 6 p.m. after 8 reprieves and 12 years in jail. A disgrace to modern civilization. [*Chessman – convicted in 1948 – was executed in the gas chamber of San Quentin, California for kidnapping and sexually assaulting two Los Angeles women. A late petition on his behalf from, among others, Marlon Brando, Albert Schweitzer, Pablo Casals, and Brigitte Bardot was of no avail.*] Saw 'Panorama' on Algeria, Ernest Marples on Road Safety, and the Channel Tunnel.

May 5   Domiciliary visit to Ashton: female, aet 59, a spinster, suffering from pernicious anaemia, gastro-enteritis and malnutrition. Admitted to hospital.

3:0 p.m. [*Male, aged 49, assistant furnaceman*] Eighteen months ago, he was in the cellar of a 'soaking pit', boring a hole through some slag with a 'red-hot' rod, when the rod broke in his hand; part of it fell and burned the lower end of his right leg above the ankle.

He made a great song to me about the extent (1¾″ x 2″) and degree of the burn, but he was not detained in hospital, and returned to work the next morning, working successfully for a week. He told me with some satisfaction, and even relish, that small ulcers have subsequently formed from time to time at the site of the burn; though it is cruel to think it, I suspect him of scratching the skin to produce the ulcers himself, in order to perpetuate them for the purpose of a claim he is pursuing. (I have occasionally come across this before.)

When I asked him about his medical history, his answer was a strange one. He said that he had had rheumatic fever 'three times' – though there was no evidence of valvular heart disease – and that this had 'made a man of' him.

May 6   Medical Out-patients: an unsatisfactory and harassing afternoon, including interviews with relatives. Domiciliaries: paramyoclonus multiplex (Denton), and broncho-pneumonia (Hyde). At 9.30 p.m., watched wedding on TV of Princess Margaret, to Antony Armstrong-Jones. Serious news of the shooting down of an American plane by the Russians.

May 7 [*Saturday*]   Bought suit from Jackson's the Tailors, £7.17s.od. Flowers, 5/6d. Watched Cup Final: Blackburn Rovers 0, Wolverhampton Wanderers 3.

May 8   J.K. [*private patient*] rings, seeking changes to the medical certificate I have given him [*for restitution claim, as a war victim, against the West German Government*]. But I will not issue it in any modified form. The ruthless dishonesty of these people is alarming, although God knows they are entitled to restitution for their sufferings at the hands of the Nazis. 6 gallons of Esso Extra, £1.8s.9d. Listened to Haydn and Mozart.

May 9   4:30 p.m. [*Male, aged 43, company director*] He complained about fatigue, 'breaking out in a sweat', and 'difficulty in swallowing'. He has a feeling of inadequacy, smokes too heavily, and cannot cope with his work. His father committed suicide at the age of 72. I could find no physical abnormalities in any of his systems, but he is grossly overworked and highly strung, and living under considerable nervous tension. Perhaps a tranquillizer like Meprabamate would help him.

May 12   Ward rounds; reports dictated; St. John St., 4 cases. Ali Khan killed in motor accident on outskirts of Paris, aet 48. International situation tense. Wrote to Dawson's [*booksellers*] of Pall Mall, about Addison and Hunter.

May 13   Lecture to the Nurses, on anuria and agranulocytosis. Medical Outpatients a dreadful experience. Large numbers, including lymphatic leukaemia and polyneuritis, with frequent interruptions and phone-calls. Finished at 5.45 p.m. Unhappy and tiresome day; driven up the wall. Watched Mortimer Wheeler, on Ancient Rome.

May 15 [*Sunday*]   Russians launch a 4½ ton space ship, with alleged dummy inside; it is probably a live man. Lazy day reading: Dr Beatty on Nelson's death, Lindforth on his journey from Liverpool to Salt Lake City and George Herbert's *Temple* (1633), including his poem on the Jews.

May 16   Domiciliary visit: severe epistaxis (Audenshaw); admitted. Ward Round, 7. St. John St., 5 cases, including a bearded printer at the *Manchester Guardian* with a poor physique, who smokes 40 cigarettes a day. Bad news about the Paris Summit Conference, disintegrating before it starts.

May 17   By car to St. Anne's-on-Sea [*to see private patient*]. A fine day, sunny with pleasant breeze; walked on Pier. Purchased pair of black suede shoes, £2.13s.od. Set off home at 5.50 p.m., but lost my way back and came in through Salford. Summit talks wrecked by Khruschev.

May 18   Two domiciliary visits in Hyde: solid dullness in left base, and cor pulmonale with deformed chest, both admitted to Ward 15. To St. John Street; 6 cases.

4:45 p.m. [*Female, aged 54, married, former cotton-mill worker*] She says that she recently 'went short of breath' and has 'never had anything like it before'. When she had this attack she went to bed, but her doctor told her to get up, and 'put it down to the weather', she says. Paroxysmal tachycardia [*palpitations*] keeps her awake. She has no cough; her menopause was ten years ago. I have sent her for investigations, including an X-Ray of the chest and electrocardiogram.

May 19   St. John St., 5 cases.

2:15 p.m. [*Male, aged 65, married, 12 years an asbestos-weaver, up to 1958*] He was a thin, sickly-looking man, whose height was 5'3" and who weighed 8 stones. (Average weight for height at this age should be 11st. 8lbs.) There was prolonged expiration, with evidence of fibrosis of both lungs. Two of his 'mates', aged 63 and 45 respectively, who worked in the same 'shed' as he for some years, have died of pneumoconiosis. During the period when they worked together they had no dust extractor and no masks were issued. He complains of a cough, shortness of breath and expectoration. He thinks his condition is stationary. He is suffering from pneumoconiosis of moderate degree, and is grossly underweight. With great care and rest he could live for another 5 or 6 years – as a maximal figure – in relative discomfort. If, of course, he were to get pneumonia or some acute infection, he would have very little resistance.

Listened to the world premiere of *Tobias and the Angel* by Sir Arthur Bliss; unmusical.

May 20   Lecture to the Nurses, on iron-deficiency anaemia; showed a case. Ward Rounds. In Ward 6, saw sick nurse with either encephalitis or schizophrenia; in Ward 3, a diabetic with ascites [*fluid in abdominal cavity*] and cirrhosis of the liver.

May 21 [*Saturday*]   Fairly easy day, but correspondence sadly neglected.

May 22   Urgent call at 11.20 a.m. to private patient in Rusholme: aet 72, seriously ill, uraemia(?), carcinoma of stomach(?). Went to hospital with his son, and arranged admission forthwith. At 6.45 p.m, visit to Ashton to see patient in Ward 12. To bed exhausted at 11 p.m. prompt. Ulcer on roof of mouth.

May 23   Examination of 6 cadet nurses. St. John St., 4 cases. Severe earthquakes in Chile, in an area 1½ times that of England.

May 26   Further earthquakes in Chile, tidal waves in

Japan and New Zealand. Anti-American demonstrations in China. Watched programme on Tonga, and prepared lecture to the nurses.

May 27 Lecture to Nurses, on asthma; case shown. Medical Out-patients, many relatives interviewed. Revolution in Turkey, Mendères arrested. The military have taken over for the time being.

May 30 Ward Round, 12: pregnant Polish woman, 33, died of pulmonary embolism.

May 31 Domiciliary in Dukinfield: aet 68, left basal pneumonia and thyrotoxicosis; admitted. St. John Street, 2 cases, including B.S., *Manchester Guardian* journalist and BBC 'Points North' interviewer. Called on Sherratt and Hughes [*Manchester booksellers*] after finishing St. John St. Purchased Arthur Bryant's life of Samuel Pepys and Victor Gollancz, *From Darkness to Light*.

June 1 Ward Round. Lunch at Masonic Temple, 7/6d; paid for 3 coffees. Gave Miss James [*receptionist*] 10/-. St. John St., 5 cases. Bird-nest in garden below the library. Thrushes probably. Geoffrey [*son-in-law*], Ruth [*daughter*] and Golda S. [*friend*] to dinner. Gave Geoffrey £20. Walk with M., after all had gone.

June 4 Very fine warm day. Temperatures in the 80s. Finest Whit Sunday since the War. David's [*son's*] birthday, 23 today. Purchased Works of Sydenham [*1697*], 2 vols, and Blackmore on *Consumptions* [*1724*]. 6/6d for charwoman's wages; a case of senile cerebral changes, who wanders about aimlessly from room to room. 'Salad Days' at the Opera House: indifferent play, with bright patches.

June 5 General inactivity. Read 'superwoman' case of chromosomal anomalies in *The Lancet*. Thunderstorm this afternoon. Walk with M. in the evening. Much hooliganism on the roads, speeding, overtaking. It was even dangerous to walk on the footpath. The human species is degenerating.

Teddy-boys up to no good in Palatine Road.

June 6   Complete round of Ward 12, including case of cryoglobulinaemia with myelomatosis, aet 66. Discussed case with Geoffrey later. Spoke to Mrs. T. Unhappily married, husband coarse and vulgar; she has to work for a living, while he loafs about.

June 8   Ward 12: case of epileptic girl of low intelligence, aet 23, with impacted chicken-bone in oesophagus which perforated her aorta. Lunch at hospital, 3/-. Home early. To Sadlers Wells Opera, 'The Marriage of Figaro', with Gwyn Griffiths as Figaro, Marion Studholme as Susanna, Raimund Herincx as the Count and Ann Edwards as the Countess. Excellent performances.

June 10   Domiciliary in Hyde: aet 67, haemoptysis [*coughing blood*], to be admitted. Ward rounds, 12, 14, 15. Met Dr. P. on way out, visited Mrs. Toon's [*pub*] at corner of Mossley Road. Lengthy boozing session, depression much relieved.

June 11   No [*Whitsun*] processions encountered.

June 12   Rooting amongst old papers. Read *BMJ* [*British Medical Journal*] and *Lancet*; and, in Sunday press, of Montgomery's visit to Mao Tse-Tung. 'Face to Face' with Stirling Moss. Slack day. Inactivity is somewhat soul-destroying.

June 14   Medical out-patients, 10.30 a.m. Miss Walton [*hospital secretary*], back from holidays, reports on exploitation of tourists at Oberammergau, and on anti-British attitudes and sentiments among Germans and Austrians. Ward rounds, and St. John Street. England beats S.Africans in First Test Match, by 100 runs.

June 16   Ward round, 14; snack in the Ward. St. John St., 3 cases. Purchased at Shaw's Bookshop T.H. Huxley's *Lectures on the Origin of Species*, 1863, first edition. 7 p.m. to

Lecture at City Library on 'The Cryptographic Books of the Bacon Theory'. Returned to hospital at 9.30 p.m. to see L.M. [*private patient*], and to Mrs. Toon's thereafter for C2H5OH [*alcohol*], £1. [*My father often uses this term in his diary in reference to the medical condition of alcoholism and, as here, when having a drink.*] Eisenhower's visit to Tokyo cancelled, owing to serious riots and anti-American demonstrations. Lovely evening. M. has lost her voice; gave her hot drink at 11.45 p.m.

June 19 [*Sunday*]   Guests with children to tea in the garden. The children raced round the house, and all the rooms. No more patience with young children. Listened to John Barbirolli reminiscing on Radio about his career. To upstairs lumber-room [*where books were kept*] making a start, after 11 or 12 years, on reorientation. Removed downstairs: Quaker Tracts and Pamphlets of some rarity, and *A Defence of the Apologie of the Church of Englande*, by John Jewel (1567).

June 20   Lunch at Masonic; thence to Shaw's Bookshop: purchased *An Inquiry into the Nature and Causes of the Wealth of Nations*, by Adam Smith, 3rd edition in 3 volumes (1784), 25/-. Thereafter, to St. John Street, 6 cases.

3:0 p.m. [*Female, aged 55, former shopkeeper*] She was of slender build, with accentuated reflexes due to her nervous state. She has recently been in hospital with a nervous breakdown [*her second*], and depression. Ten years ago she left her husband; they had slept apart for ten years before that, since her husband thought it was 'more healthy' to sleep apart. He was also 'mean with money', used bad language and told her to 'get out' or 'bugger off', and said that if she 'got away' he would give her £100. Dressed up in 'hiking clothes', he used to go hiking every Sunday, and continued to do so, she said, 'in all weathers; even in the snow and rain, any weather, it did not matter'. On one occasion he struck her in the face because she had come in late from shopping. In the past, I once wrote him a letter and asked him to come and see me so that I could discuss his wife's health with him, but he refused to come. She said that she saw him read this letter, which he threw down on the table saying he was 'not afraid of any Doctor'. After she left her husband, she went to work in a shoe-shop, and then did housekeeping for an elderly gentleman, who has since died. She is now on Public Assistance. She is chronically depressed, and suffers from bouts of weeping.

Finished late, at 6.20 p.m.

June 21   Warm and beautiful day. Domiciliary visit in Stalybridge: severe iron deficiency anaemia, 29% Hb., admitted. Ward 15: eleven coronary thromboses in Ward at present. No lunch. Domiciliary visit in Ashton: aet 55, severe anaemia, refuses admission. Dr. K. makes an impossible request for me to stand as surety for an overdraft. His affairs are chaotic, and unwarrantedly so.

June 23   Heavy thunderstorm during the night, heavy rain in the morning; nevertheless we left for a day in Blackpool. 4 gallons of Esso Petrol, at 4/8d per gallon = 18/8d. Walked on North Pier. Siesta, tea, 4/6d. Hat for M., 15/11d. Home for supper by 7.30 p.m. To bed at 10.30 p.m.

June 24   Lecture to Nurses, on jaundice. Basket of strawberries from fruiterer. Five domiciliary visits: left cerebral thrombosis (Gorton), anorexia nervosa (Ryecroft), bronchogenic carcinoma, aet 67 (Audenshaw, refuses admission), coronary thrombosis (Audenshaw), and infective hepatitis (aet 30, Denton, advice given, not admitted). Ward 15, to see L.M. [*private patient*]. Medical out-patients; large numbers. Very hectic and busy day.

June 25 [*Saturday*]   End of the day unpleasant; M. bickering with Geoffrey and Ruth, over trivialities.

June 26   Beautiful, sunny, summer's day. Read *Observer* article on D.H. Lawrence in the garden, and listened to Berlioz's *Romeo and Juliet*. Evelyn Waugh in 'Face to Face' with John Freeman; a magnificent interrogation. Felt very shivery and cold, with the temperature falling. C_2H_5OH+ [*took alcohol, '+' signifying above average amount, but not as much as '++'*].

June 28   Domiciliary visits: post-puerperal swollen feet (aet 22, Mossley); Paget's Disease (aet 78, Mossley, p.r. [*per rectum examination*] performed); and interim diagnosis of involutional insanity (aet 65, Stalybridge, admitted).

June 29   Domiciliary visit in Haughton Green: aet 39, chronic bronchitis and emphysema, *in extremis*, urgently admitted. Reports; Ward rounds. Told Sister A. of my decision not to lecture any more to this group of nurses. They are unworthy of my time.

July 2 [*Saturday*]   Domiciliary visit to Godley: senile gangrene of right foot and congestive heart failure, aet 87, to be admitted. Watched Wimbledon women's singles finals, won by Maria Bueno of Brazil. To Arnold G.'s [*friends*]. Mr. G. very self-confident and self-satisfied, with a blend of generalized egotism and bonhomie.

July 3   No breakfast, and light lunch. Outburst of rudeness from Judy [*daughter*] to M. and I. There seems to be no reward for parental sacrifice. Attack of lumbago today. Exhausted and depressed. Saw 'Monitor' film on Picasso.

July 5   Arnold G. calls with a carp, which he caught. The 12th anniversary of the National Health Service passed unnoticed in the Press or by the Public.

July 6   Ward Round; St John St., 2 cases, including J.I., [*a fishmonger patient*] who gave me some fish: salmon, hake, mackerel. Heavy rain, rain, rain all day. The death of Aneurin Bevan announced this evening.

July 7   No cases in St. John St. Purchased Homer's Odyssey, translated by E.V. Rieu, 3/6, James Thurber's *Is Sex Necessary?*, 2/6, and D.H. Lawrence's *Women in Love*, 5/-. Bad news from London of my brother Jack's collapse. He is in the Middlesex Hospital. [*He was himself a doctor.*]

July 8   Domiciliary in Hurst: aet 57, osteo-arthritis of spine, to be admitted. Previously seen on many occasions by Drs. V., B. and Uncle Tom Cobley and all. Ward rounds. Discussed case of phoeochromocytoma. Appointment of Indian doctor, as house physician.

July 9   Left for London at 7 a.m., the first time along the M.1. Gave lift to young lad, aet 20, studying engineering at Rugby Polytechnic. He was from Kenya; his parents are pulling out of there, trouble brewing. The M.1 has reduced the journey-time to London by 2 hours at least. However, there were not many people on it; but those on it exhibited some appalling driving. Visited Jack at Middlesex Hospital, and discussed his condition [*coronary*] with his doctors. Excellent lunch with David [*son*] at 'Chez Auguste', Soho; £2. 8s. od, with 4/- tip. London not a pleasant place, too noisy, expensive, and in parts blatantly immoral; not the place for a young female adolescent who wishes to remain virginal. Sat up talking for a long time to Clara [*sister-in-law*]. Her expressions of affection for Jack were completely unexpected, in view of her demeanour over the past years.

July 10   Wakened by Clara after only an hour's sleep: Jack's condition had deteriorated. Went forthwith, at 1 a.m., to Middlesex Hospital. Jack very poor: fibrillating, appeared in severe state of collapse, blood pressure fallen. Returned, and slept till 5 a.m. To hospital again at 6.30 a.m. Jack slightly improved. Left hospital at 7.15 a.m., and set off in heavy rain and mist to Manchester. Total expenditure of London journey, £6.18s.2d. Gave Geoffrey a Baskett Bible, Psalms, Common Prayer (1715).

July 12   Severe sore throat, difficulty in swallowing. Domiciliary visit in Ashton, but patient absent. He had gone to Blackpool, although he had sent urgently for his G.P. earlier. St. John St, 5 cases. To bed early, deglutition acutely painful. Took tetracycline, aspirins, tab. codein, vitamins and emulsio achromycin. Probably an adeno-viral infection.

July 13   Severe sore throat throughout the night, sleep intermittent. Phoned London. Jack no better, but holding his own, just about. Domiciliary visit in Ashton: aet 70, coronary thrombosis(?), admitted. Phoeochromocytoma removed by Mr. H. [*surgeon*]; patient comfortable. Lunch, with acute pain in throat. 4 cases at St. John St. Judy apologizes for her rudeness nearly 2 weeks ago. Severe and excruciating pain throughout the evening. To bed early.

July 14   Night of agony in the throat. Cheque for £4.15s.3d received from Henry Shaw [*Ashton debt collector*], for bad debts. [*In Nigel Gray,* The Worst of Times, *1985, a book which includes descriptions of Ashton in the 1930s, an informant tells the author: 'You'd go to the doctor. He had your name and address. And, after, you got a bill . . . If you couldn't pay it, which very few could, each doctor had his own collector. The collector used to come round each week and you'd pay sixpence . . . When the National Health Service came in all them doctors' bills were written off. The collectors used to be the same type . . . they were always little wizened fellers.' In 1977, a former patient told me that my father 'used to have a collector, Miss Goodwin of Pickford Lane [Dukinfield]. She never married. She was a fussy little body. We paid what we could afford, sixpence or a shilling.' My father was pursuing new debtors, private patients, in the 1960s. Henry Shaw's letter-head describes him as an 'Accountant, Estate Agent and Incorporated Trade Protection Agent, established 1878'.*]

Decided to see E.N.T. [*Ear Nose and Throat*] surgeon this morning. Reassuring news: it may be TB, or cancer of the throat!! Proceeded to District Infirmary, for barium swallow and X Rays: chest, sinuses, epiglottis, etc. 4 cases at St. John St., including one of pneumoconiosis, with hypertension. I phoned the E.N.T. surgeon, who postulated burning of the epiglottis, and reiterated the possibility of malignant disease. French Bastille Day. Kennedy nominated Democratic Presidential Candidate, USA. He is aged 43, and a Roman Catholic. To bed at midnight; how I have managed this week, God alone knows, with anguish in the throat like a mediaeval torture.

July 15   Acute discomfort, heavy rain. Gave Miss James [*receptionist*] £1 pocket money. Domiciliary visits: congestive heart failure, *in extremis*, admitted at once (Ashton); and coronary ischaemia (aet 43, Dukinfield). Ward Round: saw phoeochromocytoma man making excellent progress. Collected spray for throat. Medical Out-patients. Exhausted, broken down, pain in throat, feel a wreck.

July 16 [*Saturday*]   Better night after sedation, but pain in throat severe on waking. 41 miles this afternoon making visits. Acute pain in lumbar region. Am getting an old crock.

July 18   Awoke at 5.30 a.m., to find that David had already left for London. He leads a rather tense and hectic life, and appears to be getting involved in clandestine liaisons of an unwholesome nature. I trust I may be wrong.

July 19   Overslept – woke at 8.20 a.m. – so hurried onwards. Domiciliary visits: pernicious anaemia with or without carcinoma of stomach (aet 72, Denton, refuses admission), and left Bell's Palsy (aet 54, Ashton). Medical Out-patients the heaviest since the introduction of the Health Service. Rainstorm. St. John St., 3 cases. Went to bed at 7.30 p.m., but wakened by repeated phone calls. Read from *Island of the Lotus-Eaters*.

July 20   Letter from Dr. D. [*Nigerian doctor*], asking if I wish to go to Nigeria in October, to witness the independence celebrations. Will decline; first, because Ruth [*daughter*] is expecting her baby about then, and secondly because there are more exciting places to go for one's money. Hair-cut and razor-blades, 4/3d. Domiciliary visits: congestive heart failure and carcinoma of stomach (aet 70, Ashton, admitted), chronic uraemia(?) for investigations (aet 63, Ashton, to be admitted), and Wernicke's encephalopathy (aet 55, Denton, admitted). [*The latter patient died three days later*]. Jack better.

July 22   Dictated large number of reports and letters. Very cold, heavy rain and thunderstorms. Temperatures November average. Watched Michaela and Armand Denis in Japan, and film of the Resistance in Denmark. Dr. M. [*friend*] visited, to inquire about my health.

July 23 [*Saturday*]   Watched 1st Promenade Concert of 66th Season, Clifford Curzon playing Beethoven's 4th Piano Concerto.

July 25   Deposited £99.15s.9d. in bank; credit balance, this a.m., £613.2s.5d. Ward 15. Lunch at Masonic. At luncheon-table, talk to man just back from holiday in Eire, which he found too expensive and too insanitary. £450 provisional payment to the Commissioners of Inland Revenue. St. John St., 5 cases. To the Opera House: Robert Bolt's *The Tiger and the Horse*, Michael Redgrave, Catherine Lacey, Vanessa Redgrave, Kynaston Reeves and Alan Dobie. Programme 1/-.

July 27   Gargantuan lunch with Leslie C. [*friend*] at Midland Hotel, £2.11.0d. St John St., 4 cases.

3:0 p.m. [*Male, aged 48, garage proprietor*] He complains of blackouts, and for the past year has had recurring feelings of apprehension as if he is 'going to fall on his face'. He also has a 'feeling behind the eyes'. Occasionally he finds himself 'gasping for breath', and when this happens he tries to 'keep moving'. He has not had a holiday for two years, works very hard, and smokes 40 cigarettes a day. (Terrible!!!). He sleeps well, his appetite is good and his urine is normal. I do not believe there is much the matter with him, but will send him for investigations. He said, 'it's determination which stops me from falling'.

3:45 p.m. [*Female, aged 43, housewife*] She has pains in the chest; when she goes out she gets 'worked up', and has 'bad nerves', headaches, etc., etc. She has no children, and said that she leads a lonely, frustrated and empty existence. She is an attractive woman who has no sex life, and whose symptoms are psychosomatic. She said that she could feel her heart 'pumping away'.

Heavy rain and cloud. The worst July that I think I can remember. Overdose of food today.

July 28 Ward rounds; letters dictated; St. John St., 4 cases, and thereafter domiciliaries: severe angina and nutritional anaemia (aet 52, Mossley, not admitted); angina and small coronary(?) (N.O., aet 54, Denton, admitted to private ward); and rheumatic mitral disease with congestive heart failure (aet 46, Glossop, admitted). Forty-eight miles of visits, after St. John St. Home by 11.5 p.m., very exhausted. Rates £119.0.0.; paid, with protest.

July 29 David arrives from London, mentally pre-occupied.

July 30 [*Saturday*] Cheque received from Regional Hospital Board for £467.13s.5d., including a sum of £226.16s.0d. for domiciliaries. Inept letter from Dr. H. [*consultant*] asking for information [*about a patient*] which I have already given him, and giving me information I did not ask for. Ward rounds; letters; reports. David glum and uncommunicative. Out to dinner with the Youngs; they showed a remarkable lack of interest in cultural matters. M. enjoyed the evening, although God knows that the truth is I would rather have stayed at home. To bed by midnight, but got up at 1.30 a.m. to make this entry.

July 31 Gave David £1, and Judy 7/6d. Geoffrey and Ruth for supper; M. drops a jar of cherry jam, and cuts Ruth's leg. To bed early.

Aug 1 To private patient in Droylsden: R.S., aet 76, congestive heart failure, respiratory infection, senile decay. Made arrangements for her to be admitted immediately. Ward 11: N.O. [*private patient*] making good progress, but nursing appalling. (Not a soul in sight.) Visited R.S. in afternoon. She has withstood the journey.

Aug 2 Received advice from brokers, re investments in Leyland Motors and Lonsdale Investment Trust. Medical out-patients, Glossop; Ward 11; St. John St., 5 cases. 9.30 p.m., returned to hospital, to see R.S.; telephoned her son, who seemed a nasty piece of work.

Aug 3   R.S. died today. Ward rounds; took Dr. F. to lunch, and gave him £10.10s.0d. for services to private patients. Pre-holiday rush. Promised to visit Hewkin [*former employee at Sherratt and Hughes, booksellers*] on my return from Yugoslavia. He is 86, almost blind, and lonely.

Aug 4   Ward round, 15; reports; domiciliary visit (aet 55, M/c 11, hysterical paralysis, admitted). To Dr. J. for lunch. Cancelled theatre seats for Ralph Richardson and John Gielgud. To St. John St.; Jackson the Tailor's man waiting with new suit. Farewells and preparations for departure [*to Yugoslavia, by rail, for 16 days*].

Aug 20 [*Saturday*]   Woke up about 6.30 a.m. in sleeper, fine morning, hurtling through Belgian countryside. Bruxelles at 7 a.m., and thence to Ostend. Large crowd on the boat and frightful red tape at Dover: pushing, shoving and milling about for fatuous passport and customs inspection. Much in favour of air-travel after this performance. Clara [*sister-in-law*] met us at Victoria, worried about Jack. She has reason to worry. Arrived in Manchester at 11.30 p.m. Found on arrival that I had won £25, in a Premium Bond draw. Good supper, and so to bed. I thank God that we are safely home.

Aug 21   Awoke at 7.0 a.m. Wonderful bath; 2 weeks of dirt removed. Dispatched letter of application for membership of Manchester Literary and Philosophical Society. Trying to get organized for tomorrow. A hectic week approaching.

Aug 22   Memorial light purchased for my mother: may her dear soul rest in peace. Dictated letters to Mrs. Faulkner [*secretary*]; gave her daughter a present. To Mrs. K. Dukinfield: p.v. [*per vaginam examination*] and ring [*for prolapse*] removed. Ward 11; N.O. has been allowed up. Lunch at Masonic, 7/5d. Handed in 1200 dinars for cashment at bank. Checked up on share purchases. Gave Miss James present, which she appreciated. St. John St., 7 cases, including Lecturer in Chemistry. Much writing and administration today. Letter to Jack's doctor at the Middlesex.

Aug 23 Heavy rain. Judy [*daughter, aged 15*] goes to London on her own for the first time. Ward 7, full round,. Domiciliary visit: congestive heart failure (aet 61, Stalybridge, admitted). St. John St., 5 cases, including 14-stone former district commissioner in Rhodesia. Dinner with M. alone. Spent the evening in the lumber room. Many interesting items uncovered.

Aug 24 Car steering heavy; great strain on pectoral muscles.

Aug 25 Twenty-fourth Wedding Anniversary. Awakened at 3.0 a.m. by Dr. F., re N.O.: a severe allergic reaction has developed. Reports: Ward round, 15, and St. John St., 2 cases. To cinema with M: 'Psycho', murder by schizophrenic, 13/-. Nuts and ices, 3/-.

Aug 27 [*Saturday*] To Manchester University Medical Library. The librarian, Wilson, informs me that very few people in Manchester are interested in the history of medicine. Professor Mitchell, Sir Geoffrey Jefferson and Wm. Brockbank are the exceptions.

Aug 28 Read slating article in the *Sunday Times* by Ian Fleming on the rapaciousness of Italians during the tourist season. Ward 11, to see N.O., and to explain the prognosis in her case to her husband. Returned home to write to Harry W., Jr. [*friend*] of my desire to visit him in Virginia next year; and to apply for membership of the Faculty of the History of Medicine and Pharmacy of the Worshipful Society of Apothecaries of London. Summoned back to the hospital, by Mrs. G.: her husband [*a medical colleague*] was seized by a pain in the chest on lifting a suitcase, prior to leaving for holiday. Drove through the heaviest rain and storm I have yet seen in England. David left for London. He strikes me as a lonely figure.

Aug 29   Returned my Will to the bank, for their safekeeping. Lunch at hospital, 1.35 p.m.–1.45 p.m. St. John St., 3 cases.

3:0 p.m. [*Female, aged 60, housewife*] She says that she cannot sit down, because she has pains in the buttocks (which she described as 'the bottom of her ribs'), has no confidence, 'cannot eat and cannot sleep'. When she does a 'bit of walking', she has to stop, she said, and be taken home. She told me that she was 'a complete wreck'; in fact, she claimed she was quite unfit to come upstairs to my consulting room, so that I had to go down to the waiting room to see her. (She was accompanied by a lady friend, who helped her to dress and undress.) When I asked her to hold out her hands to see if there was any tremor, she kept dropping her arms down. I had to be rather firm, and told her that there was no earthly reason why she should not hold her arms out. When she eventually did so, there was no tremor to observe. She went through all kinds of other capers, was tender wherever pressed upon, had strapping all round the upper part of her abdomen, and made noisy eructations throughout the examination, swallowing a considerable amount of air. (Bloody awful situation.) It also proved impossible to examine her fundi [*floor of the eyes*] with the opthalmoscope, since she kept screwing her eyes up. She is dragging her anchor very heavily, and it could take months, if not years, for her to improve. It may be necessary to invoke psychiatric treatment. There was no silver lining to be seen.

Assassination of Premier of Jordan.

Aug 30   Woke up later than usual, 8.0 a.m. Dark and gloomy outside. Made no breakfast for M. Lost my way to Glossop. Medical out-patients at Woods Hospital very full. Domiciliary visit in Glossop: aet 84, heart failure, bronchopneumonia, *in extremis*. Cider at Junction Inn, Glossop, with Dr.R. No lunch today. St. John St., 4 cases. To bed at midnight.

Aug 31   To Arnfields and domiciliary visits: paresis of one leg, lymphadenoma (aet 56, Ashton), and respiratory infection, chronic bronchitis and emphysema (aet 74, Stalybridge, admitted). Ward 12: Mrs. J. very ill, but condition misjudged by Sister, and I did not examine her because of pressure of work. St. John St., 5 cases. Dr. F. telephoned in the evening to let me know that Mrs. J. was moribund; she died later.

Sept 1   Heavy rain, no hat. Head steaming on walk to St. John St.

Sept 2   Bought fish in Shude Hill [*Manchester market*], £1.10s.0d; fruit and vegetables, £2.1s.0d. Private visit in Dukinfield: probably steatorrhea [*diarrhoea*] and malnutrition, paid one guinea. Visited Indian doctor from Calcutta, Dr. H., in his room at the hospital; running a temperature. Medical out-patients, long session, dealt with efficiently.

Sept 3 [*Saturday*]   Fidel Castro announces his solid alliance with Russia and Communist China in defiance of the USA, and severs relations with the Formosan Chinese Government. To St. John St. for letters; much mail. Further visit to Dr. H. at the hospital; X-Ray shows right-sided consolidation. 8 p.m., The Opera House: Sybil Thorndike, Marie Lohr and Lewis Casson in Noel Coward's *Waiting in the Wings*. An excellent play, generally approved. Spoke to Sir Wm. Fletcher Shaw in the interval, who complained of his deafness.

Sept 4   'Be virtuous and you will be eccentric' (Mark Twain). Read my diary of 1935, and destroyed the day's entries as I read them. It is better to relegate to oblivion details which are of no interest to others. It was an eventful year of the disintegration and fulfilment of romances: Beryl Bailey, Eva Weaver, Rita McMahon, Noreen O'Connor and a Miss Todd, whom I cannot remember, are names which keep recurring. Much alcohol was consumed; boredom at Lewisham Hospital [*where he was Resident Medical Officer for 3½ years, from 1932 to 1935*] was the reason. Three gallons of petrol cost 4/3d; the price of petrol went up 1d, to 1/6d a gallon, on May 1st, 1935.

Two dress-shirts, white waistcoat and a pair of flannels were purchased by me on April 3rd [*1935*] for £3. I insured my car in those days for £5.18s.0d., and paid £18 for a cruise on the 'Doric'. May 6th 1935 was King George Vth's Silver Jubilee; there was a Bank Holiday. The death of Dr. James Collier, a great neurologist and teacher, is also noted in the pages I have been reading; and that I spent a delightful day in the country on Easter Monday, with Rita.

Sept 6   Medical Out-patients lengthy and complicated. Ward Rounds, 7 and 11. Rapidly to St. John St.; 6 cases. Invited to the Fays [*neighbours*] for the evening; C_2H_5OH++. The lack of modesty of Leslie Lever [*solicitor and friend*] about his Papal knighthood in the Order of St. Gregory, and about his audience with Pope John XXIII, was very striking. His devotion to the Catholic cause, although laudable, amounts to a pathological obsession.

Sept 7   Hangover from yesterday, disturbed night, milk at 4.0 a.m. Promised Judy [*daughter*] 10/- a week, henceforth. Domiciliary visits: coronary thrombosis (aet 52, Ashton; admitted), and pneumoconiosis (aet 74, Ashton; X-Ray of chest). Dr. H., Indian doctor, seen in Ward 15. Improved. To St. John St., 7 cases, including young man with high BP, both of whose parents died of strokes, and a solicitor's clerk of 47 who smokes 20 cigarettes a day, and has prolonged expiration with some of the early features of emphysema. His chest expansion was ½″ below the average.

4:15 p.m. [*Male, aged 24, fire insurance clerk*] He was rather thick-set, height 5′8″ and weight 12 st. 2 lbs., and is going out to Rhodesia. His blood pressure was 140/100 sitting, and 140/96 lying down. The reading was somewhat high for a man of his age, but perhaps could be accounted for by the stress of his decision to go abroad, and the fact that he is somewhat overweight for his height. However, it was not ominously high, and in warm climates blood pressure sometimes has a tendency to fall.

Sadlers Wells Opera: *Tannhauser*, with Ronald Dowd as Tannhauser, Victoria Elliott as Venus, and Peter Glossop as

Wolfram. Conductor, Reginald Goodall; a magnificent and pleasing performance.

Sept 8 Domiciliary visit to Hyde: aet 20, a lad who lost one leg in 1957 in a motor cycle accident, and now complains of weakness in the other; referred for physiotherapy. Wards 11, 12: saw Mrs. C.R. [*private patient*]. St. John St, 5 cases. Dr. L. presented me with 3 Havana cigars, Ramon Allones, this evening.

Sept 9 Mrs. N.O.'s husband acquainted me by telephone of his wife's extravagance and his despair. Medical Out-patients, including an undertaker's assistant, aet 74. Depressed since retirement, after disposing of 40,000 corpses in his working lifetime, he related the recovery of one such corpse, which began to move. Quite a rational conversation.

Sept 10 [*Saturday*] M. has fibrositis and lumbago. Purchased 50 Upmann Petit Coronas, 25 Flor-de-Lancha, 10 Burma Cheroots and matches: total, £22.9s.9d. To Miss James, 10/od. Domiciliary visits: malarial attacks (aet 37, Ashton, has worked in Africa, and is returning), and anastomotic ulcer, with melaena [*blackened faeces, probably from internal bleeding*] (Glossop, to be admitted). Wards 11, 12 and Woods Hospital; 50 miles since leaving home this morning.

Sept 11 1.55 p.m. Had serious accident in car; M. taken to Withington hospital. Independent witnesses seemed of doubtful reliability. Severely shocked. Thereafter to bed, but many phone calls and inquiries. Everyone asks the same questions, and the whole business has to be recapitulated *ad nauseam*. Death of Mrs. Toon, cerebral embolism.

Sept 12 Policeman called to take a statement. Felt very shaken, bruises to right hip, stiff shoulder and swollen middle finger of left hand. Phoned M. to enquire about her health: to be discharged today. St. John St., 3 cases, including otosclerotic [*deaf*] carrot merchant. Difficulty in concentrating today, and vain attempts to go to sleep.

Sept 13   Medical Out-patients at Woods Hospital; Ward rounds; and domiciliary visit: aet 51, Denton, iron-deficiency anaemia and congestive heart failure. Advice given. St. John St., 5 cases. Witnessed slanging-match between car dealers in street. Depressed feeling; like vultures fighting over carrion. Garage people tend that way.

Sept 14   Ward Rounds; St. John St, 3 cases.

4.00 p.m. [*Female, aged 47, secretary*] She was an intelligent woman of good type who has been married 13 years and has no children. She said that her husband has always been a drinker, but that since his father's death last year it has grown worse. She told me her husband has 'gone to pieces'; that he comes in at 2 in the morning, 'more often than not totally drunk'; and that 'the smell of the bedroom is like a tap room'. Even when he is sober, she said, 'he barely talks to me'. He has not been home for a meal all this week, and has not taken her out for nearly 12 months. Two weeks ago she found a shirt of his in the washing with lipstick on it. For the last five years she has had sexual intercourse with her husband 'on average three times a year'; the last time was six months ago. Today, she complained of poor appetite, insomnia, and palpitations. On examination, there was a tremor of her outstretched hands, and her pulse was 84, rapid but regular. She is having an appalling time; a young woman still, who does not love her husband and feels that the future holds very little for her.

Had anginal pain.

Sept 15   Very tired this morning. Ward Round, 7. Discharged Mrs. N.O.; she hates going. St. John St., 6 cases, and straight home. Dr. F. phones about Mrs. N.O.: she has now developed a rash on her legs. Will try to get rid of her tomorrow morning. Battle of Britain Day today, when alleged number of German planes shot down was 185. It turned out, after investigations following the war, that the number was 56, approximately.

Sept 16   Visited garage, to inspect damage to my car.

Proceeded to hospital, Ward 15. Talk to Sister B. about her first foreign trip: to Spain. Saw Mrs. N.O., Ward 12. She is in a highly nervous state, and has had many troubles and tribulations with her husband and children. Very lengthy Medical Outpatients. Home by 7 p.m. Listened to Beethoven's Choral Symphony on wireless. On TV, Sir Brian Horrocks questioned by Dimbleby, and 'News Extra' on Angola.

Sept 17 [*Saturday*]   Ward Rounds. Home by 1.15 p.m. Siesta. Later watched farrago of nonsense on TV: viz. last night of Promenade Concerts, Constance Shacklock, Rule Britannia etc., conducted by Sir Malcolm Sargent. He made a poor speech; old Basil Cameron very much in the background. Up at 4.30 a.m., tidying my room until 5.45 a.m. Returned to bed until 8.0 a.m.

Sept 18   Read Shinwell on Attlee in the Sunday paper, and Donald Fish on crime at London Airport. At 7.30 p.m. went to Steel Memorial Hall to hear Professor David Daiches on 'How to Read a Novel'. Too academic for the majority and sometimes tiresome, but interesting.

Sept 19   To Dr. M. [*hospital radiologist*], for X-Ray examination of my fingers and cervical spine. Examination of Nurses; Ward rounds. Received a piece of fresh salmon from Dr. P. My B.P. 190/110. 7 cases at St. John St., including introspective accountant, aet 41, short of breath, 'depressed and tired', who complains of 'feeling stiff after getting out of bed'. He said that he had had a 'faint' in his office, but he has a tendency to hypochondriasis. To do investigations.

Sept 20   No lunch today; glass of milk on Ward 15; St. John St., 6 cases.

4:30 p.m. [*Female, aged 17, single, a laboratory assistant*] Ten months ago she was knocked down by a car on her way home from work at about 5.30 p.m. She came round in the roadway as the ambulance arrived, and later had 14 stitches in a laceration to her forehead. She is fit now, but the scar makes her feel depressed. It was conspicuous, but not unsightly. She is a pretty girl and tells me she has a boyfriend; the scar does not appear to have interfered with her happiness to any great extent. Even with the scar she is considerably prettier than some people without scars.

Sept 21   Domiciliary visits: bronchogenic carcinoma (Houghton Green, to arrange bronchoscopy), and coronary thrombosis (?) (aet 70, Stalybridge, ECG arranged). St. John St., 5 cases. Eve of the New Year. Blessed M. and the children.

Sept 22   To synagogue this morning. Excellent sermon against materialism and money-chasers. Listened to 'The Magic Flute' after supper. To bed by 8.45 p.m.

Sept 23   Awoke at 1.0 a.m., and looked at my copy of Ketham's *Fasciculus Medicinae*, 1522. Disturbing news from United Nations: Khruschev like a bull in a china-shop.

Sept 24 [*Saturday*]   Attended marriage at St. Vincent's, Altrincham, and nuptial mass thereafter. Home by 3.30 p.m. My B.P. taken: 144/96, slight improvement.

Sept 25   Severe chill. St. Vincent's was very cold yesterday. Dictated 9 reports to Mrs Faulkner [*secretary*]. She was not in good humour at having to do them on a Sunday. How easy it is to forget good deeds done! Saw U.T. [*patient and old friend*] in Dukinfield: she tells me she has been left a house in St. Anne's-on-Sea and over £30,000. To bed early, but I will be more exhausted thereby in the morning.

Sept 26   Inquired as to hire of car: demand for £10 a week. Watched 'Panorama' on the coal situation, on the United Nations, with Khruschev leading the circus, and Iain Macleod on the Central African Federation. Thereafter, 'Face to Face', John Freeman interviewing Floyd Patterson.

Sept 28   Arose at 4 a.m., and did some administrative correspondence until 5 a.m. Returned to bed and woke up very tired. Reports; ward rounds; and 7 cases at St. John Street, including sulphuric acid burns in work accident, and case of pleural effusion. Listened to Saint-Saens' Piano Concerto on radio, with Colin Horsley, and to bed at 10.30.

Sept 29   Wards 11 and 14. Browsed around Sherratt and Hughes, and lunch at Masonic. Purchased Irish Sweepstake ticket from Head Porter, £1. 5 cases at St. John St.

2.30 p.m. [*Male, aged 36, aircraft engineer*] There was a great deal about this case, more than met the eye at first sight. His GP believes he is suffering from an anxiety state, but he complains of a burning, stinging, tingling sensation at the tip of his tongue. He said that it had been present for about 18 months to 2 years and that he is aware of it 'most of the time'. He said that he had lost about a stone during this period. There was some nystagmus [*reflex scanning movement*] in the left eye and his abdominal reflexes were diminished. He also told me that he was more irritable than he used to be. His GP has referred him to me as an 'intangible complaint', and wrote that 'the basis of all his trouble is his sense of inadequacy'. I have to give careful thought to this case and satisfy myself that there is no organic lesion of the brain system; I have seen early cases of D.S. [*disseminated, or multiple, sclerosis*] develop a tingling sensation in the tongue, while the nystagmus and diminished abdominal reflexes, even if slight, cannot be disregarded. I am not satisfied with a diagnosis of an anxiety state, and will admit him. [*An MS note reads: 'Very urgent, please'.*]

Sept 30   Signed reports; purchased stamps, 3/9d. General survey of wards. Burnley Building Society passbook collected. Total entry, £2,973. 6s. 4d. Home by 4.30 p.m.; siesta. I had much praecordial pain. Only 13 domiciliary consultations this month.

Oct 2 [*Sunday*]   Gave David a set of Shakespeare, and books on Wilde and Max Beerbohm. Gave Judy 10/- and M. £15. Read *Observer* and *Sunday Times*, and listened to Verdi's *The Force of Destiny* on the Third Programme.

Oct 3   Letter from Harry W. Jr. of Virginia, inviting

me to lecture to the Virginia Bibliographical Society, and to the Chesapeake and Ohio Railway Employees Hospital Association on the present system of medical practice in England. To Mrs. K, Dukinfield; ring [*for prolapse*] removed. Ward Rounds, and 2 domiciliaries: asthma (aet 52, Mossley; admitted), and acute sciatic neuritis, moaning with pain (aet 52, Mossley, admitted). 5 cases at St. John St., including mongol child, and asthma, aet 53. 'Panorama' on the Scarborough Labour Party Conference dilemma with Cousins' unilateralists, and on stiletto heels in women's shoes.

Oct 4   To Mrs. K., Dukinfield; ring inserted. Domiciliary in Ashton: psychosis or psychoneurosis. Hectic Outpatients' clinic, and 6 cases at St. John St., including colitis. Jack telephoned from London. He has just returned from convalescent home, but did not sound well. In congestive failure.

Oct 5   Home by 10.50 p.m.; watched Gaitskell's fighting speech about defence [*at Labour Party conference*].

Oct 6   Made breakfast for M. To Mrs. Faulkner: dictated reports of yesterday's cases, including Mongol details. Two domiciliaries: appendicular colic and moniliasis (aet 32, Clayton, to have barium meal), and mitral stenosis, with hypertension and vertigo (Gorton, to be admitted). Five cases at St. John St. My B.P. 160/95. Watched magnificent *Henry VI* on television.

Oct 7   Mrs B., Ward 11, improving daily. Domiciliaries: congestive heart failure, auricular fibrillation and C_2H_5OH (Audenshaw), and coronary thrombosis, with severe shock (aet 56, Ashton, urgently admitted). Medical Outpatients for 3 hours: reprimanded a patient for his complaint about the length of time he had been waiting.

Oct 8 [*Saturday*]   Arose at 6.40 a.m. Three domiciliaries: paresis [*a partial paralysis*] of both legs (aet 61, Hyde, admitted); angina (aet 50, Glossop, ECG arranged, no admission); and post-traumatic subdural haematoma (aet

20, Woodley). Ward 12: aet 39, carcinoma of breast, with secondaries in brain. Home by 4.30 p.m., dead beat. On arrival, learned that V.W. [*private patient*] had worsened. Returned at 6 p.m. to see him: Cheyne–Stokes breathing, pneumonia, and left ventricular failure. Received membership card today of Manchester Institute of Contemporary Art. Further visit at 10 p.m. to see V.W.; stayed until 11.

Oct 9   A quiet day. V.W. slightly improved. Bathed at 1 p.m. Read two stories from *Memoirs of Sherlock Holmes*, first edition.

Oct 10   V.W. very ill, an uncontrolled diabetic. Ward Rounds; and to St. John St., 5 cases, including T.B. meningitis. 6.0 p.m., proceeded again to hospital to see V.W. To bed at 9.15 p.m., exhausted.

Oct 11   8.15 a.m., phone-call from hospital announcing death of V.W.: broncho-pneumonia, left ventricular failure, hypertension, diabetes of unusual type, and C_2H_5OH. Adjoining house to ours for sale for £4,900. To see private case in Glossop: aet 79, ascites and cardiac asthma. Admitted to Ward 15. Proceeded to St. John St.: 3 cases, including M.W., who can't micturate. Home by 5.40 p.m. Rating Officer (date of birth, 25.2.06) [*his own was 28.2.06*] awaiting me. Showed him round; he will reduce amount of rates to £80 rateable value, i.e. less by £6 p.a. Gave party at 8.30 p.m. at home for 16 doctors and nurses. Striking tendency to C_2H_5OH observed; Dr. H. prefers slivovic and Dr. P. whisky. 1 bottle of whisky, 1 bottle of gin, ⅓ of bottle of plum brandy and ¾ of a siphon consumed.

Oct 12   Arose very tired. Ward 15: A.N. [*private patient*] very ill indeed. Loaned Cope on *Chest Diseases* to Dr. F. To St. John St., 6 cases. Afterwards, gave lift to Miss James, horrible woman. Fog settling down for the night; and frost.

Oct 15 [*Saturday*]   A letter from C.C. [*former nurse at his hospital*]. She writes of her harassed life as a Nigerian hospital matron, in the lonely bush country. Geoffrey [*son-in-law*] taken ill with colic at 4 p.m. Later, severe abdominal pain, acute appendicitis. Mr. A. [*surgeon-colleague*] won't come, Mr. B. [*another surgeon-colleague*] out boozing; got Mr. C. at 12.45 a.m., who came promptly. Appendectomy performed in hospital. Home at 2 a.m.

Oct 16　Cancel my intention of going to the Bourne wedding in order to avoid over-indulgence, and to obtain sufficient leisure. Did not dress today. Listened to *The Marriage of Figaro* on the radio, and to bed by 9.15 p.m.

Oct 19　Domiciliary visits: subarachnoid haemorrhage or cerebral thrombosis (aet 63, Audenshaw, admitted), bronchial pneumonia and congestive failure with ascites (aet 54, Audenshaw, refuses admission). Medical Out-patients until 12.45 p.m. Hurried to Manchester, without lunch; ran out of petrol on the way, car pushed. 7 cases at St. John Street.

4:30 p.m. [*Male, age 57, retired policeman, Lancashire constabulary*] He was grossly overweight, 19 st. 6 lbs., and 6′4″, with extensive varicose veins and a very high blood pressure, 210/130. He has applied for a job as a temporary filing and postal clerk, and these are serious disabilities for a man who will have to stand on his feet a great deal, or run errands.

Glass of beer at 'The Princes', then Hallé and BBC Northern Orchestras in Mahler Centenary Concert. His Seventh Symphony (1905) and Nielsen's Symphony No. 5 (1922). Geoffrey has temperature this evening.

Oct 20　Very tired on rising. Unable to make breakfast for M., or take Judy to school. 5 reports dictated; Ward Rounds; 4 cases at St. John St. Ink purchased, 1/6d, and Paul Scott's *The Chinese Love Pavilion*. 7.40 p.m., domiciliary visit to Glossop: aet 70, myocardial failure and paroxysmal supra-ventricular tachycardia; admitted. Afterwards adjourned for drinks at the home of one of Dr. R.'s patients in Glossop.

Oct 21   Gave Miss James 10/- today. She has lost her cat; it has run away.

Oct 22 [*Saturday*]   Letter from Capt. J.F. [*patient*], announcing that in addition to his gift of apples the other day, I am to expect a wooden Chinese idol which is arriving by rail. Ward Rounds: J.I. [*fishmonger husband of private patient*] gave me a packet of fish. Purchased some flowers from Mr. Cole, 4/-. [*A mortuary attendant from whom some doctors purchased deceased patients' flowers.*]

Oct 23   Geoffrey has tantrums about his temperature. Dr. M. [*former junior colleague*] was pleased with my testimonial, in contrast to the one given him by Dr. O., that poor fish. £1 to gardener. To bed by 9.0 p.m.

Oct 24   M. made breakfast. Proceeded to old Mrs. W. in Stockport. She is going down rapidly, and clutched my hand with great affection. She will be 88, she said, at the end of the month. Received Chinese statue from Capt J.F. in very debilitated condition: it has a fractured left arm, and its left foot, left hand and a right finger are missing. It is otherwise perfect.

Oct 25   Asked Dr. M. [*radiologist*] to X-Ray Chinese statue. Medical Out-patients at Glossop, and Ward rounds. St. John St., 5 cases; including Jewish printer whose parents, brothers and sisters were murdered by the Nazis. Masonic meeting: I was Junior Deacon, with nothing to do.

Oct 27   Had a good old row with Mrs. Faulkner [*secretary*] over her lack of humanity, in failing to telephone to enquire about Geoffrey. She is false and selfish. Domiciliaries: mitral stenosis (aet 49, Mossley, admitted); severe iron deficiency anaemia (aet 60, Ashton, admitted). Wards 14 and 15, complete rounds. Sandwiches made for me and hurried to St. John St., 5 cases. Geoffrey better. Floods in West Country. To bed early.

Oct 28   Elected to Manchester Literary and Philosophical Society and awarded Provincial Rank in Masonry (Provincial Grand Steward). Geoffrey making good progress. Proceeded directly to hospital; Ward round, dreadful lunch, and Medical Out-patients. Row with Mrs. Faulkner appears to be settling down. In evening, discussed purchase of Provincial regalia with S.G. [*mason*]. Randolph Churchill wins his slander action against Gerald Nabarro, M.P., £1,500 and costs. *Lady Chatterley's Lover* case continues.

Oct 30 [*Sunday*]   Geoffrey returned from hospital. In the evening, exhausting delay waiting for the Josephs [*friends*] to get ready to come out to dinner. Probably due to Mrs. Joseph's pathological preparatory titivation.

Oct 31   Pay slip from Regional Hospital Board, £443.13s.2d. Sent telegram to poor Mrs. W. [*see Oct 24*] in Stockport. She is dying of cancer. Owing to fog, unable to get to Ashton: turned back at Denton. Purchased *Petit Larousse* from Sherratt and Hughes, and ordered 100 Xmas cards. Lunch at Masonic Temple, Lord Derby present, 7/-. St. John St., 6 cases, including M.L., aet 55; the poor man has bronchogenic carcinoma, and is to be admitted. Watched report on American Presidential campaign on 'Panorama'.

Nov 1   Phoned Geoffrey, who is not very well. Domiciliary: rheumatic valvular disease and congestive heart failure, *in extremis* (aet 30, Stalybridge, admitted). Medical Out-patients, St. John St., 3 cases. Home early; no one in, except kitten. Violent gales and storms. To bed early.

Nov 2   Ward 15. Gave Dr. F. [*a junior house doctor*] *Current Medical Research*, H.M.Stationery Office, 3/6d. Domiciliary visit: cor pulmonale (aet 66, Audenshaw, admitted). St. John Street, 4 cases. Thereafter, proceeded to Sherratt and Hughes. Ordered Penguin edition of *Lady Chatterley's Lover*. Case settled in favour of the publishers Penguin: this evening's news. Indifferent Hallé concert, conducted by George Weldon.

Nov 3   1.15 p.m., personal medical examination re car accident [*see Sept. 11*] for my insurance claim.

[*Excerpt from Medical Report by Dr. M.J., on Dr. Hugh Selbourne, aet 54, Consulting Physician*] 'He was thrown against the steering wheel, was shocked, hurt his left hand and sustained bruises over the abdominal wall, right leg and iliac crests. A fracture of the left middle finger was found: this finger is painful, particularly in the mornings and when he has to use it for percussion purposes. The same evening he had a severe attack of anginal chest pain, radiating to the right arm. He tells me that since the accident the attacks of angina have been more severe and more frequent. He had a coronary thrombosis in 1953, and has had some degree of angina of effort since then ... On examination, his general condition was good, his weight 13 st. 8 lbs, with no anaemia, cyanosis, oedema or finger clubbing. His pulse was regular and soft, 72, his B.P. 185/105, with his mitral first sound reduplicated. He had partial dentures, his pupils were equal and reacted normally, and his reflexes were brisk and symmetrical. His ECG showed signs of an old healed myocardial infarct, or coronary thrombosis ...'

2:45 p.m. [*Male, aged 30, bus conductor*] More than two years ago he fell down 12 bus stairs, after catching his heel on a metal strip, and struck his left temple. He was taken to hospital, bleeding from his left ear, and an X-Ray revealed a fracture of the skull. He says he still has head-aches which 'come on every fortnight', and that his head 'goes muzzy as if it was full of cotton wool'. He also said that he had had to give up his electric razor, since he 'cannot stand the vibration'. He was a healthy looking young man, but nervous; his hands were moist and his face somewhat florid. His blood pressure was 130/80, normal. Most of his symptoms are due to a neurosis arising from the accident, but he has gone back to work on double-decker buses. He says his brother, who also works on the buses, 'does the driving'. They work together.

Smoke belches forth from my car on the way home: smoke-bomb? Back by 6.30 p.m.

Nov 6 [*Sunday*]   Gave G.K. Chesterton's autobiography to David. Read V. Sackville-West's *No Signposts in the Sea*, and watched very good play by John Osborne [*A Subject of Scandal and Concern*], with Richard Burton.

Nov 8   Talk to Sister E. about *Lady Chatterley*. Ward rounds and Medical Out-patients at Glossop. Domiciliary: vertigo of long-standing (aet 72, Hyde, admitted). St. John St., 2 cases. Shocked by the news of the death of Dr. Barber; he died at 2.20 p.m. in Buxton, aged 48.

Nov 9   Kennedy elected President of the USA, aged 43. Immunizations for polio at Arnfields. Ward 15; lunch, 4/-. To St. John St., 6 cases, including mitral stenosis. Purchased Provincial Lodge regalia, for £6 the lot. Chief points of the day: the new president of the USA and David L.'s birthday.

Nov 11   Domiciliary visit: mitral stenosis, congestive heart failure, ascites (aet 63, Hyde, admitted). Large polypoidal mass found in stomach of S. [*private patient*]; M.L.'s [*see Oct 31*] is a carcinoma of the oesophagus. Medical Out-patients hectic; finished at 6.0 p.m. Dr. F. [*house physician*] came to dinner. Showed him Cruveilhier's *Pathology*, 1829–1835, Laennec on *The Stethoscope*, 1819, and Bright's *Case Reports*, 1827. He went home at 10 p.m.; good type.

Nov 15   To Infirmary; had 2 fried eggs and milk. St. John St., 4 cases, including Mrs. W.C. from Blackpool, very tarty looking. Ruth [*daughter*] has gone into hospital with labour pains. God bless her.

Nov 16   Three domiciliary visits: pneumoconiosis (aet 64, Ashton, to be admitted if possible); praecordial pain, probably dietary indiscretion (aet 48, Stalybridge, ECG arranged); brachial neuritis [*inflammation of the brachial nerves*] (aet 45, Droylsden, for physiotherapy). Ward 15; St. John St., 4 cases. Hallé concert, conducted by Georges Tzipine: Hephzibah Menuhin playing Beethoven's 4th Piano Concerto, and Honegger's 3rd Symphony. Then to St. Mary's

Hospital to make further enquiries about Ruth. Prof. M. gave us bulletin: ruptured membranes, 2nd stage. Death of Gilbert Harding announced.

Nov 17 Wake up a grandfather, a beloved grandmother at my side. Ruth has a son. Breakfast made for M. Arranged admission for yesterday's pneumoconiosis. First sight of my grandchild. Whisky at Toon's place, and curried chicken dinner offered by Indian residents. Excellent stuff, coffee and cigar. Home by 9.0 p.m., fog descending.

Nov 18 Purchased my ordered copy of *Lady Chatterley's Lover*, Penguin, 3/6d, and Hamilton Bailey's *Demonstrations of Physical Signs in Clinical Surgery*. Interesting Medical Out-patients and comprehensive Ward Round. Toffees, 8/11d.

Nov 19 [*Saturday*] Full day of social round. Usual spivs.

Nov 21 Told by my solicitor that police are taking proceedings against man who drove car into me. St. John St., 5 cases, including E.E., who is not in good condition, too heavy, with varicose veins, obese and sallow. Listened to Verdi's *Don Carlos* on the radio.

Nov 22 Medical Out-patients at Glossop: 5/- piece given to me for my grandson by Sister E. No lunch today; St. John St., 2 cases.

2:15 p.m. [*Male, aged 54, grocer*] He complains of acid 'rising into his mouth', which has made his gums 'all sore'. He also suffers from constant nausea without sickness. Deep pressure from the 11th dorsal to the 1st lumbar was not as painful as a light touch. This is characteristic of chronic cholecystitis, and is known as Boas' Sign. He also said that 'eggs cause trouble'. Another important feature was his slight thirst, and the fact that there was a distinct trace of sugar in his urine. He said that he had recently 'knocked off' fatty foods and potatoes. Most of his symptoms are suggestive of disease of the gall bladder.

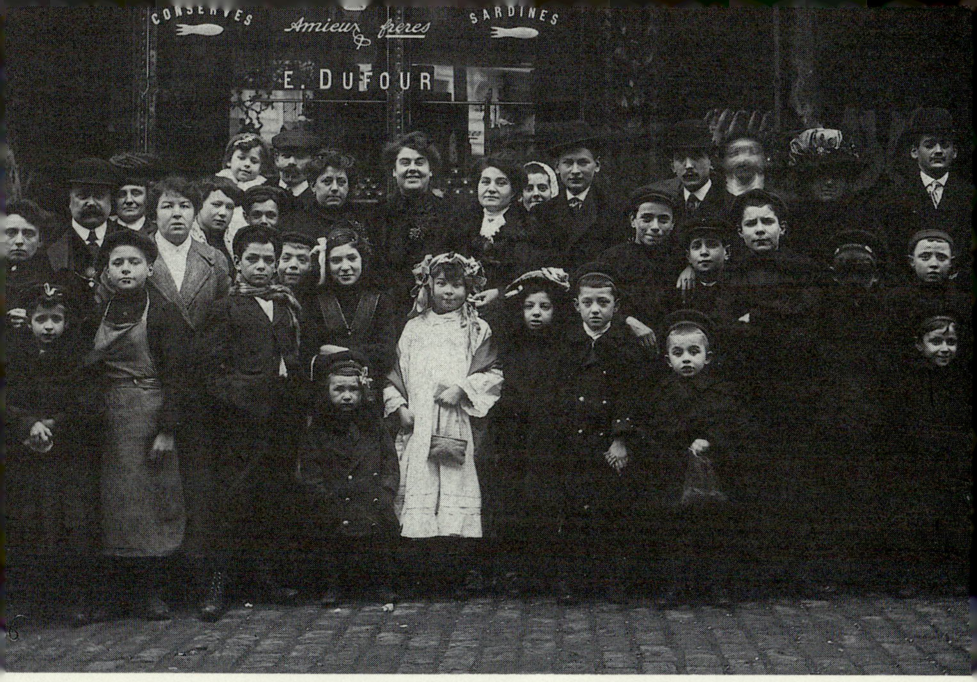

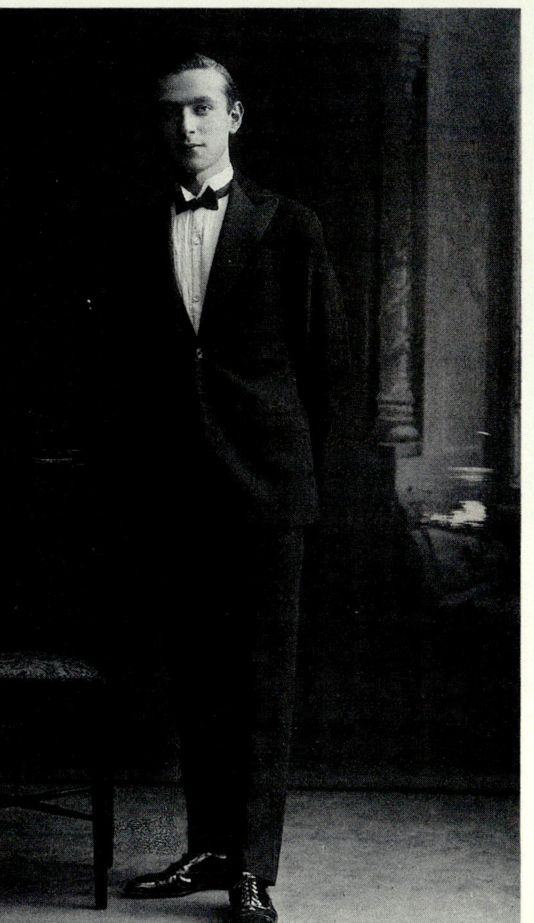
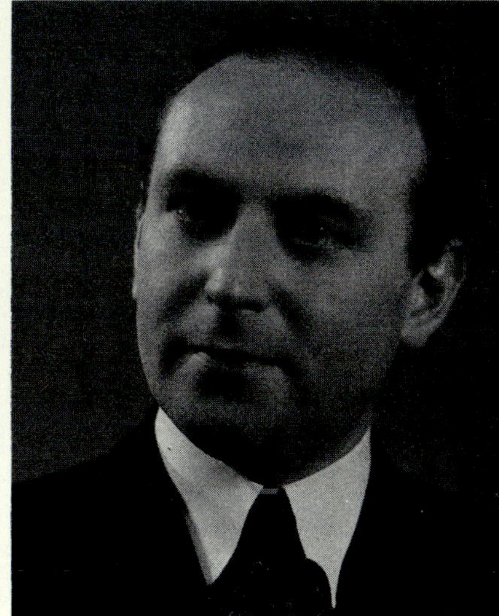

Top Montmartre, about
1910: the future Manchester
physician is on the far right
of the front row

Left The young medical
student at King's College,
London

Above Doctor Hugh
Selbourne

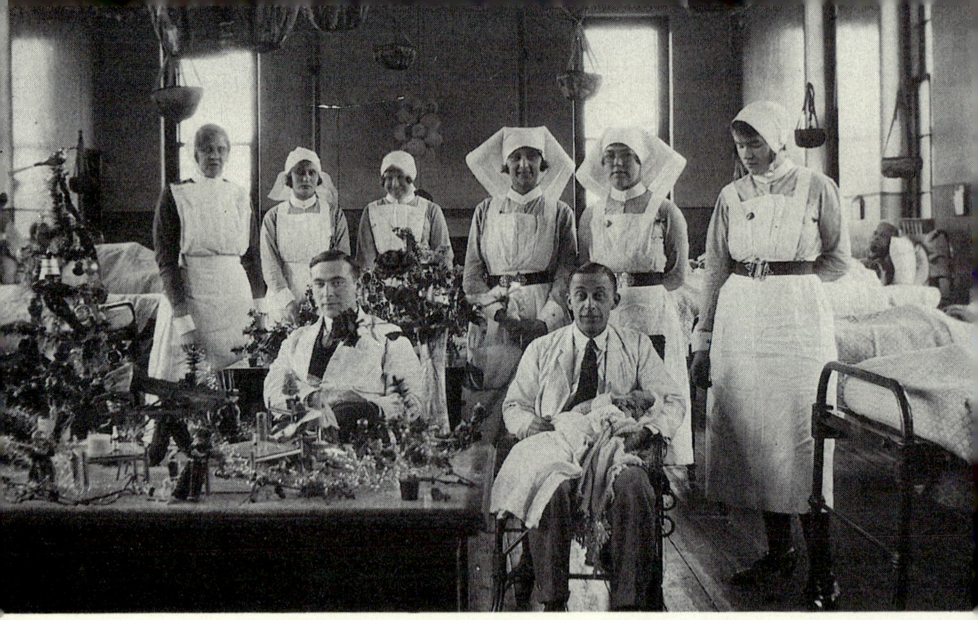

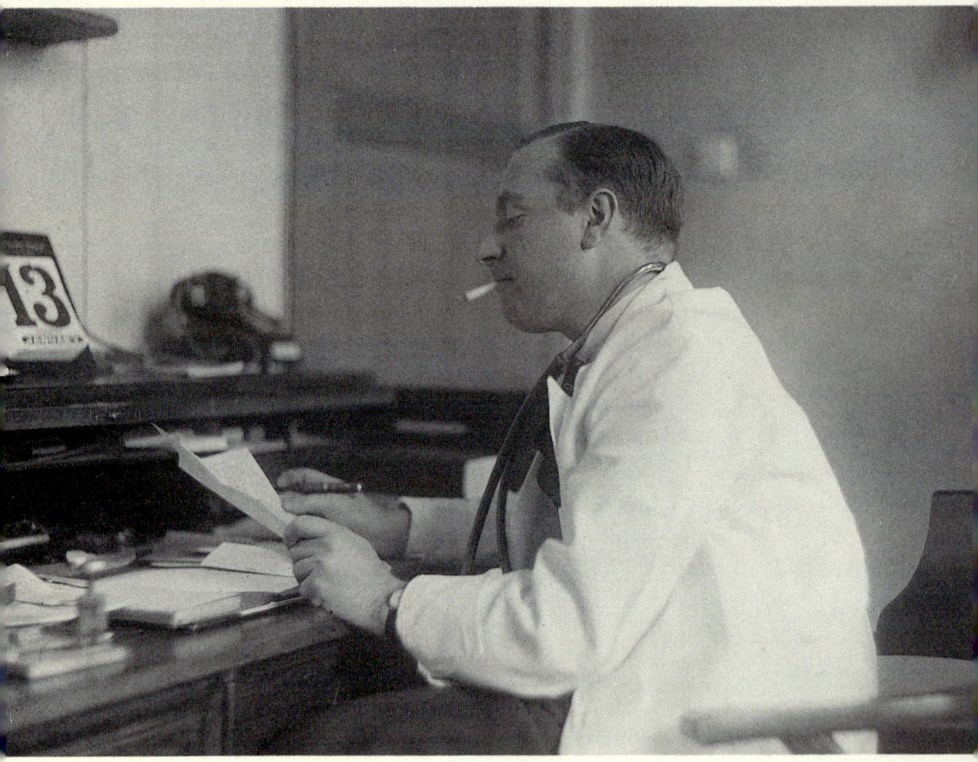

Resident Medical Officer at Lewisham Hospital, South London, at Christmas

Locum in a London general practice, 1936

Purchased new stethoscope, £1.19s.6d., and sphygmo-manometer [*blood pressure apparatus*], £7.10s.0d. Listened to Chamber Concert: Bach, Vivaldi and Handel.

Nov 23   To St. John St.; 5 cases, one of whom gave me silver sugar-tongs.

5:0 p.m. [*Female, aged 27, housewife*] She suffers from what she calls 'crying fits', nightmares and 'rheumatic attacks'. In 1943, at the age of ten, she went to Belsen, and lived through terrible experiences of hunger, physical exhaustion, and swelling of the joints, with repeated sore throats, which suggests rheumatic fever. When she left Belsen in 1945, she says she was anaemic, undernourished and 'full of fears'. Her later childhood was a continual physical and spiritual battle for rehabilitation; she came to England in 1953, when she was 20, and married two years later. I found her depressed; her pulse was rapid (96) and at the apex of her heart there was a fine systolic murmur.

Listened to a recording of poor old Gilbert Harding talking to Eamonn Andrews.

Nov 24   The man who ran into me has been summoned to appear at Manchester Magistrates Court on Dec. 14th at 10 a.m. Ward Round 12, comprehensive. Afterwards to circumcision of my grandson at St Mary's Hospital. Income tax provisional payment, £800.

Nov 26 [*Saturday*]   43 miles of domiciliary visits. Heavy rain. Mrs N.O. readmitted, with further chest pains.

Nov 27   Judy rude to me. Long talk with Arnold G. [*see July 5*], who thinks I ought to take up fishing. To the Hallé at 7 p.m: Moiseiwitch playing the Emperor Concerto.

Nov 29   Took Judy's pencil-case to school, which she had forgotten. To Medical Out-patients, and appointments committee for Registrar in General Medicine (3 applicants). St. John St., 3 cases, one ex-T.B. Home for dinner, and then called out to Dukinfield to see U.T. [*see Sept. 25*]: appalled to find that she has carcinoma of left breast involving chest-wall and glands, a frightful mess. I have asked Dr. L. to see her at the hospital on Friday morning.

Nov 30   Visited U.T.; will call for her Friday morning. Arnfields; reports; signed letters. St. John Street, 3 cases, including a nit-wit of an Irish woman who came a half-hour late. Visited Bob Walmsley's bookshop and purchased old numbers of *History Today*. Met Tomlinson there, a Salford schoolmaster, local historian and book-collector. Tea at Duncan and Foster's, 1/5d; the man sitting next to me was a telephone engineer with neuropathy. Then to the Hallé: André Tchaikovsky played Rachmaninoff's Variations on a Theme of Paganini. Home in extremely bad mood.

Dec 1   Full round of Ward 12, with cheerless sister. In Ward 11, Mrs. B. looks very ill; spoke to her militant husband. St. John St., 4 cases. Watched Leoncavallo's *Pagliacci* on television: Charles Mackerras conducted, with Peter Glossop. Ford shares fall, take-over of Dagenham now doubtful. It serves the gamblers right.

Dec 2   Letter from Judge Laski congratulating me on the birth of a 'grand-daughter'. To U.T.: took the poor woman to hospital, to see Dr. L. (X-rayed, no hope, very advanced, infiltrating the lungs and lymphatic system.) Took her home thereafter. Ward Rounds 12, 14, 15. Purchased white gloves, 8/6d, for Provincial Grand Lodge meeting at 4 p.m. in the Albert Hall [*Manchester*]. Lord Derby presided. Invested with collar of Provincial Grand Steward. Henry Wade, a horrible and dreadful creature, is Provincial Senior Grand Warden. Whose boots did he lick?

Dec 3   Day in bed. Food poisoning of mild degree, following dinner at Masonic Temple.

Dec 4   To Bournemouth, for a week's holiday. Many roads flooded, particularly at Kenilworth and Warwick.

Dec 11 [*Sunday*]   Paid bill, £57.8s.3d.; £1 tip to waiter at table, and 10/- to chamber-maid. Total cost, £70 for one week, including petrol. Fine day, roads fairly clear. To bed at home at 8 p.m., and read Sunday papers.

Dec 12   Ward 12, complete round; cholecystectomy [*removal of gall bladder*] performed on Mrs. B. U.T. again visited in Dukinfield; she is going into hospital for radium treatment next Wednesday. Domiciliary: praecordial pain (aet 50, Stalybridge, ECG arranged). Fog descending. St. John St., 3 cases, including a Catholic born in Bethlehem with a large family and fibrous nodules. Multiple demands for tax from all sources, surtax, schedule A, arrears etc. Called out to Glossop tonight, but impossible owing to fog. What a dreadful life!

Dec 13   Heavy fog. Temporised to see how things were shaping; then set off. Medical Out-patients. Private visits: right basal dullness, haemoptysis, semi-comatose, incontinent (aet 73, Glossop), paid 10 guineas; and chronic alcoholism (aet 59, Glossop, to be admitted), paid 10 guineas. Straight to St. John St. without lunch; 4 cases. Miss James gave me two boiled eggs and coffee.

3:0 p.m. [*Male, aged 55, clerk*] He has had high blood pressure, he says, for more than ten years, but has had no treatment for it. Eight weeks ago he woke up from his sleep at about 2.0 a.m. and found that he had 'lost the power' in his right arm, and then found that he could not walk. His speech, he said, 'went', but by 10.0 p.m. of the same day 'things began to get better'. His doctor told him he had had a stroke, but the rapid recovery suggests an attack of cerebral spasm. He said that his right foot swells, but this was not evident. His blood pressure was 190/115 in the left arm, and 200/120 in the right. I told him to resume light work and to keep his mind occupied while under treatment.

Dec 14   [*see Nov 24*] 10 a.m., attended City Magistrates Court with M.: Police v. F.W., with P.C. Cordingley,

45. W. pleaded guilty and we were out by 10.30. Lunch at Masonic Temple, coffee with Col. Rothband. St. John St., 5 cases.

3:45 p.m. [*Male, aged 48, former press operator, now nightwatchman*] He was a thick-set, pleasant man of good colour, with a slight tremor of his outstretched hands. Sixteen months ago a steel girder being lifted by a crane slipped and dropped on his left foot; severe injury was caused to it, including three fractured metatarsals. Later the foot went septic and amputation was seriously considered. Two weeks after his final discharge from hospital he started to complain of intense thirst, and diabetes was diagnosed. He is now working as a nightwatchman, feels 'fit' – he said that his foot was 'quite good', considering that he 'nearly lost it' – but his urine contained an appreciable amount of sugar. In predisposed individuals an accident can precipitate symptoms of diabetes which were already lying latent. It is a fairly common occurrence.

To Hallé Concert, Sir John Barbirolli, Chetham Boys' Choir singing Carols. Left at interval.

Dec 15   Letter informing me that F.W. was only fined £5 for driving without due care and attention, and his licence endorsed; a light sentence indeed. Patchy fog. Domiciliary visit: loss of weight (aet 60, Ashton, for investigations). Ward Round 15, and saw Mrs B. in Ward 11.

12:30 p.m. [*Male, aged 52, businessman*] For seven or eight months he has noticed a change in his bowel action. As soon as he gets up he has a loose, windy, noisy evacuation, and this is repeated once or twice during the day. When he has the desire to stool he has to move quickly. He has not noticed that his stools are particularly pale, but on one occasion at least there was some red discolouration; he could not decide whether it was blood or tomato. He has a certain amount of intermittent abdominal pain, but he finds it hard to differentiate this from a long-standing duodenal ulcer. There has been slight weight loss, but abdominal examination disclosed no tenderness or tumour. There was nothing abnormal on rectal examination.

However, the symptoms seem like those of carcinoma of the colon. [*It was.*]

Much fog this evening. King Baudouin married Fabiola today, the King of Nepal sacked his Prime Minister, and the Ethiopian Crown Prince deposed his father Haile Selassie [*the attempted coup failed; the Emperor's position was secured 4 days later*]. Listened to the *Messiah*.

Dec 16   Three domiciliaries: loss of weight, fatigue, Koch's disease(?) (aet 16, Hyde, admitted); probably cerebral haemorrhage (aet 45, Hyde, admitted); pulseless, with acute pulmonary oedema (aet 57, Hyde, admitted). Ward 12, full round; Mrs. N.O. once more reluctant to go. Gave Dr. V. [*fellow consultant physician*] £7.17.6d. as contribution to Xmas gifts for medical residents. Medical Out-patients long-winded. Home by 7.15 p.m. Frightful air-crash over Brooklyn; at least 126 dead, and only one survivor, a boy of 11. Watched Japanese films on television, with irrationally gruesome themes.

Dec 17 [*Saturday*]   Visited U.T. [*see Dec 12*]; some improvement. Ward 3; case of carbon monoxide poisoning. Ward Round, 14. Massive income tax demands confirmed by the accountant: Surtax for 1959–60, £787.10s.0d. Too many appointments for next week; exhausting prospect.

Dec 19   Gave M. £15 housekeeping money. Bought gift tokens (7 x £1.1s.0d.) from Boots. Domiciliary visits: congestive heart failure, oedema (aet 68, Audenshaw, to be admitted after Xmas); cor pulmonale (aet 64, Droylsden, to be admitted after Xmas). Gave Sister G. £2.2s.0d. as Xmas box. Purchased Kingsley Amis, *Take a Girl Like You.*

Dec 20   No lunch. St. John., 5 cases.

5:0 p.m. [*Female, aged 45, confectioner*] She was a well-built woman, tired-looking, with bad varicose veins, who says she has been wakened up in the middle of the night for the last 12 months with acidity and heartburn. The discomfort is relieved by food, but returns about 1½–2 hours thereafter. She had marked epigastric tenderness, particularly to the right of the umbilicus. She does not smoke, but has an 'occasional gin and tonic'. I have no doubt that she has an active duodenal ulcer and needs a good rest from her small confectionery business.

Various Xmas presents and packages, including one containing an eider-down, had been delivered to St. John St. Miss James already seemed to know their contents.

Dec 21   Ward rounds comprehensive; St. John St., 6 cases.

3:0 p.m. [*Female, aged 76, retired cotton worker*] She was a pleasant old lady, accompanied by her daughter, who had difficulty in walking because of osteo-arthritis in both knees, but was otherwise in a reasonable state for her age. She says that seven weeks ago, and the day after having a 'cold perm' at J.'s, a 'rash' broke out 'all over' her scalp. From her account it was in the nature of a weeping chemical eczema, which spread down to the ears and corner of the left eye, and later crusted over. (For 20 years she had had her 'perms' done at another local establishment, but the hairdresser there had retired. It was the first time she had been to J.'s) Her scalp was still extensively crusted over. She herself thinks that the 'rash' was 'due to the lacquer'. Old people's skins are of course prone to the development of eczematous conditions.

Delivery of alcohol to house, for Xmas party: whisky, gin (Booth's), brandy (Courvoisier), sherry (Harvey's), Martini and ginger ale. Eight more cards dispatched = 71 total.

*

This is the last entry for 1960: on the evening of Dec 21, after writing up his diary, he suffered an attack of anginal pain and was admitted to the Manchester Royal Infirmary with a diagnosis of 'acute coronary insufficiency', and 'probable further occlusion'. An electrocardiogram taken on admission showed evidence of 'myocardial ischaemia'.

1961

Jan 11   Left Manchester Royal Infirmary at 11.30 a.m. after completion of three weeks' stay. Paid rent for St. John St., £31.15s.0d.; note increase. Read *A Zoo in My Luggage*.

Jan 12   Many telephone calls, including from Mrs. M.L. on her husband's cancer of the oesophagus, and visitors. Road vehicle licences sent off, £25.0.0d for the two cars.

Jan 13   Restful and inept day. Television out of order. Read a lot of tripe, including Henri de Montherlant's *A Jew-Boy Goes to War*.

Jan 15   Read Sunday papers: including favourable reviews of Ludovic Kennedy's *10 Rillington Place*, Harold Nicolson's apologia [*about, among other things, his pre-war association with Oswald Mosley*] in the *Observer*, Trevor Philpott on Judge Laski, and Noel Coward on beatnik playwrights.

Jan 16   Received road licences: they have a new pattern on them. Phone calls about my health. Bored to death by inactivity. Reading Alan Moorhead's *White Nile*. Edith Summerskill made Life Peeress!

Jan 17   Wakened from sleep by feeling of pressure on upper part of sternum: pulmonary embolism (?), small coronary thrombosis(?), cardiac asthma(?). At 5.20 a.m., extreme *angor animae* [*fear of death*]. Eased off after hot tea. Vol 57 of *Book Auction Records* received this morning, £4.16s.0d. Many down with flu at Arnfield's. Phone call from Mrs. N.T.: she is in a bad way, has had a hysterectomy and is neglected by her husband, whom she claims to be unfaithful, etc. She is 51, she stated.

Jan 18   To MRI [*Manchester Royal Infirmary*] for check-up. Wrote to accountant about punitive taxation; no incentive. Purchased Graham Greene, *A Burnt-Out Case*.

Jan 19   Reading on about the White Nile, and Somerset Maugham short stories. Visitors and phone calls. Took choledyl, 400 mgms, chlorothiazide and Marcoumar, 3 mgm. Last day of Eisenhower administration. Dr. Ramsey of York is the new Archbishop of Canterbury, the 100th.

Jan 20   J.I. [*fishmonger-patient*] called with present of fish. Finished *The White Nile*. President Kennedy inaugurated; a brilliant address.

Jan 22 [*Sunday*]   Total of 14 visitors. Very exhausted.

Jan 23   Dressed today and drove car. To Sherratt and Hughes: purchased Field-Marshal Montgomery's *Path to Leadership*, Collins, 21/-. Request sent off for Persantin, new drug for ischaemic heart disease.

Jan 24   Letter from BMA: an autocratic and useless trade union. To bed early.

Jan 25   Letter from the Regional Hospital Board, telling me not to hurry back. Phoned hospital and talked to telephonist and Sister G. Blood collected from me this a.m., for prothrombin estimation. [*An estimation of the clotting, or coagulation, time of a blood sample.*]

Jan 26   Anti-coagulant therapy chart sent me by the Manchester Royal Infirmary Out-patients department. Baby-sitting for Ruth: the first session in my life, this evening.

Jan 27   Nil of note. In bed most of the day, with throat infection.

Jan 30 Days drag on wearily. Tidied up my study to some extent. Useless papers, circulars, periodicals ejected. Two visitors today. Watched 'Panorama' on Krupps, the consultant-patient relationship in hospitals, and the Iraq problem.

Jan 31 Heavy rain today, cold. Regional Board salary cheque, £460.1s.8d., £20 sickness benefit deducted. Took M. to lunch at The Midland. Not good at walking. Dismal month of inactivity and discomfort ending.

Feb 1 Dosage of Marcoumar increased. Harry L. [*friend*] brought me six Havana cigars. Cancelled visit of Josephs this evening.

Feb 2 Ordered first number of the *Sunday Telegraph* for the coming Sunday. Dictated letters and report to Mrs. Faulkner [*secretary*]. Went to Masonic Temple, for Past Masters' meeting. Refreshments. Home at 2.30 p.m. Found two copies of *Captains Courageous* in lumber-room.

Feb 3 R.R. [*fruiterer*] seriously ill, *in extremis*. Fruit purchased, £2.4s.6d. Heard with regret of I.H.'s death [*former private patient*]; he saved a lot of money, but never spent it. Visited hospital; saw Dr. V., Sister H., the new house-physician and others. Returned home by 3.30 p.m. Siesta. Watched extraordinary film on Elsa the Lioness.

Feb 4 Letter from Reuben M. [*cousin*]. His sister has died in Istanbul. Another link with the past severed. The Gouldings [*friends*] came in the evening, and stayed too long. More spring-cleaning. David arrived at 1.15 a.m.; long talk with him on work, health, prospects etc, until 2.30 a.m.

Feb 5 [*Sunday*] *Sunday Telegraph* appeared today; not satisfactory for my purpose. To continue with *Sunday Times* and *Observer* as usual. Days passing more pleasantly in spite of inactivity. Visited by the Harrises: good friends, I believe.

Feb 6 11.30 a.m: Saw Dr. W.F. [*heart physician*] at

Manchester Royal Infirmary for consultation. ECG taken; my B.P. raised today, but labile. Therapy: Marcoumar, Deserpidine, Persantin, Peritrate. Lunch at Masonic, 7/- (increase in price). St. John St., 4 cases. Feel better for getting back to old routine. Cancelled *Sunday Telegraph*.

Feb 7   Lunch at Masonic, very pleasant session. Proceeded to Sherratt and Hughes, and purchased *The Last of the Just* by André Schwarz-Bart, le Prix Goncourt.

Feb 8   Visited Manchester Royal Infirmary: my prothrombin 33%. Dictated two reports, and thence to Arnfields. Palpitations, probably due to Deserpidine.

Feb 11 [*Saturday*]   Feel very tired. Trying to rest. More spring-cleaning, and a little more order out of chaos.

Feb 13   *Laennec: His Life and Times* given me by Leslie C. [*friend*]. St. John St., 2 cases.

3:0 p.m. [*Male aged 56, crane driver*] He was a sallow man of average build, and was very slow in giving his story. It seems that six months ago, while reaching out of the cab of his crane, he was struck on the forehead and 'knocked dizzy' by a ladder swinging from his own crane-hook; he also appears to have strained his pectoral muscles in twisting round to try to steady the ladder. Two hours later he 'felt rotten' and asked to go home. He says that he went to bed thinking that he would be 'all right in the morning', but in the night 'started with pains all over the chest, right across'. (His wife added that during the night he was 'talking funny'). In the morning, the doctor concentrated on the bruise which he had on his forehead, and told him that he had concussion. But after 4 weeks at home, he 'came over queer', his legs 'gave way' and he collapsed, although he did not 'go unconscious'. This collapse was diagnosed as a coronary thrombosis. But his account suggested that he had had a coronary thrombosis earlier, precipitated by the pectoral strain in the crane-cabin: a strenuous rotatory movement of his body probably led to the sequence of events. I have seen this happen before. Today, he said he felt 'weak', has 'zig-zag patterns in front of the eyes', and 'head noises', but his pulse, blood pressure and reflex systems were normal. The shape, size and sounds of his heart were also normal. The sooner he starts work again, the better.

Home by 5.15 p.m. Mentally tired, searching helter-skelter for things put away yesterday, which I cannot find.

Feb 14   Called on Dr. I. [*general practitioner with hypertension*] to enquire about his health. Purchased nail-brush, 1/11d. To hospital dispensary, for Marcoumar and Peritrate to take away with me. Heard of the death of M.L., cancer of the oesophagus. Went for a short walk this evening; some sternal discomfort about half-way round. Trinitrini taken.

Feb 16   Judy's birthday; she is 16. God bless her. Watched TV from 7.15 a.m. to 8.0 a.m. of total eclipse of the Sun by the Moon's shadow. (The next one will be on Aug 11th, 1999). Excellent pictures from the South of France, Firenze and Yugoslavia. To Manchester Royal Infirmary; arranged schedule of my anti-coagulants. Farewells at Arnfields. To Mrs Faulkner to sign letters; she gave me a small bottle of brandy. At 4.0 p.m. to Ark Lodge: the first time I have worn the red regalia of Provincial Grand Steward. Terrible crash of Boeing 707 today, at Brussels. 73 dead, no survivors.

*

Until March 20, entries are perfunctory and infrequent, and seemingly made after the event. In this period – after complaining of the 'slothful and desultory' arrangements made by the travel agent – he visited the Middle East (including Tel Aviv), Greece and Italy. On Feb 28, his '55th anniversary', he wrote of 'feeling grim in Tel Aviv, with fairly severe angina of effort'. On March 9 he was at the Temple of Poseidon in Sounion 'in magnificent weather'; then at Delphi, with 'much walking to the site of the oracle', followed by a journey back to Athens 'in a coach of inferior construction with a dangerous driver'. He was 'sorry to leave Athens'; the same evening, after a flight in a Comet 4B, he took a walk in the Forum of Trajan. In Rome he also visited Keats' house, the Villa Borghese, the Ghetto, the Vatican ('watched Procession') and the Church of St. Mary Major, where he 'met a priest from Newton-le-Willows'.

On March 19 he was at a concert, in a 'very fine auditorium', given by the St. Cecilia Orchestra ('Beethoven's 4th and Benjamin Britten'), conducted by Fernando Previtali.

*

March 20   Rome air terminal to airport, near Ostia; 3,000 lire for the journey. Flying time, by Boeing 707, 1.25 hours: amazing flight. Low cloud over London, and somewhat tense landing. Manchester dreadfully cold and windy.

March 22   Very cold and windy. Angina moderately severe. Presents given to Mrs Faulkner and her daughter. Lunch at hospital; talked to Sister G. and residents. To Hallé Concert, Schubert's 9th, Barbirolli.

March 23   Correspondence sorted out, and blood collected by Geoffrey. To Manchester Royal Infirmary for check of sample: prothrombin 18 seconds, about 30%, satisfactory.

March 26 [*Sunday*]   Watched TV play about Charles Darwin. Trouble in Laos.

March 27   In my absence there has been a botch-up of appointments, and loss of work in St. John St. Called at hospital: spoke to Dr. F., Sister J., and Mr. Cole, of the post-mortem room. Noted that too many coronary cases have been admitted over the weekend. Wedding of Michael D. [*brother of colleague*]: he is suffering from pituitary sarcoidosis.

March 28   To Northern Hospital, to see Abraham P. [*friend*]. Poor A. looked acutely ill with his grave malady: carcinoma of bronchus, with metastases. Thence to Lodge meeting; at festive board seated next to Lord Rusholme.

March 29   To Arnfields: 19 polio immunisations. St. John St., 3 cases. Dr. Ellis [*the landlord*] offers me a ground floor room after June. To Wilson [*the librarian*] at Manchester Medical Library: he mopes about in an atmosphere which is dust-laden and untidy.

March 30   2.30 p.m: to Dr. W.F. [*heart physician*], ECGs taken. He told me to cut down work by 50%, etc. Purchased Graham Greene's *The Power and the Glory*, and *The Book of Modern English Verse, 1900–1950*, at Sherratt and Hughes; *Byron's Last Journey to Greece* by Count Peter Gamba (1825), and J.O. Westwood's *The Butterflies of Great Britain* (1855), at Walmsley's.

March 31   Mainly restful day. Passover; and all my children gathered together.

April 2 [*Sunday*]   David left for London; he is rather silent and uncommunicative. Feeling much better today. Listened to Haydn's *The Seasons*. Short walk in Fletcher Moss gardens; looking forward to more activity next week.

April 4   Resumed duties. Domiciliary visit: angina and myxoedema (aet 64, Denton, ECG arranged). Ward Rounds, 14 and 15. St. John St., 1 case. Snow, sleet, wind, rain; foul weather. Insomnia. Read excellent short story 'Tahiti Waits', by Alec Waugh.

April 5   Arnfields. Domiciliary visit: angina pectoris, coronary thrombosis(?) (aet 63, Audenshaw, ECG arranged). To Shaw's Bookshop. No cases at St. John St. To bed by 7.30 p.m. Would like to visit the Far East or the West Indies.

April 6   Three domiciliary visits: cerebral arteriosclerosis and uraemia (aet 65, Clayton, admitted); haemorrhoids, etc (aet 53, Dukinfield, admitted for investigation); cor pulmonale (aet 70, Audenshaw, for investigation). Wards 5, 12 and 15. Slipped over, while at hospital.

April 7   First Medical Out-patients clinic since my illness in December. Tragic death of Mrs. R. [*neighbour*]: carcinoma of the cervix.

April 8 [*Saturday*]   Cancelled *Punch*. Domiciliary visit: 'fainting attacks' (aet 19, Glossop, ECG normal; hysteria). Presented with ½ bottle of whisky and Manikins by Dr R.

Saw Miss H. [*daughter of former patient and friend*], now teaching at St. John's School, Dukinfield, aet 30. I had not seen her for years. She is going grey.

April 9   Restful day. Read *Sunday Times* and *Observer* in toto, excluding adverts.

April 10   Third week since return from Rome. To Larmuth and Bulmer, wire-rope makers in Salford: 17 people immunized against polio. Home for lunch. St. John St., 4 cases, including lazy, indolent fellow with C_2H_5OH problem. Watched 'Panorama': Trial of Eichmann, threatened school-masters' strike, and meeting in Washington of Kennedy and Macmillan.

April 11   Eichmann's Trial begins today. Medical Out-patients in Glossop: walked in the grounds with Sister E., in bright sunshine. Wards 14, 15: saw Dr. H.C. [*colleague*], who was coming out of anaesthetic after surgery. Purchased sweets and crisps, 11/3d.

April 12   Russia puts first man into orbit and returns him to Earth: orbit 180–187 miles maximum, 101–109 miles minimum, speed 25,000 miles an hour. Epoch-making day in the History of Mankind.

April 13   Domiciliary visits: praecordial pain (aet 68, Audenshaw, ECG arranged); auricular fibrillation (aet 60, Droylsden, to be sent for Out-patient investigation). Ward Rounds 12, 14; St. John St., 3 cases. This evening found Mark Twain's *Roughing it* (1872) and Hazlitt's *Lectures on Poetry*, first edition (1818), in lumber-room.

April 14   Medical Out-patients heavy-going, with many interruptions. Watched transmission from Moscow of first cosmonaut's welcome. Single-engined Auster crashed outside Withington Hospital. Pilot killed.

April 15 [*Saturday*]   David arrived from London: uncommunicative and introspective. Yesterday's domiciliary patient died before admission. £1.10s.0d. to Judy, to entertain her friends.

April 16   'The less we deserve good fortune, the more we hope for it' (Molière). Eleven guests to tea. Afterwards studied American maps, with view to visit in May 1962. To bed at 8.30 p.m. 'People who cannot find time for recreation sooner or later have to find time for illness.'

April 17   Death of Abraham P. [*see March 28*]; dreadful news. May he have everlasting peace. St. John St., 4 cases, including an invisible Irish hernia.

3:45 p.m. [*Female, aged 62, housewife*] She had angina pectoris for some 2½ years, before suffering a broken left rib and lacerations as a front-seat passenger in a car collision. She said that she may have knocked her head on the windscreen. While in hospital she became unable to grip with her left hand, and her speech became slurred. Today, there was some weakness of the left hand grip, twitching of the muscles of the left side of her face and an upgoing toe in her left foot (Babinski Response), all residual symptoms of a cerebral thrombosis, or small cerebral haemorrhage; her speech, however, was normal. She also said that since the accident, six months ago, her attacks of angina pectoris have become worse and more frequent. It is not unusual for this to happen; I have personal experience of it. Given such aggravation of her condition, her expectation of life has been diminished. How long she will live is a matter of guess-work. In angina pectoris sudden death may occur at any time.

Budget Day: some surtax concessions, car road-tax rise to £15, and closer watch on expense accounts. Eichmann Trial proceeding. Invasion of Cuba [*by U.S.-backed mercenaries*].

April 18   Ward Round, 12. Medical Out-patients lengthy and tiresome. Lunch at Midland. Anginal attack on way to Sherratt and Hughes, suppressed by large doses of Trinitrini. Home by 5.0 p.m.

April 19   Ward Round, 15: met Rev. Paul Guinness

of Christ Church, Ashton. Arnfields: 2 polio vaccinations and case of breast abscess. St. John St., 3 cases.

4:30 p.m. [*Male, aged 59, letter-press printer*] He was struck in the back by a motor cycle 2 months ago; he did not see it coming, as it was dark. The noise, he said, 'brought the neighbours out'; he picked himself up, he added. He was in bed for 17 days with various bumps and abrasions, and some bleeding into the tissues of the right leg; he went back to work only two days ago. He was wearing a deaf-aid and was accompanied by his wife, who did most of the talking. 'It has upset his nerves', she said; 'he jumps at the least thing'. There was some induration over the calf due to a resolving haematoma, but there should be no permanent ill-effects. He was still a little apprehensive.

Watched 'Tonight' on the Cuban Revolution, and Diane Cilento.

April 22 [*Saturday*]   Completed Census Form, E90; census reference 525/3, District 35. Talked to Harvey Rhodes [*Labour M.P. for Ashton*] at annual nurses' prizegiving. Bad weather, cold and rainy.

April 24   Domiciliary visit: gross oedema, congestive heart failure, (aet 61, Ashton, admitted). Ward Rounds, 14 and 15. St. John St., 3 cases. Reading Lord Russell of Liverpool's *Scourge of the Swastika*. Mutiny in Algeria against de Gaulle.

April 25   Letter from David Colley, City Librarian. [*'We have missed your cheery company at the Book Collectors' meetings this year . . . I am looking forward to your descriptions, in your own inimitable style, of what it feels like to be on the receiving end of medical treatment'*.] Medical Out-patients, Glossop. Ward 18: Mrs. E., aged 38, old TB, mitral stenosis, cerebral embolism, puerperium [*after childbirth*]. To St. John St., no cases. To Sherratt and Hughes; much anginal discomfort. Home, very fatigued.

April 26   No news from David; M. depressed. Blood

collected at hospital for prothrombin estimation, by finger-prick method: clotting time 40 seconds, 16%. Arnfields, 19 polio injections. Domiciliary visit: haemoptysis, cor pulmonale (Ashton, admitted). Chat to Dr. M.L., re anti-coagulants; tried new drug for angina. St. John St., 3 cases. Algerian Fascist rebellion collapses.

April 27 Received instructions from Manchester Royal Infirmary re anti-coagulant therapy. Gloomy, dark and overcast day, like mid-November.

April 28 Domiciliary visits: congenital deformities and paresis of arms (aet 31, Ashton, refuses admission; visited him twice, dangerous alsatian); black-outs and heavy falls (aet 55, Ashton, admitted); albuminuria (aet 69, Hyde, admitted); cerebral embolism and mitral stenosis (aet 55, Ashton, admitted). Medical Out-patients, including peptic ulcer with gross deformity of duodenum, and nun with colitis.

April 29 [*Saturday*] Morning off; walk with M. Anginal pain and discomfort less severe when taking Sustac and Gina together. President Tshombe of Katanga incarcerated by Congolese. Anti-nuclear demonstration in London; over 800 arrested for obstruction.

May 2 Appointments picking up again.

May 4 Cheque from Lancashire County Council for 39 polio injections, £9.15s.0d. Wards 7, 12; full rounds. St. John St., 4 cases.

2:30 p.m. [*Male, aged 23, printer's assistant*] He was a healthy young man, who put his left hand (three months ago) through a toilet window at work while trying to close it. He said that it was a 'tilting type of window' with a metal frame, but the frame was stiff and rusty. Five stitches were inserted in the resulting laceration to his left thumb. Today, there was some anaesthesia to pin-prick on the outer surface of the thumb, corresponding to the distribution of the superficial branch of the median cutaneous nerve. It may take as long as

6 to 9 months to disappear, and is quite common after the division of one of the nerves to that part of the skin. 'It soon goes blue', he said of his thumb. He already has 3 children, aged 3½, 2½ and 1 year.

Dinner with M., Geoffrey and Ruth. Very happy evening.

May 5   Withdrew £25 from bank for living expenses. Domiciliary: hypertensive heart failure (aet 67, Audenshaw, admitted). Long chat with the Matron, an intelligent woman. Ward 15, full round, and Medical Out-patients. Discussed with Dr. V. [*consultant physician colleague*] the setting up at the hospital of an Anti-coagulant clinic. Americans send man up into space (sub-orbital), and recover him.

May 6 [*Saturday*]   Gave Miss James 2/6d for 6 eggs. Private visit to Glossop: lung cyst and hypertension. Signed reports. Quiet evening at home, and early to bed.

May 7   Read *Sunday Times*: Elizabeth Nicholas on Peru, book review on slavery in Timbuctoo, and Cecil Beaton on the Windsors. Also excellent editorial in the *Observer* on the Congo. Thunder and heavy rain showers. To hospital in the evening, with M., for dinner made by the Indian doctors.

May 8   No letter from David; very worried. Medical examination of 9 student nurses. Lunch with Leslie C. [*friend*] at the Midland. Attack of angina on way to St. John St., 7 cases. Watched 'Panorama': De Gaulle's speech to the French people in Algeria.

May 9   David telephoned this morning. To Miss A. [*private patient*], Dukinfield. She looks ill. Offered her admission to hospital. Ward 12, full round. David telephoned again.

May 10   St. John St., 4 cases.

2:30 p.m. [*Female, aged 62, housewife*] She was a thick-set, florid woman of short stature with a very high blood pressure (230/110); she has been a widow for 2½ years and has had ten children, seven of whom are living. She has what she called 'bad heads first thing' (frontal in location), and also feels 'wobbly' when she gets up in the morning. Two weeks ago she fell down stairs, and a few days ago 'fell into the wardrobe'. Her nose 'keeps on bleeding'. Although very obese, she is not on a diet. The type of headache she described – which occurs on rising and disappears in the afternoon – is characteristic of high blood pressure. The nose bleeding and dizzy spells could also be attributed to it.

May 12   Ward Round, 7. Four domiciliary visits: senility (aet 70, Hyde); congestive heart failure (aet 78, Hyde, ECG arranged); congestive heart failure, with old gummatous lesion [*tumour of syphilitic origin*] and tabes(?) [*syphilis of spinal cord*] (aet 60, Hyde, admitted); chest fibrosis, malnutrition, Belsen-like appearance (aet 65, Hyde, admitted). 'The Organ' for lunch. Medical Out-patients, 2.30 p.m. Further domiciliary thereafter: anxiety state, with hirsutism [*increase in hairiness*] (aet 38, Droylsden, admitted). To bed at 8.30 p.m; listened to 'Scrapbook for 1940'.

May 13 [*Saturday*]   Did not go to the hospital. Siesta in garden. Warm, sunny day. £1 to gardener. 'Eminent positions are like the summit of Rocks, only vultures and reptiles can get there': a correction of Madame Necker's version.

May 14   National Coal Board, 10 bags of coal, £4.11s.8d. Read newspapers: corruption in Soviet Union, death penalties introduced; arrest of leading generals and cabinet ministers in Persia, also for corruption; Cuba going Marxist; Tshombe still incarcerated in Congo; S. Africa on verge of Racial Riots; Angola and Nyasaland in trouble; Eichmann Trial continues. The Wickedness of Mankind is manifest in all its works, activities and aspirations.

May 15   Vaccinated four nurses. Wards 7, 14; full rounds. Private patient in Ward 11: aet 55, neurotic type, pain in the neck, and cystitis. One case only at St. John St. Home early. Sorted out some scarce early travel books: Pitcairn Islands, Australia, and East Indian archipelago (New York, 1855). Watched 'Tonight': shop-lifting in self-help Super Market stores; the 'Vasa' (1628) lifted from Stockholm Harbour; rise in Property and Land values in Green Belt and London (e.g. £6,000 to £276,000 since 1945). 'Panorama': James Mossman interviews white blimps (unpleasant types, who probably deserve to have their throats cut) in Natal and Durban.

May 17   Arnfield's and domiciliary visit: epilepsy (aet 67, Hyde, admitted). St. John St., 5 cases.

3:30 p.m. [*Male, aged 70, self-employed engineering contractor*] He was a healthy looking man, accompanied by his wife, who came into my room walking with two sticks. Seven months ago, in the middle of the afternoon, he was knocked down by a car while crossing the road, and suffered a fractured pelvis, fractures to his left leg, and internal haemorrhage. He claimed that he had been 'off business' for the whole period since (which I did not believe), and would be obliged to sell up as he is 'unable to walk about'. He also said that he 'cannot sleep', and that he has pain on the outer side of his left thigh which radiates to the toes. In fact, he is improving. But I found that there was some wasting of his left thigh and calf muscles, foot-drop, and analgesia in the distribution of the anterior tibial nerve; and reflexes were absent both at the left knee and the left ankle. His partial disablement is likely to last for an indefinite period, but he is financially comfortable enough to do without his business.

Finished late. Many appointments made for next week.

May 20 [*Saturday*]   To the Opera House at 7.0 p.m.: Sadlers Wells' *Barber of Seville*, with Julian Moyle as Figaro and Catherine Wilson as Rosina. Outstanding.

May 21   Gave David some first editions of D.H. Lawrence and Walter Pater.

May 22   Ward rounds, 12, 14, 15: place fairly deserted. News of racial riots of some severity in Alabama; American Nazis and Ku Klux Klan in action. Watched 'Panorama': interview of Archbishop of Canterbury by Richard Dimbleby,

James Mossman in Basutoland, and Robin Day on the American President's forthcoming meeting with Khruschev.

May 23   Medical Out-patients at Glossop; Ward round, 15. St. John St., 2 cases. Met Mr. C. [*surgeon and friend*], who discussed his recent trip to the French West Indies and Haiti. Called at Sherratt and Hughes and Walmsley's. To Library Theatre, with M.: *The Same Sky*, by Yvonne Mitchell; M. enjoyed it and wept. On return, listened to the 'Great' Symphony, Schubert's 9th.

May 25   Ward round, 7. My prothrombin time estimated: 34 seconds before clotting = 19%. St. John St., 4 cases. Home early. Watched 'Tonight' on Venezuela: the few grow fat on oil, while 95% of the people on the land are poverty-stricken. Paid £15.17s.0d. account to A. Sherman and Co., for wines and spirits.

May 26   H.G. [*private patient*] happy and contented in Ward 11, to be discharged on Sunday. (Do not delay account at the height of her gratitude). Dr. D. [*Nigerian opthalmologist and friend*] to dinner. He has been appointed Senior Lecturer in Opthalmology at Ibadan. The Ibadan Principal rejected the London University applicant (jobs for the boys again), quite rightly. Took him to the station.

May 28   Complete rest, reading books on India, and *L'Espion Juif*, by the Marquis D'Argens, 1738. Then 'What is a Saint?', by Christopher Mayhew, on BBC television.

May 31   Knocked dog on the head in Gorton. Domiciliary visit: uraemia (aet 63, Hyde, to be admitted). Ward 12, full round. Prothrombin test: my coagulation time has fallen to 17½ seconds = 33%. Phoned Dr. O. [*pathologist, Manchester Royal Infirmary*] and saw him after lunch, for thumb-puncture test. St. John St., 3 cases. Watched very good programme on 'Falling In Love', Independent television.

June 2   Toffees, 10/11d; stamps, 4/-. Three domiciliaries: subarachnoid haemorrhage, with history of hypertension (aet 73, Dukinfield, admitted); cor pulmonale with gross oedema (aet 65, Audenshaw, admitted); acute pulmonary oedema with cerebral anoxia, *in extremis* (aet 70, Denton, admitted). Hectic afternoon's Out-patients; case of stridor [*harsh vocal noise caused by bronchial or trachial obstruction*] admitted. Watched film on the animals of Madagascar by David Attenborough, and J. Kennedy's Press Conference in Paris.

June 3 [*Saturday*]   Ward rounds, 14 and 15. Domiciliary; gout and severe anaemia, on Butazolidine for years (aet 69, Mossley, admission arranged). To St. John St., for letters. 8.0 p.m. to 'Bye-Bye Birdie', with Chita Rivera, Marty Wilde, Angela Baddeley and Peter Marshall. Frightful nonsense, fit for morons.

June 5   Ward rounds, 7, 12, 14. Appointments Committee, 12 noon: new Indian house-physician, Dr. B., appointed. Heard extraordinary story that Dr. X. had stolen a ticket of admission to see the Queen when she visited Belle Vue [*Manchester Zoo*]. St. John St., 5 cases.

4:20 p.m. [*Male, aged 44, textile traveller*] Ten weeks ago he fractured his right kneecap in a road collision; he said he had 'sat down in the road to recover from the shock'. He complained today that he 'can't sleep without tablets' and has 'terrible, fantastic dreams', in which he participates in funerals. In addition, 'bangs and flashes' come before his eyes when he wakes up in the morning. He was a thin, worried looking man, who came in limping, is still not working, and who moaned most of the time about his 'bad nerves' and about how he had 'gone to pieces'. There was not much swelling in his right knee; its circumference was about ½″ more than the left one, though flexion of it was 40% limited. This accident has fallen on poor soil.

Called out at 9.0 p.m. to see private patient: aet 51, Hyde, probable diagnosis phoeochromocytoma, paid £10.10s.0d.

June 6   Dr. C. has died suddenly of a cerebral embolism, aet 71.

June 7   Deposited £500 in bank; discussed 'scrip issues', whatever that may mean. Domiciliary visit: cor pulmonale (Hurst, admitted). To optician, for eye-testing and 2 pairs of spectacles. No cases at St. John St. To Bolton Town Hall in afternoon, for Provincial Grand Lodge Meeting: a frightful experience of concentrated boredom.

June 8   Phoned Walter S. [*friend and insurance Company manager*] on behalf of Dr. M. [*Indian house-physician*], about discrimination against Indians seeking to take out life policies. This was denied. Lunch at 'The Organ', Hollingworth. St. John St., 4 cases, including Pakistani businessman with glycosuria.

June 12 [*Sunday*]   Optician called to deliver reading glasses; he recounted adventures of his son in London with a homosexual. Two domiciliaries: psychopath with spastic colon (aet 60, Ashton, admitted), and acute asthma (aet 54, Ashton, admitted). Phoned bank, re Hudson Bay shares. Ward 15, several attempted suicides admitted. St. John St., 3 cases, including one of right-hand amputated in machinery.

June 13   Domiciliary: coronary thrombosis (aet 60, Dukinfield, admitted). Medical Out-patients. St. John St., 3 cases, including pulselessness in paroxysmal heart block. Listened on radio to one-hour reading on life in Auschwitz by Anthony Quayle, from *If This Is A Man*, by Primo Levi.

June 14   Ward 12, full round. Masonic Temple, restful lunch, £1.2s.0d. St. John St., 2 cases. 6 guests to dinner, 7.30.

June 15   Tried to get passport application form. Post Office girls told me to go to Withington Town Hall. The latter told me to go to the Ministry of National Insurance Offices in Wilbraham Road, and there they told me to go to their offices in Burton Road, and so on. The general deterioration of efficiency is increasingly manifest in civil service occupations. Wards 12, 14; 15, full round. Had mangoes with Indian doctors.

June 16   Things getting under way for planned visit to India. Ward round, 7. Lunch at Masonic Temple: Eric B. asks me fatuous questions about the trial of Eichmann. Medical Out-patients in afternoon. F.E. [*friend and patient*] to dinner. Showed him some books: Volume of Nelson manuscripts, George Herbert's *Temple*, Thomas Wise forgeries, and Tagliacozzi [*De Curtorum Chirurgia, Venice, 1597*].

June 17 [*Saturday*]   Lazy day. World events depressing. Bad news about Jack [*brother*]. Heavy rain.

June 19   Ward rounds, 12, 15. Severe angina today. St. John Street, 5 cases. 'Panorama': Archbishop Makarios interviewed in Cyprus, schoolmasters' rejection of Pay Award, question of export licence for Goya's 'Duke of Wellington' (sold for £140,000), and Lord Beveridge on old age and old people.

June 20   Medical Out-patients and ward round at Glossop: case of pneumococcal meningitis in woman of 60, good recovery. Gave prints on religious themes to Staff Nurse K. Examination of nursing cadets. Saw N. [*hospital administrator*]: his personality has improved since his illness. No lunch. Three domiciliaries: auricular fibrillation precipitated by respiratory infection (aet 52, schoolteacher, Audenshaw, ECG arranged); cerebral haemorrhage, dying (aet 71, Hyde); coronary thrombosis (aet 63, Droylsden, admitted). St. John St., 4 cases, including twice-divorced woman from Wigan, and furrier's widow.

June 21   Dreary session at Arnfields. 2lbs of cotton wool purchased from chemists, 2/-. Ward round, 12. Spoke to Dr. V. [*consultant colleague*] in Eye Department re Dr. H. [*Indian doctor*]. He was in paranoidal mood of fundamental prejudice; unpleasant atmosphere created. (Noted his religious fervour, and the hypocrisy of it.) To wedding of Patricia S. [*daughter of friends*]; Mrs. S. [*bride's mother*] vomits all over me. 2/6d tip to waitress, for assistance.

June 22   Ward rounds, 12 and 14. Dr. V. cancels his

earlier acceptance of my invitation to dinner; feel relieved at turn of events, after yesterday's conversation. St. John St., 3 cases.

3:0 p.m. [*Female, aged 60, fish and chip shop owner*] She was very obese, and accompanied by a lady-friend. Among other things, she recently sustained a fat burn while frying; 'a lot of colour comes up in my face for the slightest thing', she said; and she has pain in her back which, she claimed, 'never' leaves her. (She also complained of 'sore buttocks', after a fall). She was a homely, kindly sort, talkative and cheerful, who described how she stands on her feet 'all day' working and serving chips, helped by her husband and several women. To relieve the back pain, she has to 'stand up against a wall' with her hands in the small of her back; some nights it wakes her, and then she lies reading 'till 4 o'clock in the morning'. Apart from the obesity of her chest, abdomen and buttocks, I could find very little the matter with her. She was making heavy weather.

June 23 Two domiciliaries: anorexia, ascites, carcinoma of colon or stomach(?) (aet 66, Hyde, admitted); and praecordial pain (aet 36, Ashton, ECG ordered). Medical Out-patients, easy session. Watched TV with a vengeance: Tony Hancock as a blood donor, animal film on Madagascar, Part II of 'Magnolia Street' and the Test Match. Today, 50th domiciliary since April 1st successfully completed.

June 26 Watched 'Panorama': Fidel Castro interviewed by Robin Day; and Mr. Nyerere of Tanganyika, interviewed by James Mossman.

June 27 Medical Out-patients, all peptic ulcers. Illness of Dr. L. [*Indian house doctor*]; visited her in Ward 17. St. John St., 3 cases. Watched enthronement of the 100th Archbishop of Canterbury, Dr. Michael Ramsey, D.D. Impressive ceremony, and so to bed.

June 28 Arnfields; talked to managing director re salary increase. Domiciliary visit: recurrent jaundice, four

attacks in 5 years, gallstones(?) (aet 15, Ashton, admitted).
Called to see private patient in Denton: aet 69, arthritis, for
some years on Prednisone. Now she is going pale and is
generally weak; it may be osteoporosis [*bone weakness*] and
other complications of long-term steroid treatment. Lunch,
3/–. Visited Dr. L. again, Ward 17. St. John St., 3 cases,
including snooty sort of fellow, probably fascist-minded, with
rheumatic history and heart murmur.

June 29   Received postcard from Sister G. in Lourdes.
Domiciliary visit: coronary thrombosis (aet 53, Ashton,
admitted). Ward 15, full round; Ward 17, to see Dr. L.,
gave her a book. Lunch at Masonic; eating too much of
late. St. John St., 4 cases.

3:0 p.m. [*Female, aged 17, accountant's clerk, Salford*] She
was riding pillion on a Lambretta motor scooter, with her
boyfriend, when she was flung off in a collision and lacerated her left leg. Fifteen stitches were put in it, and she
stayed off work for 5½ weeks. (Her grandmother who
had come with her – and was most youthful-looking – did
most of the complaining on her behalf. I had to reprimand
her for interrupting the conversation). She said that she had
'face-ache' and had been sick last Thursday when she 'went
out dancing'; she also suffers from headaches, but only when
she is 'nowty'. I asked her jocularly how often she was
'nowty', but she did not answer. She was healthy, and, apart
from the residual scars, $1\frac{3}{8}''$ and $2\frac{1}{8}''$ long, there was
nothing wrong with her. However, since an insurance claim
has been made against the other driver, neither she nor her
grandmother was anxious to minimize her disabilities, which
are non-existent.

Hudson's Bay Company rights issue, £53.19s.6d. Phoned
Leonard A. [*friend*], to defer tomorrow's lunch appointment.

July 1 [*Saturday*]   Masterly article by James Morris
on Colombia, in the *Manchester Guardian*.

July 2   Watched 'Monitor' interview with J.B.
Priestley.

July 3   Ward 7, full round. Sister G. has returned from Lourdes. Quarterly rent paid for St. John Street, £33.5s.0d. Bad news of Mr. A. [*surgeon and friend*]: cerebral haemorrhage. Saw ITV film on Borneo and Sarawak, and the lives of orang-outans.

July 4   Beginning of anti-coagulant clinic at hospital; supreme chaos. Owren's Method [*of measuring coagulation*] causes consternation over results obtained, as compared with Quick's Method. St. John St., 6 cases, including G.I. bride.

2:5 p.m. [*Male, aged 49, linotype operator*] He had a coronary at 39 and his work is sedentary; he said he sits down 'all the time' at work. (His father died at 63 of 'heart failure', probably a coronary also). He now has pain down the left arm when under stress or walking. He plays bowls and snooker; if he is 'getting beat' at bowls, he becomes tense and gets pain in the left arm. An unfavourable feature is that he drinks 5 or 6 pints of beer a night and smokes '10 a day'. The prognosis is quite unsatisfactory. The heart sounds were toneless and his face congested from the nightly intake of alcoholic fluid. He needs to abstain from alcohol and have urgent treatment for his angina.

July 6   Wards 7, 15; visited Dr. L. in Ward 17. Domiciliary visit: diabetic gangrene, foot nearly dropping off (aet 63, Ashton, admitted). Lunch, 3/-. To St. John St., 4 cases, one a man of 30 whose wife has TB and three children; another a voluble and exhausting neurotic. To dinner with the Livingstones [*friends*]; angina thereafter, with nausea.

July 7   Anti-coagulant clinic; Wards 12 and 15. Talked to Rev. Guinness, Ward 15. Lunch at The Organ Inn with Leonard A. 2.30 p.m: Medical Out-patients, heavy-going, Dr. F. [*colleague*] indisposed with bronchial asthma. Talk to Dr. M. [*consultant radiologist*] about the G.P.s in the area. Many of them are incompetents, dangerous men.

July 8 [*Saturday*]   Watched T.V. Angela Mortimer beat Christine Truman in Women's Finals at Wimbledon.

Saw England beat Australians in 3rd Test Match at Leeds; Fred Trueman took 5 wickets for 0. To bed at 9.0 p.m., angina.

July 11   Anti-coagulant clinic becoming more controllable: to cut down on use of Ambulance Service, and to use Quick's Method. St. John St., 2 cases. Major Gagarin, first Astronaut, comes to Soviet Exhibition in London; Manchester tomorrow.

July 13   Purchased Premium Bonds, £30. Voted in municipal election for Mrs. G. [*friend*], Liberal candidate. Domiciliary visit: acromegaly [*enlargement of hands and feet*] and hypertension (aet 58, Audenshaw, admitted). Lunch at Masonic Temple; J. gives me Havana cigar, and then has a 'kerbside consultation' about his paraphimosis [*painfully retracted foreskin*]. St. John St., 3 cases.

3:0 p.m. [*Female, aged 21, indexer*] She was a pleasant girl, of good type and appearance, who lives with her parents but came with her married elder sister. She is moody and has constant backache, for which she takes as many as six tablets a day, but there was no evidence of sciatica, she could stoop fully and there was no muscle spasm. Her sister described how she 'sits and broods in a depressed sort of way', and how 'the slightest thing upsets her'; she often 'snaps back', she added. (I gathered that their parents are rather severe and puritanical; the elder sister said she had had to leave home because of it.) She also suffers from insomnia and headaches. Her main problem appeared to me to be the constantly recurring frustration of having rigorous parents, and the severity of her upbringing. If there is deterioration in her mental state, which I think unlikely, she might even have to be referred to a psychiatric physician.

Purchased bottle of brandy, £2. 6s. 0d. Heavy rain most of the day.

July 14   Dr. V. tells me of Dr. F.'s disloyalty to me and double-dealing. A strange world; I kill everybody with kindness and they turn on me. Evening visit from medical insurance broker: I had to admit my own illness to him, and doubt whether I will be accepted. Heavy rain all day. Watched interview by Malcolm Muggeridge of Kingsley Amis.

July 15 [*Saturday*]   Further excellent article by James Morris, on Peru, in *Manchester Guardian*. Reading *Lucky Jim*.

July 16   Sunday papers: Lord Boothby on Iron Curtain Central European States, article on lousy British restaurants, piece by survivor of train journey to Auschwitz, and Elizabeth Nicholas pushing Sicily as a holiday resort. Growing economic crisis: Selwyn Lloyd, Chancellor, to announce measures on July 26. Railway accident at Weeton, outside Blackpool, 6 dead so far, 120 injured. Concluded Amis' *Lucky Jim*: not as funny as critics made out.

July 19   To Miss James, £2. os. od. gift, for her holidays in Bournemouth. Mort Sahl on television; poor stuff.

July 21   Had to interrupt Outpatients because of attack of haematuria [*blood in urine*]. My Prothrombin taken by Dr. Y.: 36 seconds, 18%. Dr. Y. ordered vitamin K1, Konakion, 10mgms. Went to Manchester Royal Infirmary. No haematuria there but again present in the evening, after defaecation. Walk with M. after supper. Watched TV film on the Life of Termites.

July 22 [*Saturday*]   Drs. M. and L. ring to inquire about my health. No further haematuria by 6.0 p.m. To the Opera House, 8.15 p.m.: Albert Finney in 'Luther', by John Osborne. House packed; I liked it in parts.

July 23   Further haematuria on defaecation, brownish blood. Pleasant, short walk in Hale. My visit to India may have to be abandoned.

July 24   Haematuria at hospital, residual clots passed. Full rounds, Wards 7, 12. St. John St., 6 cases. 'Panorama': discussion for and against the Common Market; impressions of Russian students on visit to England probed unsuccessfully; resumption of atomic bomb tests contemplated by USA. Sixteenth anniversary of Hiroshima.

July 25   Visited Union Castle offices re possible trip to South Africa. Severe Budget tax increases by Selwyn Lloyd: 10% purchase tax, and customs and excise increases. Watched David Attenborough's 'Savage Men of New Guinea'.

July 26   Arnfields: polio injections. Obtained Marcoumar tablets from hospital dispensary. Ward 15, full round. St. John St., 4 cases.

4:15 p.m. [*Female, aged 56, school meals assistant*] A year ago she was knocked off her bicycle on the way to school, and suffered a fractured skull with concussion. (She was totally unconscious, critically ill, and on the hospital danger list). Today she reported that she feels 'all right really', but has 'dizzy do's', and headaches 'off and on all day, any time'. She does not know what 'brings them on'; 'perhaps the weather has something to do with it', she added. These are essentially minor symptoms of a post-concussional state. They usually wear off in time.

On TV, watched President Kennedy's speech last night to the American people, on the Berlin Crisis. King George Vth cup for horse-jumping won by an Italian.

July 27   Phoned accountant about excessive and punitive taxation. 7.0 p.m., to see Pinter's *The Caretaker*. Ice cream, 3/-. Not as boring as I thought it would be. Went to the stage door, and invited cast home for tomorrow night.

July 28   Ward rounds, and follow-up clinic; discharged a few 'stickers'. Lunch at 'The Organ'. Medical Out-patients. Car cleaned, 5/-; parts of the car disarticulated by the cleaner. 10.30 p.m. – 1.0 a.m., visited by the cast of *The Caretaker*: Daniel Moynihan (Mick), Dudley Jones (Tramp) and Grahame Mcpherson (the schizoid Aston), an Australian. Pleasing.

July 29 [*Saturday*]   'Marriage has many pains, but celibacy has no pleasures' (Samuel Johnson). Hospital board cheque: £512.9s.9d., including £244.13s.0d. for domiciliary visits. Basic salary = £3,286.13s.0d. p.a.

July 30   Read in the *Observer* of dreadful atrocities committed by the French on the Tunisians at Bizerta; favourable reports of 'Luther'; Britain likely to ask to join the Common Market. Discussion of the Eichmann Trial on television, with Patrick O'Donovan as the chairman.

July 31   Macmillan asks to join the Rome Treaty. Five domiciliaries in July, lowest ever.

Aug 1   Anti-coagulant clinic: too many patients, and carrying out my duties with extreme displeasure. That oaf of a pathologist should be doing it. Woods Hospital out-patients, including poor Miss G.D.; she needs 'hymeneal exercises', as William Harvey [*1578–1657*] put it. St. John St., 2 cases.

3:30 p.m. [*Male, aged 70, tool-room hand and grinder*] He stumbled over a duck-board at the end of the day's work eight months ago, after the lights had been switched off for the night by the charge-hand; he fell head first, got up in the dark, and saw that his hands and knees were bleeding when he 'got to a light'. One of his mates with a car took him home, and he stayed in bed for 3 weeks on the advice of his doctor. He has not worked since. (He said that he had served in the First War, had never been out of work, had never been in hospital, and 'would start tomorrow' if his doctor would let him. If he could get his 'discharge', he was sure that his foreman would take him back). He was a man of good average build, with a worried expression and a gross-ly irregular pulse characteristic of auricular fibrillation, due to degenerative changes in his heart muscle. His hands and knees are better, but he 'goes dizzy', he said, when walking; he seems to be 'out of balance'. He was short of breath, his lips were cyanosed [*bluish*], and there was prolonged expira-tion, with evidence of emphysema. (He is a non-smoker, and has one stout nightly). It would help him if he could get back to some sort of work; although he needs a fair amount of rest, his anxiety would be lessened. There are many people with auricular fibrillation who are actively employed; but at 70 he is very much out of the labour market.

England loses the Ashes after exciting 4th Test at Old Trafford; Australia has not won a match in Manchester since 1902. Dr. W.F. [*heart physician*] phoned, advising me to cancel India.

Aug 2   Arnfields: loaned Simone de Beauvoir's *The Second Sex* to Miss Lambert [*managing director's secretary*]. Domiciliary visit: cerebral vascular lesion and hypertension (aet 56, Audenshaw, admitted) and bronchogenic carcinoma(?) (aet 48, Ashton, admitted). Watched 'Tonight' on TV: on crofters in the Outer Hebrides, and guns in Houston, Texas. There are 9,000 murders in the USA annually; 135 in Britain.

Aug 3   Cancelled Indian trip and confirmed S. African one. St. John St., 3 cases; including Italian head-waiter, originally from Venice, who is marrying a Lancashire girl, and an overweight salesman, aet 45, with gross hypertension. Home at 6.30 p.m. 'He makes no friends who never made a foe', Tennyson.

Aug 4   Watched 'Tonight': hairstyles amongst the native Indians of Ecuador, and a discussion on 'New Town Blues'. Also, a poor speech by Prime Minister Macmillan.

Aug 6   Read *Observer* and *Sunday Times*: Russians put up another man, Titov, in orbit for 24 hours; due to descend tomorrow. Bit my tongue at lunch, bled profusely. Clearing in lumber-room. To dinner at hospital, given by the Indian residents: tough and inedible chicken.

Aug 7   Bank Holiday, restful day. Sat in the garden and read Oscar Wilde's *De Profundis*.

Aug 9   Gave Ruth [*daughter*] £5 and a Bank Book with £25 savings, for her 22nd birthday.

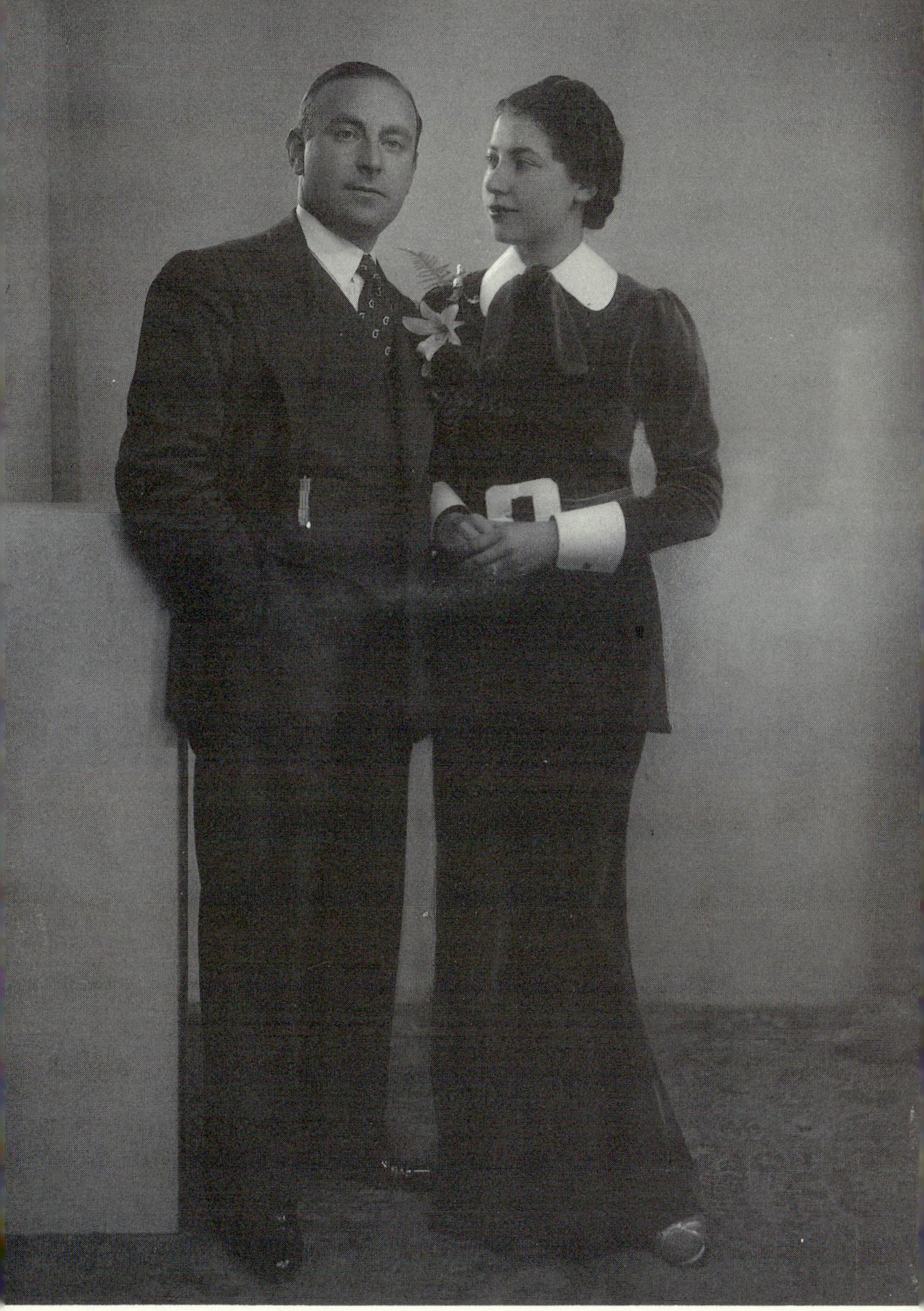

Engagement photograph: Hugh Selbourne M.D. and Sulamith
Amiel ('M.') of Antwerp, 1935

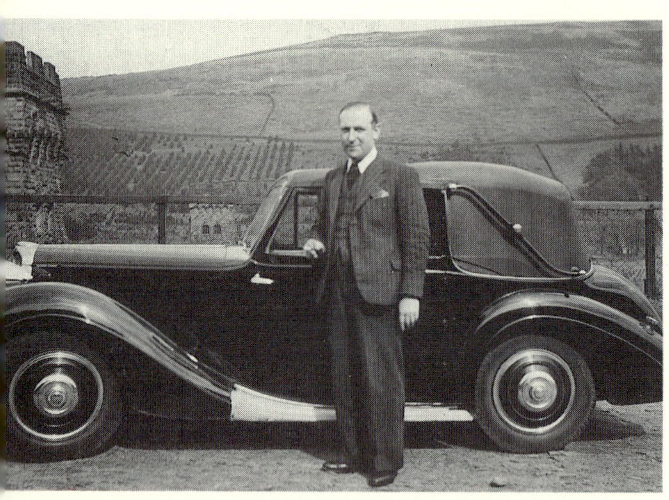

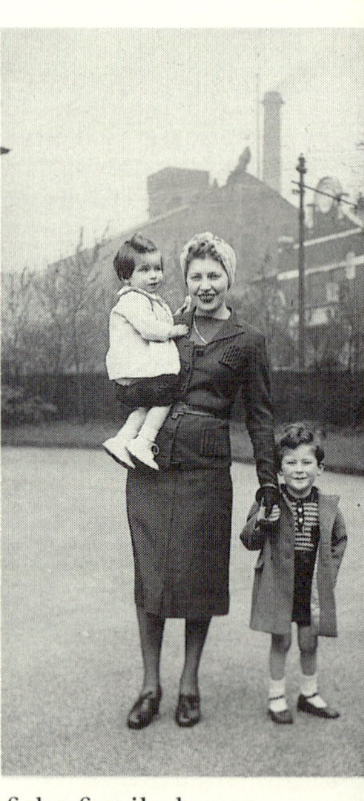

Above On an outing to Derwent Water in
his Sunbeam Talbot, May 1940

Above right Ruth, 'M.' and David in the drive of the family house,
Dukinfield, Cheshire; in the background, Buckley's Mill

The wartime general practitioner, with 'M.', at Dukinfield

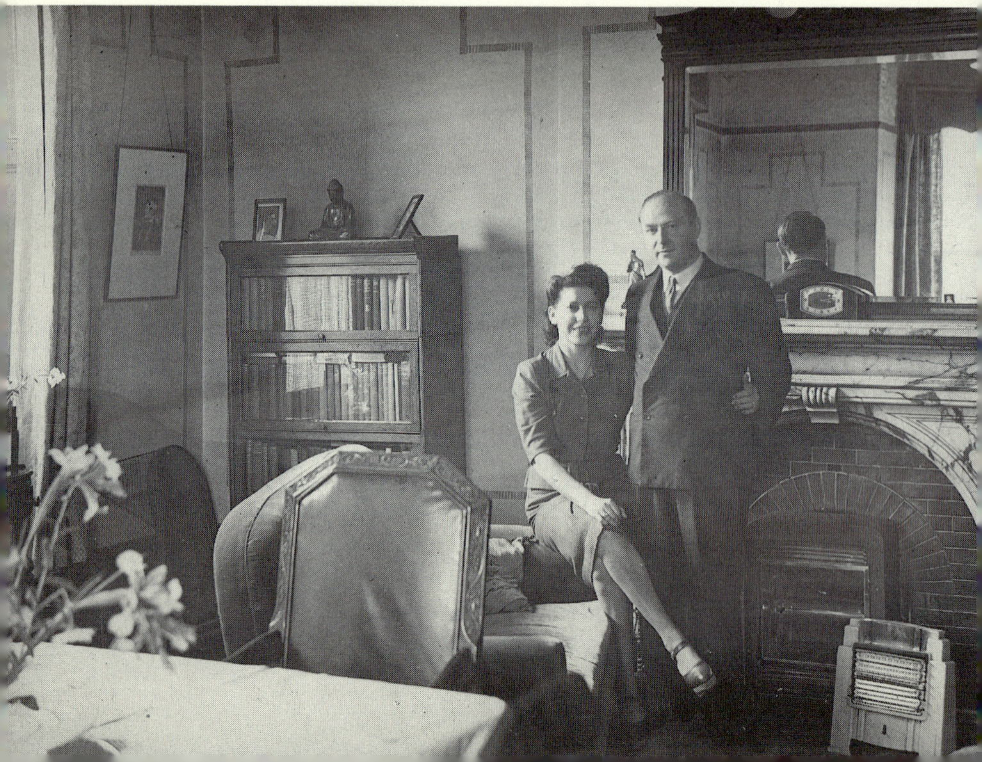

Aug 10   Crash of Cunard-Eagle plane confirmed, with loss of 39 passengers, near Stavanger. Visited Miss A. [*private patient*], injection. Ward rounds, 14 and 15: some good people very ill, whilst rogues flourish.

4:15 p.m. [*Male, aged 6, schoolboy*] He was an alert and sensible child, rather thin and slender in build, accompanied by his parents. He made no complaints about himself; the complaints were made by his parents. He has been bedwetting, and, according to the parents, 'has to sleep with the light on' because he is easily scared. I asked him why he liked the light on, but he just smiled back at me in a friendly sort of way, without giving any specific reason. His parents appear to have spoiled him.

'Tonight': on Texas (Dallas), with overcoats at £230 and rings at £30,000; on Christopher Isherwood; and on performing dolphins in Miami.

Aug 12 [*Saturday*]   Day of my Mother's death, 1950; may her soul rest in peace. Awoke at 4.30 a.m. and read until 6. To University Medical Library; St. John St., for letters; and Colam for Manx Kippers. Also 3 melons, Shude Hill, 9/-. Ward rounds, 12, 15. Domiciliary visit with Dr. R.: acute cystitis and haematuria (aet 18, married, Glossop, admitted). This was the 12th domiciliary in 12 days; compare July. Gave Dr. R. *Lucky Jim*.

Aug 13   Read good book review by Hugh Trevor-Roper on the Crucifixion. Further tidying in lumber room: heavy dust deposits, lack of space, chaotic, extraordinary number of engravings. Walk with M. in Cheadle: poor quality housing, streets depressing. Cold, almost wintry, wind.

Aug 15   Anti-coagulant clinic and 4 domiciliaries: severe anaemia (aet 74, Hyde, admitted); probably Herpes Zoster [*blisters caused by same virus as chickenpox*] (aet 71, Ashton, unpleasant dirty fellow, lives alone, admitted because of pain); psychogenic headaches (aet 25, separated from husband, Ashton, for observation); and mitral stenosis

with renal pain (aet 55, Dukinfield, admitted). Home by 3
p.m.

Aug 16   Judy goes to London. St. John St., 3 cases;
including life insurance examination, not completed after I
discovered very high B.P.: 200/140. Gave appropriate advice.
Further severe income tax demand for 1959–60: £314. 1s. 6d.
No incentive at all.

Aug 17   Comprehensive ward round, 14. My B.P.
taken by Dr. H: 170/100. 'Tonight': the Brigitte Bardot cult,
and interview with fat man, aged 59, 32st. 10½ lbs. Berlin
Crisis deepens. House lonely without Judy.

Aug 18   Awoke depressed. Anti-coagulant clinic, and
Ward round, 7. Watched 5th Test Match at the Oval in
Residents' Room; poor play by England. Lunch, food deteriorating. Domiciliary: chest pain (aet 81, Glossop). Medical Out-patients, to 5.35 p.m. Talked to Dr. V. about 33
applicants for house-job. Six short-listed, all Indians and
Pakistanis. Home for dinner, alone with M. Cloud, wind
and rain. Gloom and despondency: Berlin crisis, Rhodesians'
clash, salaries of £12,000 being paid to railway executives in
England, Macmillan grouse-shooting.

Aug 19 [*Saturday*]   Further sabre-rattling over Berlin,
things looking serious. Read James Morris, 'Sunday on the
River Plate', excellent writer. Dusted and rearranged my
limited edition set of G.B. Shaw's *Works*, 33 volumes: only
1,000 sets printed. (Mine is no. 46.) Also found a signed copy
of Barnum's Autobiography [*1855*], printed in Buffalo. Phone
call from Dr. F. about a dreadful case of a diabetic woman,
brought in in a coma, with a blood-sugar of over 900 mgm%
and being treated for 'gastritis' by Dr. Q. [*her G.P.*] of
Denton!!

Aug 20   Domiciliary visit: sudden attack of uncon-
sciousness (aet 46, Woodley, to be admitted). To wedding of
Robert W. and Valerie B.; hundreds of people, hot and stuffy.
Attack of angina tonight, when walking hurriedly in the rain

with M. Fairly severe and long-lasting, attributable to heat of the wedding reception, alcohol, too much food, hurry and bustle: all bad.

Aug 21 Phoned Town Hall, re rodents in the house. 'Tonight' on Berlin and its crisis.

Aug 22 Anti-coagulant clinic, 10 a.m. Proceeded to *Manchester Guardian* office and placed silver wedding announcement for 25th inst.

Aug 25 Our Silver Wedding day: many telegrams, cards, flowers. Medical Out-patients; coffee with colleagues. Domiciliary: rheumatoid arthritis (aet 51, Denton, admitted). Complete family assembly at dinner. Felix C. [*friend*] has given me his score of Verdi's *Requiem*.

Aug 26 [*Saturday*] Cards, telegrams, messages, flowers, in continuous stream. Gave David 17-volume set of Byron's *Works*, poems of W.H. Davies, and Martial's *Epigrams* (Paris, 1531). His dour behaviour makes me wonder whether he is deserving of such beneficence.

Aug 29 More cards arriving. Went to appointments meeting of Regional Hospital Board, to speak on behalf of Dr. N. [*seeking appointment to local general practice*]; saw the half-literates around the table who now determine these matters. Returned to hospital to do Dr. V.'s out-patients: he has been taken ill with suspected coronary. Lunch at hospital; food gets worse, did not pay for it. Very hot day, temperature in the 90s.

Aug 30 Domiciliary visit: paranoia (aet 60, Ashton, to be admitted). St. John St., 3 cases. Watched Johnny Morris in Venice and Naples, and read James Morris on Brazil in *Manchester Guardian*. 6 killed in Mont Blanc cable-car disaster; about 40 people left suspended in the cold. M. tired out.

Aug 31 Rose early. More and more cards. Breakfasted at hospital. Domiciliary visits: coronary thrombosis, *in extremis* (aet 60, Droylsden, admitted) and congestive heart failure with enlarged liver (aet 50, Stalybridge, admitted). Phoned Regional Hospital Board, seeking extra help with clinics. To Benton's cigar shop: 2 boxes of Henry Clay, 2 boxes of Bolivar (5 in each), 1 pocket ash-tray and 1 box of matches = £22.0s.10d.

Sept 1   Death of yesterday's coronary thrombosis. Letters dictated; lunch and siesta for half-hour. Medical Out-patients interesting. The hospital at present is a morass of petty feuds and backbiting. Watched beautiful film on Zen Buddhism. Mid-air explosion on flight from Boston to Chicago, 78 dead, no survivors; believed to have been a bomb on board. Russia has resumed atom-testing today. International situation appalling. A quiet, serene night, with M. and Judy.

Sept 3   Thunderstorms throughout the night and early morning: kept awake by continuous downpour, rain coming in on top floor. After lunch, slept till 3 p.m. At 4 p.m. Sister G., Dr. and Mrs. F., Mr. and Mrs. Faulkner and Miss Lambert came to tea: a painful experience. There were long silences, in which no one spoke, not even after alcohol. I made a desultory attempt to entertain them with talk of my travels, etc, without avail. At 6.15 p.m. the party broke up, with generalized sigh of relief from our household.

Sept 4   Rang insurance company about storm damage. Ward rounds, 7, 15. Wrote to gramophone company for record of heart sounds. Domiciliary visit: jaundice, pain in right groin, enlarged liver, clubbing of fingers (aet 51, Ashton, admitted). St. John St., 3 cases. ETU expelled from TUC. Watched the Durrells in Patagonia, and 'Africa Now' on the Advance of Islam.

Sept 5   Did Anti-coagulant clinic. Gave tea-cosy, embroidered by my mother, to Dr. F. Talk to catering officer to improve amenities for Indian and other Commonwealth resident doctors. Ward 15, and St. John St., 2 cases. Home

5.30 p.m. Sister G. phones to tell me of the death of Dr. R. of Glossop: a dreadful shock to me [*see Aug 12*]. He died suddenly doing a crossword puzzle in his dining room. A charming and eccentric character whom I liked very much. Russia explodes 3rd bomb in current atom-testing.

Sept 6   This morning, heavy rain and occasional thunder. Union Castle has allocated us Cabins 171 and 173. To the Livingstones [*friends*] in Hyde: met a relative of theirs from New York, an obese, bawdy violinist who has come over here as music critic for American newspapers. Heavy rain all day.

Sept 8   Arose at 5 a.m., and read H.E. Bates short story: *Grapes of Paradise*. 9.30, Arnfields. Thence to Anti-coagulant clinic. To recommence lectures to Nurses on 18th inst. Domiciliary: left ventricular failure and hypertension (aet 55, Ashton, admitted). Medical out-patients. Jack and Clara come from London for a short stay.

Sept 9 [*Saturday*]   Spent whole morning at St. John St. tidying up book-cases. Lunch at home, with Jack and Clara. Jack taken ill this evening: coronary thrombosis. Dr. W.F. [*heart physician*] summoned; Jack admitted to Manchester Royal Infirmary.

Sept 10   Visited Jack this afternoon; gave ½ bottle of whisky to Ward Sister. £3 to M. Watched TV programme, introduced by Kenneth Kendall, on the films shown this year at the Edinburgh Festival, including one about a girls' public school in Athens. Air-crash (Dusseldorf to Chicago) in Shannon Estuary, 83 dead. Speed-car runs into crowd in Italy; 14 dead, including driver. War clouds gathering.

Sept 11   Attended Dinting Church for funeral of Dr. R.: visited the house before the funeral, and spoke to mourners. Called at Woods Hospital. Thence to synagogue for New Year service; excellent sermon. Jack much better. Heavy storms in USA, especially Galveston, Texas. Winds at 180 mph, floods and snakes.

Sept 14   Visited Jack; improving further. Ward rounds, 7 and 14. Lunch, 3/-. St. John St., 5 cases, including flatulent dyspepsia. 'Tonight' on H-Bomb shelters being constructed in Los Angeles.

Sept 15   Heard of parlous state of Dr. R.'s housekeeper, who has been left nothing in his will and has to get out on Monday, 18th inst. Watched Japanese Noh play on TV: very strange. Mendères condemned to death by hanging; takes overdose of sleeping pills.

Sept 16 [*Saturday*]   Tidying up in Library seems an endless task. TV programme with commentary by Patrick O'Donovan, on the German Elections tomorrow: Adenauer and Willy Brandt. Last night of Promenade Concerts: customary performance, Constance Shacklock, Rule Britannia and the rest.

Sept 17   Awoke at 4.30 a.m., and read until 6. Visited hospital: saw case of diabetic coma, aet 56, with broncho-pneumonia and athetosis [*uncontrolled, purposeless movements*].

Sept 18   Wards 12, 15; and lecture to the Nurses on angina and coronary thrombosis, with patient Mr. E. as demonstration. St. John St., 5 cases. Dag Hammarsköld killed in plane crash near Ndola, Northern Rhodesia; probably sabotage. Mendères hanged in Turkey.

Sept 19   That bloody woman Miss James sulking, because of telling-off.

Sept 20   Visited Jack in Ward M4M, and Dr. V. [*consultant colleague*] in M6M. Day of Atonement.

Sept 21   Woke at 5.45 a.m. Jack returned from hospital by taxi; farewell to him and Clara. Domiciliary visit: sulphonamide drug-rash (aet 20, M/c 11, admitted). Arnfields; Wards 12 and 15. St. John St., 4 cases, including epileptic. Watched 'Tonight' on Macchu Pichu, the lost city of the Incas, on Wm Randolph Hearst, and on Hiroshima post-Bomb.

Sept 22 Brutal treatment of Demonstrators by the Police; questions to be raised in the House. [*On September 17, the police arrested 1,314 people during an anti-nuclear demonstration in Trafalgar Square.*]

Sept 23 [*Saturday*] To the Opera House at 7 p.m: Sadlers Wells' new version of *Carmen*, conducted by Colin Davis; some good singing, but Carmen (Patricia Johnson) not 'sympatique'. Walked with M. at midnight; saw black cat.

Sept 24 To St. John St. for letters: Miss James still gloomy. Watched programme with Bishop Reeves on apartheid. Discussion with youth group, and rabid South African nationalist. Dreadful row this evening between Judy and M.: Judy at fault, refuses to wash-up, etc. What a household! Sought comfort in my books: Owen Feltham's *Resolves* (1677) [*a work of moral homily*]. A real shindy later but all's well that ends well. It is miraculous that I survive all this hysteria.

Sept 25 Urgent domiciliary visit: praecordial pain, melaena (aet 60, Stalybridge, admitted). Vaccinated 8 nurses. Second lecture on coronary thrombosis and angina. Visited the housekeeper of Dr. R., poor man. His BP apparatus and stethoscope given to me. Further domiciliary: coronary thrombosis (aet 58, Ashton, admitted). No lunch today. St. John St., 2 cases. Home early.

Sept 26 Full ward rounds, 14 and 15; Anti-coagulant clinic. St. John St., 3 cases. Thereafter, Mr. P. called from the Halifax Building Society; £2,000 cheque given him, to open account in my name. A verbose man who started telling me his symptoms.

Sept 27 Arnfields; Ward 12, very full round. Miss G. [*hospital radiographer*] is ill with food-poisoning; something eaten on a train. Proceeded to St. John St.; 2 cases, including a woman of 35, with a son of 17, who has had fourteen years of asthma, and complained of shortness of breath, fatigue and wheezing. Her latest series of attacks followed a cold and 'running to do an errand.'

Sept 28   Yesterday's case of asthma to be admitted, Ward 12. St. John St., 3 cases.

3:30 p.m. [*Female, aged 50, secretary*] She is unmarried and has suffered from rheumatoid arthritis for 16 years. (Both her parents suffered from rheumatism). It began 'on September 3rd 1945' – she remembers the exact date – with groin pains, and 'fleeting pains' in the hands and knees. Since then she has had many forms of treatment: aspirin (16 a day), Spa treatment, and Plaquenil. She now has very stiff knees and ankles, and swelling of the hands with the wrists virtually fixed, though in good position. Her feet are inflamed and rigid. Despite this, she has remained healthy and able to manage her work. I have referred her to a rheumatologist, to see what further can be done for her.

To Lodge meeting: very dull, only 41 present, anginal attack. Proceeded at 9.30 p.m. to hospital, to see F.E. [*private patient*]; had to give unpleasant news to his son.

Sept 29   Made breakfast for M., and reestablished routine abandoned a month ago. Also had lunch at home with M. To St. John St. for letters; no cases. Proceeded to Sherratt and Hughes, to order new book on the Renaissance. Purchased Irving Stone's *The Agony and The Ecstasy*, Dennis Wheatley's *Vendetta in Spain*, and Lin Yutang's *The Importance of Understanding*, translations from the Chinese. F.E.'s anxious sons came about their father: a prolonged and tiresome consultation, until midnight.

Sept 30   [*Saturday*]   To St. Anne's for the weekend, with M. Walked on St. Anne's Pier; tea, 3/-. Driven by Arnold S. [*friend*] to see the Blackpool Lights: garish. The town was crowded with youths; all Beer and Bingo, their behaviour rough, and deteriorating. Stayed at the Majestic.

Oct 2   Lecture to Nurses, with 2 cases demonstrated (Stokes-Adams syndrome, and sub-arachnoid haemorrhage). Visited Miss N. [*housekeeper of Dr. R. of Glossop, and still in situ*], who asked me to help dispose of Dr. R.'s medical books. Wards 12, 15; partial rounds. St. John St., 4 cases.

4:15 p.m. [*Male, aged 38, lorry driver*] He was a tall, hefty-looking man with an alcoholic aroma from his breath, who weighed 13st 8lbs without his jacket. There was a faint tremor of his outstretched hands and his blood pressure was 200/110, considerably raised for a man of his age, with evidence of left ventricular enlargement. He admitted to drinking 'up to 4 pints of beer' a day, and said that he had been a bus-driver for years, but had given it up for lorry driving because of 'boredom'. He complained that he has 'dizzy spells' when he is shaving, and even when lying down; and that he has to 'jump out of bed' when he feels dizzy. He is suffering from uncontrolled hypertension. The large intake of fluids is in itself sufficient to cause a rise of blood pressure. He also smokes 20 cigarettes a day. Moreover, his personality is such that I think he will not cooperate with my recommendation to him of a salt-free diet, or with any other form of therapy recommended. He looked at least ten years older than his age and had a bulbous nose associated with excessive alcoholic intake. His wife is a hospital-cleaner, and they have 5 children.

Watched 'Tonight': the silver jubilee of the dictator Franco, Kenneth Allsop's *Bootleggers* (about Chicago and Al Capone), and a new book criticizing the war bombing strategy of Bomber Command under Harris. Then 'Panorama' on anti-British trends in Ghana, Hugh Gaitskell and the Labour Conference in Blackpool, and overcharging by butchers.

Oct 3   St. John Street, 4 cases, including two of cyanide poisoning in the same work accident. Earldom for Armstrong-Jones (Earl Snowdon), with viscountcy for any future son. 'Tonight': Alan Whicker on crime in San Francisco, with twice as many murders (40) p.a. in a population of 800,000, as in the British Isles with a population of 50 million.

Oct 4   Called on Dr. N. [*G.P. and friend*] at his surgery: coffee and Equanil [*tranquillizer*]. Domiciliary visit: uraemia, moribund (aet 60, Ashton). Full Ward round, 15. Lunch at Masonic Temple, 16/9d. St. John St., 3 cases; including a florist, aet 61, with no children, who had a tubercular left kidney removed ten years ago. (She now complains of 'constant' headaches, has a raised blood pressure and angina of effort. She said that her chest was 'troubling' her. To be admitted, as private patient.)

Oct 5   Wards 14 and 15: Dr. A. [*local G.P.*] in Ward 14, with fractured forearm. Examination of nurses, 1¾ hours. Visit to Masonic Temple to see Harold S. [*Masonic Official*]: amazing nonsense this Freemasonry.

Oct 7 [*Saturday*]   Heavy rain and cloud. Read about the philosopher-poet Su Tung-Po (1036–1101), in Lin Yutang's *The Importance of Understanding*. Toffees and melon purchased, 12/3d. Resumed reading: Shen Fu (1763–1808), 'In Memory of his Wife', and Shen Chun-Lieh, 'In Memory of a Child' (1624), very touching and tender. Also read article by Alan Ross on 'The Pitcairnese Language' in vol. 103 of the Manchester Literary and Philosophical Society's transactions. Started Ernest Bramah's *The Wallet of Kai-Lung*. To bed at 9 p.m. Dreadful air disaster: flight from Gatwick to Perpignan, 34 passengers killed, including 23 women and the Town Clerk of Paignton.

Oct 9   Up at 4.0 a.m: read yesterday's book reviews in the Sunday papers, including Cyril Connolly on the last of the Bourbon Kings of Naples, and Trevor-Roper on Cross, *The Fascists in Britain*. Lecture to the Nurses on barbiturate and coal-gas poisoning. St. John St., 3 cases.

4:15 p.m. [*Female, aged about 30, former bakery cleaner*] She was a single Jamaican woman who said she was 'about 30', but was 'not sure'. I thought she was at least 40; whatever the case, the eldest of her four children is 16. She has been in Britain 'close on two years', she told me, for some of the time cleaning and sweeping up in a bakery. She was a bulky woman, obese, with a large abdomen, who was knocked down seven months ago on a pedestrian crossing: she was struck in the back and over the left buttock. From her account, which I had some difficulty understanding, she picked herself up and 'held on to the Belisha Beacon'; the motorist involved took her to the police station, and from there she went by ambulance to hospital, where she fainted. However, she was not detained, because there was 'nothing broken', and for three weeks she visited the hospital for dressings to her buttock, and electrical treatment.

On examination today, there was a well-marked and extensive scar, 9″ by 5″ (over a rather large buttock), with discolouration and linear streaking of the skin, due to abrasive contact with the vehicle which struck her. The scar, eight months after the accident, was still tender. She was also unable to straighten her left knee when lying on her back. It is clear that she received a violent blow on the back, and still registered intense pain over the sacro-iliac and lumbo-sacral regions. There is no doubt in my mind that she is a genuine case, and that she needs to go back to hospital for further X-Rays.

She also told me that after the accident she was off work for three weeks, and then went to work for another bakery. She 'stopped', she said, because she 'could not stand' on her feet, and because her new employers told her her work was 'too slow'. She is now signing on at the Labour Exchange, for which she gets £2.12s.0d. a week, with £1.4s.6d. National Assistance. She pays £1.10s.0d. a week for a single room in Moss Side, for herself and her children.

Paid annual subscription, Literary and Philosophical Society, £3.3s.0d. Walk with M. and Judy tonight.

Oct 10   St. John St., 4 cases.

3:0 p.m.[*Male, aged 62, light labourer*] He was a man of slender build and myopic, who appeared very distressed with his breathing when he came into my room. However, this shortness of breath was itself short-lived, and he began to settle down; but after a little time he started once more to breathe deeply, and complained of shortness of breath.

He said he was 'going worse', and 'getting more do's'; that is, increasingly frequent attacks of dyspnoea. He told me he was depressed, 'cannot lift any weight' at work, and sleeps propped up with three pillows. But apart from a fortnight off last winter for flu – he said he had 'had a bad winter' – he has worked fairly consistently, with the aid of tablets from his doctor to make him 'breathe better'.

On examination, he had a markedly barrel-shaped, emphysematous chest with only 1″ expansion, and expiration was prolonged. (His clavicles were prominent, and there was some jugular pulsation. His blood pressure, however, was normal.) Although I think there was some respiratory neurosis in his condition – his shortness of breath seemed erratic, and not always related to effort – he is suffering from chronic emphysema, is not in good shape, and is deteriorating; sleeping with three pillows behind his back (orthopnoea) is an indication of damage to his respiratory system. With the sort of symptoms he presented today, he is likely to develop right-sided heart failure in the near future. His job consists in picking up cotton waste and 'putting weft in boxes', but with 'no sweeping'.

8 p.m: with M. to Palace Theatre, to see Sammy Davis (Jr), and thence to Midland Hotel for supper. Home by 1.0 a.m.

Oct 11   Rose at 7.30 a.m. and made breakfast for M. To Arnfield's; thence to Miss A. (injection); and Ward round, 12. Volcanic eruption on Tristan da Cunha. Evacuated completely, 280 inhabitants taken off. To bed at 9.0 p.m.

Oct 12   Received £1.2s.6d. from Shaw's, debt collector. Dictated reports. Domiciliary: recent coronary occlusion, with right pleural effusion (aet 76, Ashton, admitted). Ward 15; Mr. B. [*private patient*] improving. Lunch 3/-. St. John Street, 4 cases, including fat lino-salesman from Hyde.

Oct 14 [*Saturday*]   Read informative article on Tristan Da Cunha, *Manchester Guardian*. Made breakfast for M. Domiciliary visits: coronary thrombosis (aet 57, Denton, admitted);

coronary thrombosis (aet 56, Ashton, admitted). Ward rounds, 12, 15. Dr. F. reports Drs. X and Y for incompetence: Dr. X lazy, indolent and stupid, Dr. Y. drunk, irresponsible and supine. I will deal with them on Monday.

Oct 15   Restful but lazy day; soul-destroying. Watched 'Tempo' film on Maxim Gorki, with David. His personality – strangely secretive – worries me. Then 'Face to Face': John Freeman interviewing Frank Cousins.

Oct 16   Unable to sleep: in library from 2.10 a.m. to 4.0 a.m. Arnfields, 10 a.m. Ward rounds, 12, 15. Talk to Dr. C., depressed about everything professionally. St. John St., 1 case, and home early. D.C. [*friend*] phones about his eyes and blurring of vision. Watched ITV film on the launching of the 'Queen Mary' 25 years ago, and Malcolm Muggeridge interviewing Iain Macleod, Chairman of the Conservative Party. Chubb locks fitted to three doors, in preparation for our departure for South Africa.

Oct 17   Dr. V. [*colleague*] is not coming back until January. He is certainly making a dish of it [*coronary in mid-September*].

Oct 18   Arnfields, and domiciliary: space-occupying lesion, cerebral tumour(?) (aet 66, Ashton, admitted). Visited hospital dispensary for holiday eventualities or emergencies.

Oct 19   Woke with a start at 8.50 a.m. Phoned Professor Z. [*Manchester Royal Infirmary*] about Miss A. [*patient referred to him*]; he adopts an astonishingly casual attitude to her. (He must be a shit, despite all the ballyhoo about him). Reports signed, and visit to Ward 7, to see interesting case of generalized bone disease. Anginal pain on way to Masonic for lunch, £1.4s.4d. A cold and bitter wind; inadvisable to go about thus, with insufficient clothing. St. John St., 3 cases. Home at 6 p.m. D.C. called for drops in the eyes, etc; I refused to take his gift of £5, but he insisted.

Oct 20   Ward rounds, 12, 14, 15; many discharged.

St. John St., no cases. To Sherratt and Hughes: purchased *Picasso's Picasso* and *Paintings of the World's Great Galleries*. Watched Graham Greene's 'The Complaisant Husband'. Later looked over my Restoration and other plays, reawakening memories of happy collecting days: Massinger, Chapman, Mountford, Shirley, Davenport, Aphra Behn, Dryden, Congreve. Severe angina.

Oct 21 [*Saturday*]   Made breakfast for M. Went to see R.B. [*friend and neighbour*] about wife's asthma, and the surveillance of the house during our absence.

Oct 22   In bed until 5.0 p.m., reading. 7.30 p.m, to Steele Hall as member of Brains Trust, with Frank Allaun, Labour Member of Parliament for Salford West, R. Du Vivier of the British Council, and the Secretary of the Anti-Apartheid Movement. Some silly questions; outside, a howling gale. Fell in a ditch on leaving.

Oct 23   Boots, 8/2d. Domiciliary visit: acute nephritis (aet 18, Audenshaw, admitted). To hospital, where Sister G. instills drops into my eyes. My blood test by venepuncture: 35 seconds. Lecture to the Nurses on auricular fibrillation, no cases demonstrated. Ward round, 15. Thence to second domiciliary visit: bronchogenic carcinoma(?) (aet 54, Ashton, for investigation). Russia drops 50-megaton bomb.

Oct 24   Strong world reaction to Russian contamination of the atmosphere. To Lodge at 5.30 p.m., for election of new Worshipful Master; gave reply to toast to Provincial Officers. Home by 9.30 p.m. TV programme on the Death Penalty.

Oct 26   Woke at 6.0 a.m. and read for half-hour; translations of Chinese poetry. Letter from Harry W. Jr. in Virginia, saying that part of his farm has burned down, with loss of cattle. News of bonus issue by Hudson's Bay Company: my holding has risen from 88 to 176 shares. Phoned Union Castle, and disapproved of cabins and provisional dining-room table-plan.

Oct 28 [*Saturday*]   Selected a short-list of books to take with me: including Graham Greene's *A Burnt-Out Case*, Richard Church's *Calm October*, and books by Errol Braithwaite and John Masters. To the Thomases [*friends*] for dinner.

Oct 29   Clocks turned back one hour. Domiciliary visit: uraemia (aet 61, Ashton, admitted). Called at hospital, home by 1 p.m. Dr. E. came to tea at 4.0 p.m. and stayed too long: I am writing this at 7.20 p.m. and he has not gone yet. Watched 'Face to Face' with Martin Luther King.

Oct 30   My Prothrombin time down to 25 seconds by finger-prick method. Saw N.W. [*private patient*] in Ward 14: he is in parlous state. Lecture to the Nurses, on multiple sclerosis and Motor Neurone Lesions. To lunch with F.E. [*friend*], and general discussion about his health. St. John St., 4 cases. Watched 'Tonight': Russian Atom Testing, Tom Mboya, and a young man who dyes his hair green. Stalin's corpse has been moved from the Red Square mausoleum.

Oct 31   Pay-slip from Regional Hospital Board, £373.5s.2d. Domiciliary visit: congestive heart failure (aet 62, Newton, admitted). Death of Augustus John, the artist, and more news of the removal of Stalin.

Nov 1   Took Miss James to her friends on my way home. Watched 'Scrapbook for 1936' on television, and 'Tonight' discussion of a new book alleging that Stalin was murdered. Paid TV and Broadcast Receiving Licence, £4.0s.0d.

Nov 2   Took Judy to school. Two domiciliaries: pernicious anaemia and cardiac ischaemia (aet 75, Denton, admitted); cerebral haemorrhage, moribund (aet 54, Ashton).

4:55 p.m. [*Male, aged 54, labourer*] He was an obese man who has already been off work for 2¼ months after 'jerking' his neck, and 'spraining his shoulders', when the taxi in which he was travelling was involved in a minor collision;

he had just landed at Liverpool after a holiday with his wife (a canteen assistant) in Ireland. He said that he had pains at the bottom of his neck and 'sometimes in the eyes'; and if he stoops down – 'like doing up my shoelaces' – he goes 'giddy'. His wife, who came with him, suffered similar injuries and manifested almost identical symptoms: though when she is dizzy she goes 'off the pavement'. He also sleeps badly and is 'bad-tempered'.

On examination, his blood pressure was 210/100, considerably raised, and the fundi of his eyes showed the 'copper-wiring' signs of hypertensive changes. His hypertension may be perpetuating his headaches and vertigo, but he is essentially bedding down into a chronic state of post-accident neurosis. In 1942, when he was 35, he was off work for nine months after fracturing his ankle; in 1952 for six months, after fracturing his left knee-cap. He had an alternately depressed and militant expression; and was not inclined to underestimate his disabilities, as I have often found with the Irish.

In pouring rain to Masonic Temple, to return Masonic Lump-of-Metal to P. [*lodge official*]. Masonry employs the mythology and symbolism of the Old Testament but is an organized racket.

Nov 3   The staff nurse in Ward 15 has broken with her policeman. Took N. and R. [*hospital administrators*] to 'The Organ': saw Michael Jeuda [*prominent member of the Manchester Jewish Community*] eating ham and eggs there.

Nov 4 [*Saturday*]   £3.16s.4d. for alcohol for visitors tomorrow. To Sherratt and Hughes: purchased Robert Jungk, *Children of the Ashes: The People of Hiroshima*, 25/- and a Penguin edition of Jerome K. Jerome's *Three Men in a Boat*, to take with me to South Africa. Also called at Shaw's bookshop. Siesta. Read *British Medical Journal*, and started *Children of the Ashes*.

Nov 5   Am I taking too many books with me to read? Difficult to decide. Thirteen guests to party this evening, 8 p.m. to midnight.

Nov 6   Lecture to Nurses on poliomyelitis, and fare-wells for Xmas. Ward 12 round, including case of tachycardia. Domiciliary visits: ulcerative stomatitis, case for diagnosis (aet 19½, Upper Mill, Yorkshire, admitted); anxiety state (aet 37, Ashton, to be recommended to the Lady Almoner). Further domiciliary: pregnancy with pancreatitis (aet 26, Haughton Green, for observation).

3:0 p.m. [*Female, aged 51, 'home help for old people'*] Three weeks ago she was travelling in a bus when the driver took a corner 'sharply' and the conductor's ticket box – which was stowed on a ledge – fell on her head. (She said that she was not wearing a hat). The bus stopped and the driver applied a bandage to her scalp – it 'bled a lot', she said – before driving her on to the local hospital. Four stitches were put in the laceration. The next day the cut was still bleeding, so she had to return to hospital to have another stitch inserted, and is now suing the bus company. Today, she said that she has headaches 'three times a day' across the frontal region; 'it is like somebody pressing on top of me', she stated, making heavy weather. She also told me that her sleep was 'not as good as it ought to be' and that her brain had been 'knocked cock-eyed'. There was a soundly-healed ½" scar on the dome of her scalp: she had actually cut the hair away to bare it, before coming to see me.

I told her that I thought she should be back at work, and that hundreds of people are knocked on the head throughout the day in minor accidents without making a song-and-dance about it. She herself postulated in a half-hearted manner that she 'might be able to go back in about two weeks' time'. (Her purpose is gain, I am certain.) She was a healthy-looking woman of heavy build, with a slightly-raised blood pressure (160/100), who had four fingers missing on her right hand – only the thumb was present – and the middle and ring fingers missing on the left hand. Severe burns as a child had required the removal of her fingers.

Nov 8   Arnfields, and domiciliary visit: right pleural effusion, enlarged liver, C_2H_5OH (aet 40, Ashton, admitted). Home early, and called on R.B. [*friend and neighbour*] with instructions about feeding the bird, lights, and central heating in our absence.

Nov 9   Up from 4.30 a.m. to 5.30 a.m.: began packing my attaché case.

Nov 10   Up again from 4.0 a.m. to 5.0 a.m. To bed again, and up at 8.30. Letters arrived late today, much fog. Deposited £155.17s.7d. in cheques and, in 2 sealed envelopes, £305, savings certificates, jewels and pass-books.

Nov 12   No breakfast. Read profile of Patrick White, Australian author, in 'Observer'. Also: the Queen in Ghana, Hoxha's attack on Khruschev, Harold Nicolson on Asquith and other prime ministers, the last days of Chamberlain, and the question of whether Singapore should be abandoned in view of new talks about Malaysia. In the afternoon, looked at George Herbert's *Temple* (1633), first edition; Thomas Shelton's *Tachygraphy, or Short-Writing the Most Easie, Exact and Speedie* (1645, printed at Cambridge by R.D.); *On the Safety Lamp*, etc., by Sir Humphrey Davy, 1825, presentation copy; and Vaccination items by Jenner. Watched 'Tempo' on ITV, about a film of Sigmund Freud in preparation, directed by John Houston, and Edna O'Brien on the Teenage Appreciation of Art. Also 'Face to Face', John Freeman interviewing Lord Hailsham. Hailsham strikes me now as a complacent member of the blimpish Tory establishment, of some degree of mediocrity.

Nov 13   In spite of Soneryl, rose at 4.15 a.m. Took Judy to school and my blazer to Express cleaners. Deposited black metal deed-box with books and policies at bank. Urgent domiciliary visit: coronary thrombosis (aet 49, Stalybridge, admitted). Presents to Miss Miller (black leather purse), Dr. F. (cheque), and Miss L. [*house physician*] (red leather purse). Full round, Ward 15; and to Dispensary for further medicines from the Dispenser. Second domiciliary: praecordial pain (aet 45, Audenshaw, ECG arranged). To Manchester; the first time I have used a 'parking meter', 6d. St. John St., 2 cases.

4:0 p.m. [*Male, aged 57, cashier*] He is an abstemious man who does not drink and smokes little, with nothing very striking in his medical history – he has had no operations, and his parents are still alive – and his only illness was tonsillitis 24 years ago. He seemed all right in every respect. However, when I examined him, I found that his blood pressure was raised to 170/100; the normal for his age and weight is 140/90, sometimes 150/95. I found also that his urine contained a significant amount of sugar. His G.P. needs informing.

Nov 14   Home at 4 p.m. Percy K. [*neighbour and friend*] called round and gave me *Angélique and the Sultan*, frightful stuff, sex, fornication etc.

Nov 15   Cancelled newspapers for the 3rd time, and informed police of our departure. Arnfields, polio injections; forgot my spectacles there. Gave Mrs Faulkner [*secretary*] Xmas gift, £3.3s.od. Many calls this evening, including someone with my glasses and R.B., who took the bird away for safe-keeping. Left with M. and Judy on midnight sleeper to London.

Nov 16   A fine morning. By boat train from Waterloo to Southampton. Sailed at 4 p.m. on 'Stirling Castle' (Cabins 49 and 51), to South Africa.

[*There are no further entries until January 1 1962.*]

1962

Jan 1   Saw Dr. V: he had a faraway look, offered no New Year wishes, must be going mad.

Jan 2   Watched BBC programme summarizing the main scientific events of the year: Gagarin in space; discovery of DNA in genetics; structure and content of meteorites indicative of extra-terrestrial organic existence; large microscope in Toulouse to study viruses and bacteria; interferon in virus diseases; attempts in the Pacific to study the Earth's crust by boring through it; and Exploration of the Moon contemplated.

Jan 4   At the hospital saw the lecherous and neurotic E.T.; investigations normal. Ward Round, 15; discharged four, in order to be helpful in making room for admissions.

3:0 p.m. [*Female, aged 55, manageress*] She is a spinster, who for 22 years has been a factory manageress, and for nine years has suffered from ulcerative colitis. Five years ago she had part of her colon removed. She says that she passes a blood-stained mucus 'about 12 times a day', has stiffness in the right thigh 'down to the toes', and 'bad nerves'. She will have to be admitted. We can only try to do what we can for her.

Jan 5   Domiciliary visit: broncho-pneumonia (aet 55, Denton, admitted for investigation). Ward rounds, 12 and 15. Talked to Dr. V. Lunch at 'The Organ Inn' with George W. and Tony T. [*friends*], £2.17s.6d; the charges appear excessive these days. I was advised to retire by the above mentioned.

Thereafter, prolonged but interesting Medical out-patients.

Jan 6 [*Saturday*]   Day in bed, reading: on Hiroshima and the aftermath; on Napoleon's Death, in the *Lancet*; an article on Rome in *Réalités*; and translations from the Chinese on the origins of foot-binding in the middle of the 10th century, etc.

Jan 7   Leisurely day. Watched 'Face to Face': John Freeman interviewing Sir Compton Mackenzie. Prepared lecture to the Nurses for tomorrow.

Jan 8   Talk to Dr. P. at the hospital; I feel regret at his leaving. Lecture to the Nurses, on Meningitis and its Treatment. Ward Round 7, with Dr. L.; saw girl of 17 with Addison's Disease and history of small TB lesion in the lung. Domiciliary visit: brachial neuritis (aet 64, Ashton, for investigation as out-patient). Home at 6.30 p.m. Dreadful railway accident in Holland; head-on collision between two trains near Utrecht. 90 dead, the worst accident in Dutch railway history.

Jan 9   Last Friday's [*Jan 5*] domiciliary case of broncho-pneumonia died today, of acute leukaemia.

Jan 10   Very bad night. Arose at 4.0 a.m., made tea, and rearranged [*books by*] Robert Boyle, magnificent items. Back to bed at 5.0 a.m., but slept badly and rose again at 8.30. To Arnfields, long session; gave some coloured prints to E.G.T. [*managing director*]. Ward Round 12, and St. John Street. Saw Barr and Mosco [*accountants*], for assessment of loss of income following my car accident in Sept. 1960.

Jan 11   Letters to secretary of Athenaeum, removing my name from the waiting-list, and to Union Castle, claiming for the loss of my Pen on the voyage. To hospital; Sister G. lachrymose at failing the driving test for the third time. My BP taken today by Dr. D.: 150/75. Too good to be true.

3:0 p.m. [*Female, aged 19, shorthand typist*] Last August, she was on her way by car for a holiday abroad with Dr. A.S., a Pakistani doctor, when their car collided in Stoke-on-Trent with an NCB lorry. The right side of her forehead struck the driving-mirror light, and she received a laceration of the scalp which required twelve stitches; the Pakistani doctor's scalp was also lacerated. After treatment in hospital, and a rest there for two hours, they repaired to the Metropole Hotel, Stoke on Trent, where they stayed the night. In the morning they proceeded to London by train, and thereafter to Paris and Geneva, in each of which places they spent a week. She said it was the first time she had been on the Continent, and despite the 12 stitches in her scalp she had a happy time. However, she claims that on getting back she began to suffer from headaches; that is, after enjoying a fortnight's holiday, headaches miraculously began on her return to England. Today, she said she still had headaches 'two or three times a week', which last 'three or four hours', and which are relieved by aspirins. I do not believe for one moment that she has any headaches whatever, or that she takes aspirin. Genuine post-concussional headaches begin immediately after a blow to the head.

Tried on a new suit in my rooms, from Jackson's.

Jan 13 [*Saturday*]   'He that falls in love with himself will have no rivals', Benjamin Franklin. Lazy day. Read the *BMJ* and set examination-paper for the Nurses on TB meningitis, barbiturate and coal-gas poisoning, smallpox, ulcerative colitis and insomnia. Learned of the death during our absence of Sir William Fletcher Shaw [*see Sept 3 1960*]. I spoke to the latter last time we were in the Opera House; he was very deaf and over 80, but looked all right. Watched TV discussion of a film which presents an adverse picture of Britain to the Americans; with Michael Frayn, Al Capp and Randolph Churchill, and Aidan Crawley as chairman. The main effect of the discussion was to reveal R. Churchill to be a most unpleasant person.

Jan 14   To Judy 10/-, and £15 to M. Nothing very

significant in the press; an article by Christopher Sykes on 'Lust' shows it to be a good thing, on the whole. Also, an irritating account of the wealth of the Maharani of Baroda and her useless 16-year-old son, designated as a 'Prince'; some work would improve their characters. Prepared to-morrow's Lecture to the Nurses; will be glad when the lectures end.

Jan 15   Domiciliary visits: emphysema and prae-cordial pain (aet 72, Ashton, ECG arranged, his wife gave me some chocolates to give to M.) and generalized allergic rash, glandular fever(?) (aet 70, Ashton). Lecture to the Nurses, on smallpox. Ward rounds; St. John St., 3 cases. Purchased 12 bottles of Hock.

Jan 16   Arose at 7 a.m., and made breakfast for M. Domiciliaries: congestive heart failure (aet 62, Clayton, admitted); congestive heart failure, *in extremis* (aet 53, Dukin-field, admitted). Vaccinated 200 people against polio at hospital, with help from Dr. A.; I am vaccinated too. Flowers from Mr. Cole of the post-mortem room. No lunch. I am very harassed and busy.

4:0 p.m. [*Female, aged 61, schoolteacher*] She was a thick-set woman and obese, with a normal pulse and blood pressure, whose 'inside goes like a machine' when she wakes up in the morning. She worries about her husband when he is out in the car, and has 'lost confidence' in herself: she said that her 'nerves' were 'bad', and that she was 'frightened of standing up in front of the class'. She eats and sleeps well, and had a motor-coach holiday in Scotland last August. I do not believe that she is half as bad as she makes out.

Hannen Swaffer died today, aged 82, and Sir William Coates, aged 102 (1860–1962). My Prothrombin time 32 seconds. Listened to Thurston Dart playing on the organ.

Jan 17   9.30 a.m., Arnfields. Domiciliary visits: rheu-matoid arthritis (aet 58, Dukinfield, to be admitted later) and suppurative purulent bronchitis (aet 56, Ashton). Lunch, 3/-. St. John St., 3 cases; two failed to attend today, very convenient. Gave David copy of Hazlitt's *British Senate*, 2 vols, 1808, first edition. Dawson's catalogue contains Thomas Stanley's *Poems*, for which they want £185; they bought it from me for £90. They also want £550 for Gilbert, *De Magnete* (1600). These are excessive prices. Listened to Beethoven's Second Symphony on wireless.

Jan 18   Exorbitant demand for surtax; phoned Barr [*accountant*] in alarm. Medical examination of Nurses, 10 a.m. Thence to Higher Crumpsall, to see private patient, aet 77, who complains of radiating pains in back, and 'difficulty in walking'. Talk to Dr. Ellis [*fellow consultant*], who attended the funeral today of Sir Wm. Coates. Dr. F. [*Pakistani hospital colleague*] returning tonight from Pakistan. Large problems have arisen over his estate. Work to rule by post-office workers continuing.

Jan 19   Haircut opposite Odeon, near Guide Bridge, 3/6d. Anti-coagulant clinic; Ward rounds 12 and 15. Medical out-patients: Sister H. eavesdropping, a jealous and disloyal woman. Much industrial unrest owing to pay-pause: postmen, GPO engineers, Equity actors, coal-miners, redundancies on Railways, etc.

Jan 20 [*Saturday*]   Dr. J. called round this afternoon. A complaint has been made against him by a patient; a reply to the Manchester Executive Council formulated on his behalf. The Livingstones [*friends*] have given M. a frying-pan for her birthday: very serviceable.

Jan 21   Paucity of news, apart from chronic strife in the world. Working up an appetite for travel to the USA, in May or June. May sell Swift's *Genteel Conversations* (1738) and an anonymous Cromwellian tract of great rarity to help pay for it. Watched 'Face to Face': John Freeman interviewing John Osborne.

Jan 22   Lecture to the Nurses, on thyroid diseases; the nurses in this class are particularly stupid, inattentive, unattractive, and lazy. Donation to Nurses' Fund, £2.2s.0d.

Watched TV programme on Immigration, with Iain Macleod and Derek Walker-Smith.

Jan 23   Heavy rain. Ward Rounds, 7 and 15: my congestive heart failure case [*see Jan 16*] died early this morning. St. John St., 4 cases, including a chartered accountant, aet 24, whose mother had a TB hip as a girl. To Lodge, 5 p.m.; I made a poor speech at dinner, but Dr. I. raised laughs only by deriding others. I find that a great deal of humour can be produced, even in averagely-educated people, by running others down. Profundity, however, is unacceptable.

Jan 24   Arose at 6.30 a.m. Vol 58 of *Book Auction Records* arrived, £4.16s.0d.; cost 25/- a few years ago. Thence, to domiciliaries: myocardial ischaemia (aet 50, Audenshaw, admitted); right basal effusion (aet 58, Denton); diabetes and cardiac asthma (aet 70, Ashton, admitted); mitral stenosis and congestive heart failure (aet 58, Ashton, to be admitted). Ward Rounds, 12 and 15. Caught speeding by radar trap on visit to private patient in Audenshaw. Aet 54, he woke up at 2 a.m., ten days ago, with pain in the sternum and left arm. In the last two days his stools have been 'pitch black', he said. Probably a small coronary; to have ECG. This evening watched Harold Macmillan on TV. He made an empty speech, full of platitudes and drivel.

Jan 25   Domiciliary visits: acute demyelinating disease (aet 24, Audenshaw, admitted); coronary thrombosis and Parkinsonism, very ill (aet 68, Ashton, to be admitted(?)). Letter typed to Chief Superintendent Stebbings re speeding, and delivered immediately by me. Mr. A. [*consultant surgeon who had had a stroke, see July 3 1961*] comes to chat. A changed man, extremely ill-looking, with bad co-ordination. He says he is hypertensive. Home at 7 p.m. At 9 p.m., the E.'s again came to discuss their father's illness. Their questions were opinionated, as if they were telling me, not asking.

Jan 26   Very bad cold. To hospital, to do follow-up clinic; a strong smell of C_2H_5OH from Dr. Z. Twenty patients seen, and seven discharged. Thereafter, did medical outpatients, and thence to domiciliary: haematuria (aet 18, Ashton, not admitted, to wait till Jan 29 and see). He passed green urine for me, in a decorated drinking-glass.

Jan 27 [*Saturday*]   Read on side-effects of Dindivan therapy, in the *Lancet*. Thick fog descended.

Jan 29   Today's *Manchester Guardian* describes Adam Faith as 'the devil's advocate'. Lecture to the Nurses, on chronic lymphatic leukaemia, with case (Mrs. D.C.) demonstrated. Domiciliary: cerebral thrombosis, unconscious, hopeless (aet 64, Mossley, unfit to move). Ward Round, 15. Lunch, 3/-; a rise in charges to 3/6d next month. St. John St., 2 cases; including menopausal housewife of 43, lachrymose and emotional, who complained of a 'lump in the throat', and anorexia. Provisional diagnosis is globus hystericus, but have sent her for X-ray of chest and thoracic inlet. Fritz Kreisler, the violinist, has died, aged 86.

Jan 30   Thirty-six cases in the Anti-coagulant clinic. My blood test, 25 seconds. Collected cough mixture for myself from Dr. N. Ward rounds, 12 and 14. Lunch 3/-. To private patient in Glossop: obesity, hypertension and ischaemia. Listened to André Navarra playing Schumann's Cello Concerto. Chaos in London as a result of yesterday's Railway Strike.

Feb 1   Cautionary letter from Ashton police re speeding; no prosecution. Ward rounds; lunch, 3/6d. To travel agent to collect literature on the USA. Thence, to Sherratt and Hughes; met a new employee, Mr. N., who used to be a teacher in Cairo, an agnostic and rationalist, and well-read.

Feb 2   M. goes in to St. Mary's for a check-up. Anticoagulant clinic and domiciliary visit: probably bronchogenic carcinoma (aet 50, Stalybridge, admitted). Ward Round and Medical out-patients; Sister H. a most unpleasant and sinister person.

Feb 3 [*Saturday*]   M. in St. Mary's. Up at 7.20 a.m. To Manchester Royal Infirmary, to see Dr. O. [*pathologist*] about my prothrombin: 20 seconds, 28 per cent. This tallies fairly well with my own Clinic estimation. To Colam, fish collected free of charge, and 6 lemons, 2/-. Thence to St. John St., for letters. There was a smell of cat's urine in the house; Miss James's atrocious cat sleeps on my couch and armchair cushions!! Home for lunch. Siesta this afternoon. Manchester United 3, Cardiff 0.

Feb 4   Took M. home from St. Mary's; 2/- tip to porter. This evening watched 'Face to Face', John Freeman interviewing Roy Thomson. His main object is profit, irrespective of his so-called conscience. He appeared in a very bad light, ruthless.

Feb 6   Did Anti-coagulant clinic. Spoke to P. [*hospital administrator*] about a period of leave. The hospital administrative staff now loaf about most of the time, gossiping and drinking tea. Ward rounds and St. John St., 2 cases. Proceeded to Lodge meeting. Afterwards, heat in dining room overpowering and felt ill. Left at 9.45 p.m.

Feb 7   Ward Rounds, 7 and 12. St. John St., 3 cases. Proceeded to Barr [*accountant*]. Takings at St. John St. show decline: 1958–9, £2,800; 1959–60, £1,500 only. Tax punitive: 1960–1, £1,016.19s.0d. in surtax. Feel depressed today.

Feb 8   Visited Miss A. and unguents given. Ward 15, and thence to Hospital Medical Advisory Meeting [*meeting of senior hospital medical staff*]: I find little of interest in it. My BP 180/100; 10 mgm of Guanethidine taken. To St. John St., 4 cases, one of whom has a serious problem with his schizophrenic and diabetic son, who has been arrested for armed robbery.

4:45 p.m. [*Male, aged 64, bachelor, electrical components salesman*] He said that his nerves were bad and that his left hand felt colder than the right one. He also complained of dizziness, cramp in the left calf, stomach trouble, chapped fingers and toes, dry lips etc. On examination, there were tortuous vessels over the temporal surfaces of both sides of his head and other signs of general arteriosclerosis. His blood pressure was moderately raised (180/105), and his chest was emphysematous with wheezing respirations. On his back there was a rash, which was that of lichen planus and which arises from anxiety. What he needs is sedation to keep his nerves quiet. He said that he 'jumps when the door opens'.

Watched 'Tonight' on security firms which are being used to prevent Robbery of Friday's Wage packets, and on cheating at Cruft's Dog-Show. Fog and mist. A cold night.

Feb 9   Judy away; her morning noises absent. To domiciliaries: praecordial pain (aet 70, Ashton, ECG arranged); lymphatic leukaemia (aet 49, Ashton, to be admitted); p.u.o. [*pyrexia, or fever, of unknown origin*] (aet 26, Hyde, admitted). Lunch at 'The Organ'. Medical out-patients finished at 5 p.m. Wrote to Dr. W.F. [*heart physician treating him*] with observations on myocardial ischaemia and angina. Toffees, 10/-. Miss F. [*radiographer*] phones to confirm that this morning's domiciliary with praecordial pain had had a coronary thrombosis. Watched Bolshoi Company in Tschaikovsky's *Queen of Spades*.

Feb 11 [*Sunday*]   Death of Lord Birkett. Read the book reviews: including J. H. Plumb on John Wilkes, and Raymond Mortimer on Thomas Cranmer. The Meirs [*friends*] called in the evening, and disturbed the 'Monitor' programme on Modern Music.

Feb 12   Lecture to the Nurses, on congestive heart failure, the final lecture; a hopeless crowd, lazy, the worst ever. Domiciliaries: pneumoconiosis (aet 63, Ashton, to arrange pension if he fails to do so himself); myocardial ischaemia (aet 53, Ashton, arranged anti-coagulants); diabetes mellitus, trophic ulcers of both legs, and incipient gangrene of one foot (aet 38, Ashton, admitted). St. John St., 3 cases.

2:30 p.m. [*Male, aged 38, motor-cycle mechanic*] He complained of a 'pain' in the pit of the stomach, which 'comes and goes', a cough 'with phlegm' and weight loss. He also said that three weeks ago he had had a 'blackout, at about 5.0 p.m'.

On examination, he had a tremor of his outstretched hands, and bitten finger nails. He is a tense and anxious fellow who fractured his skull 2 years ago in a motor cycle accident, smokes '20 cigarettes a day', and has dental caries. He is unmarried. His father died two weeks ago, aged 68, of pneumonia. My provisional diagnosis was that he is suffering either from nervous dyspepsia or a duodenal ulcer. I have sent him for a barium meal and a full blood count. He is a private patient, and paid 5 guineas.

Proceeded to Hyde, to Lodge meeting as guest of Dr. C. Lost my gloves somewhere. Home by 11.0 p.m., M. sleeping.

Feb 13 Feel exhausted today. Did Anti-coagulant clinic; my test, 20 seconds. Domiciliary: chest disease, old case of phthisis [*pulmonary tuberculosis*] (aet 42, Hyde, admitted). To St. John St., 3 cases, including a man of 16 stone who has been an Atlantic whaler, and a Rabbi with asthma. Watched 'Tonight' on Dame Edith Sitwell, and lonely young intellectual wives. Death of Hugh Dalton.

Feb 14 Arnfields and Ward rounds, 14 and 15; Mr. Y. in Ward 14 to go private. Lunch, 3/6d. To St. John St., 2 cases, including an interesting childless couple who are vegetarians, cyclists and walkers. Home early, and studied a Minute Book of the Pickwick Club (started in 1837), which I bought for £1 some years ago; also found an album with old Valentines, and Baker's *Chronicle of the Kings of England*, 1643. My life has been wonderfully enriched by this harmless and instructive hobby.

Feb 15 Judy is 17 today. She received a transistor radio. God Bless Her. To gas showrooms with M. to purchase new gas-stove. Thence to hospital, Ward 14 and 15; Mr. Y. *in extremis.*

Feb 17 [*Saturday*]   Restful day. Listened to Alan Taylor's Lecture on the Treaty of Versailles; a bit ponderous this week. Thereafter, to the Livingstones until 11.30 p.m. A short walk with M., on our return.

Feb 18   Made breakfast for M., and read the *Sunday Times* almost without omissions, except for the adverts. Sundays are helpful; they give me time for contemplation, and for preparation for toil in the week ahead. Hanratty has been sentenced to death by Mr. Justice Gorman, the longest murder trial in history. The jury was out for ten hours. To Judy, £1; an increase in allowance this week since her birthday. Watched a television discussion on Freedom of Worship between Rev. Leslie Timmins and atheist Miss M. Laski. Also 'Face to Face', John Freeman interviewing Cecil Beaton, who looked to me like a homosexual psychopath, but whose intelligence was a modicum above the average.

Feb 19   Charming little letters from Dr. J.'s children, thanking me for the books I gave them; compare Dr. N.'s children, who have received many more without thanks. Did supplementary follow-up clinic, and Ward rounds 7, 15: Mr. Y. dying. Gave out-patients' Sister H. a present, accepted with bad grace; a frightful woman. Thereafter, 2 domiciliaries: pericarditis [*inflammation of the pericardium, sometimes a complication of rheumatic fever*] (aet 15, Dukinfield, admitted); and cor pulmonale, with bronchiectasis (aet 59, Ashton, admitted). St. John St., 6 cases. Tonight's news: storm damage in Sheffield, and Lord Boothby to give up public speaking.

Feb 20   Received W.W. Greg's *Licencers for the Press, to 1640*, from Oxford Bibliographical Society. M. complaining of praecordial pain: Miss F. [*radiographer*] summoned, but ECG normal. To domiciliary visit: collapse of left lung (aet 47, Ashton, admitted). Ward rounds, 12 and 15; Mr. Y. died this morning. Lunch, 3/6d. St. John St., 4 cases. Colonel Glenn makes successful Orbital Flight. At 10.35 p.m., watched special film flown from USA about his achievement. Also a programme on the Lebanon: riches and poverty, white slave traffic, hashish and drug-dealing. A clever programme, but what a country!

Feb 21   Rose at 7.0 a.m., and read about Colonel Glenn's outer space venture. Took Judy to school, and thence to Arnfields to give 31 polio injections. Visited U.T. [*See Nov 29 1960*] in Dukinfield. She appeared much worse; she told me that her sister-in-law, who had a sharp tongue and rheumatoid arthritis, has died recently, aet 63. Thereafter, two domiciliaries: cerebral vascular lesion (aet 68, Dukinfield, to be admitted), and disseminated lupus erythematosis (most likely) (aet 60, Ashton, admitted urgently). Lunch, 3/6d. St. John Street, 4 cases, including case of old tuberculosis.

Feb 22   Rose at 2.0 a.m., made tea, and read further details of Colonel Glenn in yesterday's *Manchester Guardian*, and an account of Budapest. To Stockport Magistrates' Court at 9.30 a.m., to give medical evidence for the defendant in running-down case. Ward round, thereafter. To St. John St., 4 cases, including a hypertensive industrial chemist. The appointments are coming in again fairly rapidly. Phoned John Whittle & Co. [*solicitors*] to reprimand them for not having had the courtesy to tell me the result of the magistrates' hearing, which I read about in the *Manchester Evening News*: case dismissed, my account sent. Solicitors are mostly all alike.

Feb 23   David arrived this evening, morose as ever. Watched Michaela Denis on snakes, and the birth of chameleons; magnificent.

Feb 24 [*Saturday*]   Arose at 4.0 a.m., made tea, dusted some books and read the *Lancet*. Settlement holding has increased to 546 shares, with Lloyds Bank bonus issue. To St. John St., for letters. Thence to Wards 14 and 15. Paid 2/6d for flowers obtained from Post-Mortem room. Domiciliary visit: pneumonia (aet 51, Denton, admitted). David hints at a permanent liaison with Hazel S., which has upset us considerably. Dr. X.Y. calls. He has failed his primary FRCS three times; his tenacity is admirable, but the fault is in his grey matter.

Feb 25   Depressing day; a cloud hangs over the household. David's anxious and silent preoccupation, without confiding in us, is a painful experience. Read in the Sunday papers about Colonel Glenn's space-shot and a Committee of 100 Meeting in Trafalgar Square. Early to bed.

Feb 26   Heavy snow, temperatures below zero. Arose at 7.0. a.m. and had tea with David. No hospital today, so proceeded to the H. travel agency, to talk about arrangements for visit to USA. (F. [*another travel agent*] has gone bankrupt, and about time too). Thence to St. John Street, one case only; two others cancelled because of the weather. Watched 'Tonight': Alan Whicker, excellent and reporting direct, giving an account of Algiers as it is today; a terrifying city.

Feb 27   Received cheque for £75 for storm-damage to prints [*see Sept 4 1961*], and small book from M.F. [*private patient*] on the 'Art of Love'. Domiciliary visits: streptococcal throat (aet 13, Denton); hypertensive heart disease and angina (aet 73, Dukinfield, ECG arranged); and congestive heart failure (aet 60, Clayton, admitted). No cases at St. John St., so proceeded to Sherratt and Hughes, and thence to Masonic meeting: appalling boredom of ceremony. Too tired to read the papers.

Feb 28   56 today; going on to 60. Cards and telegrams. M. has bad cold. Regional Hospital Board statement, £255.0s.6d. To Arnfields, and thereafter called on Mrs. Faulkner [*secretary*] for conversation. She gave me a stainless steel ashtray. Ward Rounds, and lunch, 3/6d. Not much leisure for a birthday.

March 1   Disturbed night. Paid annual subscription to Medical Protection Society, £2.0s.0d. Took Judy to school, and thence to Miss A., for her injection. Domiciliary: obesity, aortic stenosis, myocardial ischaemia (aet 56, Ashton, admitted). To St. John St., 4 cases, including a gross neurotic with *pruritus ani*. Sixteen to eighteen appointments have come in for next week. Home at 6.30 p.m. Fearful air crash of Boeing 707 at Idlewild Airport, New York after take-off, 95 killed, no survivors; one hour before ticker-tape welcome to Colonel Glenn. Watched late news of it: inexplicable and depressing.

March 2 Received letter and report from Dr. W.F. on the aetiology of my ischaemic heart disease. No cases at St. John St.; called at travel agent for further literature on USA. Heard this evening that my usher at the MRCP clinical examination [*in 1931*], Dr. Geoffrey Konstam, has died. Alas!

March 3 [*Saturday*] Awoke at 2.0 a.m., made tea and had a snack. Heavy snow, garden like an Xmas pattern. To sleep again at 4.15 a.m.; cannot sleep now without sedation. Made breakfast for M. and then to domiciliary visit: cerebral thrombosis, *in extremis* (aet 76, Ashton). The house and family – ex-publicans – were prosperous and they could have paid, with flash new cars in the driveway, but nevertheless used the National Health Service.

March 4 Restful day. Read in the *Sunday Times* and *Observer* of the trouble in Algeria, and an attack by Dr. Leavis of Cambridge, in his farewell lecture, on Sir Charles Snow.

March 5 Heavy snow and cold weather. £15 to M. Ward Rounds, 7, 12, 14, 15, complete and comprehensive; measured for dressing-gown by A.P. [*private patient*]. Domiciliary visit: left ventricular failure, probably coronary thrombosis (aet 63, Droylsden, admitted) St. John St., 6 cases; also a Mr. L. who called to inquire about his son, the Rabbi [*see Feb 13 1962*]. Another dreadful air-crash, 111 dead, 101 Passengers and 10 Crew. Also a crash of a private plane; a man and two children killed. Watched 'Panorama': interviews with Whites in Salisbury, interviews with Blacks in Trinidad, and salmon-fishing on the Tweed.

March 6   Balance at bank, £894.14s.11d. Anti-coagulant clinic; my Prothrombin time 29 seconds. Lunch, 3/6d. To St. John St., 8 cases, including tall blonde with very short skirt, who came half an hour late.

March 7   Bitterly cold day. Report on Smoking and Cancer published today by Royal College of Physicians.

March 8   As I was entering the hospital, Sister G. told me that all was under control, so proceeded to Colam for fish, £1.0s.0d.; also purchased grapes, £1.2s.0d. Lunch at Masonic Temple and St. John St., 5 cases. Snack with M. at Black's, 8/–. To Opera House, to *The Lizard and the Rock*, by John Hall, his first play, about Farming in Western Australia. Poor house, poor play; earlier, destructive criticism by the *Guardian*.

March 10 [*Saturday*]   Today, sold a number of books to Michael Papantoniou [*American bookdealer from New York*], including Swift's *Genteel and Polite Conversations*, Beaumont and Fletcher folio (first condition, tall copy), Boswell on the *Douglas Case*, Robert Davenport's *City Night-Cap* and sundry Henry James' novels, first editions: £534.10s.0d. Our visit to the U.S. now possible.

March 11   Read the Sunday papers. Perception is dulled by the constant drivel of news, TV, disasters, nuclear race, political polemics, and the constant outpourings of writing in an incessant stream, good, bad and indifferent.

March 12   Insomnia is becoming irksome. Phoned Gas Board, re gas escapes, for the fourth time. Ward Rounds 7, 15; and farewell-gathering, with presentation (£1 contribution), for Dr. P. St. John St., 5 cases.

3:45 p.m. [*Female, aged 54, single, shop assistant*] She was a nervous-looking woman, with a moderately raised blood pressure, and some bowing of both legs from childhood rickets. She is single, lives alone, and is a Woolworth's shop assistant. Her father died six years ago; she said that arthritis had 'come on' in her knees after the death of her father. Her periods also ceased six years ago. Nine months ago, she tripped over some uneven flagstones in West Gorton and bruised her knees; a passer-by 'from across the road' helped her to her feet. (She said that she then walked home, and 'went to bed after tea'). She was off work for 16 days, returned to Woolworths for 3 weeks, visited Lourdes for a week in August, but spent most of the time in the hotel, since her eyes 'kept going funny'. On her return from Lourdes, she was off work for a further month – she said that she 'rested' – and was then sacked from her employment. She was out of work for three days, before finding a similar job at Lewis's as a shop assistant. Today she said that her knees are painful, that she always feels tired, and goes to bed early. She also gets a 'numb feeling on her left side', sometimes in her left arm, or on the 'left side' of her tongue, or in two fingers of her left hand. This is an unhappy situation: of symptoms most of which are essentially subjective, of grating sounds in both knees, of depression, and of feelings of tiredness quite common in cases of neurosis following accidents (however trivial). The fact that she is suing the council and may in consequence be developing an obsession about her fall, with an accompanying sense of grievance, is not helping her medical state. Instead, she is likely to go on like this indefinitely; and at least until the case has been disposed of.

On television, Mrs. Wedgwood-Benn, an intelligent American woman.

March 13   Anti-coagulant clinic. I asked Dr. C. [*consultant physician*] to do the coming weekend for me; I will do the next one for him. Domiciliary visit: cor pulmonale (aet 60, Audenshaw, to be admitted). To Committee Meeting of Manchester Society of Book Collectors, 5.15 p.m. Afterwards found that a fully-blown half-wit had parked his car a paper-breadth from my entry door. The problem was solved with the assistance of many teen-aged youths.

March 14   Heavy traffic home, because of football replay; football has replaced Christ.

March 16   V. [*friend*] phones to tell me that his wife has secondary cancer. Left for London by car at about 12 noon: Hyde, Chapel-en-le-Frith, Buxton and to Aldbourne. Lunch at 'The Green Man', £1.5s.od. Then Sudbury, Lichfield, Coleshill, Stonebridge, Coventry to M.1 and Watford by-pass to West End, via Swiss Cottage, Baker St., Park Lane, to Ritz Hotel. Arrived at 5.30 p.m. Afternoon tea, 13/-. Met Michael Papantoniou at 7.5 p.m. He purchased, inter alia, N. Payne's *Fatal Jealousie*, Charles Churchill's *Verses*, Shirley's *The Young Admiral*, and 3 Minerva Press volumes. Total, £121. os. od. Decided to stay at The Ritz, room 126, 2nd floor. 1/4 for a 3d phone call, and 6d for an evening paper. Dinner was an elaborate affair, but the dining room was deserted; very few can afford to dine in this stifling Victorian discomfort.

March 17 [*Saturday*]   Bright morning. Ritz bill, £5.4s.4d. = 10/- an hour for sleeping. Went to Kardomah in Piccadilly for breakfast, 3/9d, and homeward by same route as yesterday. Stopped for excellent lunch at 'The Swan Revived', Newport Pagnell, £1.7s.od. Home by 7.30 p.m. M. had gone with Judy and David to the Opera House, to see *The Rehearsal* by Jean Anouilh, with Phyllis Calvert, Diana Churchill, Alan Badel and Robert Hardy.

March 18   Dr. F. telephoned to inquire about my health. David gave me a cheque for £4.10s.7d., for his telephone calls during our absence. I am reluctant to put pressure on him, but he has little appreciation of financial matters and it may help him to understand that I have to work for my living.

March 20   Woke up at 3.0 a.m. for second night in succession; insomnia troubles me of late. Letter to Sir Francis Frazer re modern medicine. Anti-coagulant clinic: personal test, 27 seconds. Ward Rounds at Glossop: saw Miss R., aet 46, who has grown fat and ugly. To domiciliary visit: multiple myelomatosis (aet 59, Audenshaw, admitted). St. John St., 3 cases. Watched 'Tonight': Jimenez, ex-dictator of Venezuela in exile in Miami, discussion of next Budget, and tame

Golden Eagle. Afterwards, tidied up some plays by Dryden and Congreve, and started to read Henry Glapthorne's *The Hollander*, 1640.

March 21 Gave Dr. J. some books for his children. Domiciliary visit: hypertensive heart failure (aet 51, Audenshaw, for admission). Ward Rounds 12, 14, 15 with Dr. M. [*house physician*]. Proceeded to Manchester and lunch at Masonic Temple, 7/-. Looked briefly into Walmsley's bookshop. St. John St., 4 cases. Thereafter, visited Manchester Medical Library, where I found the librarian in his usual torpor, dozing in his chair. Pamphlets of some importance were lying about, dirty and dusty, and in the same positions as I had seen them 12 months ago.

March 22 Woke at 7.0 a.m., with intense giddiness and vertigo. To American consular office to apply for visa, but forgot to bring photographs; to Woolworth's, Piccadilly with M. and took pictures, returned to Consulate and 2 visas granted. Morning coffee with M. at Affleck's, 2/6d. To Sherratt and Hughes and long talk with Mr. N. [*see Feb 1 1962*], a tough nut with a streak of unpleasantness. Purchased D.H. Lawrence's *Letters*, 2 vols, edited by Harry T. Moore; I have had a Limited Edition of the previous collection, edited by Aldous Huxley, since 1932. Small lunch at Midland Hotel, with Walter S. [*friend*]. St. John St., 3 cases, including a woman who drank from a bottle of lemonade smelling of petrol, and has sued the manufacturer. Looked in at Walmsley's bookshop thereafter, and then to Masonic Temple for a rest and smoke, and a few drinks with Bert W. and Harry G. [*friends*]. The Opera House, 7 p.m.: Trevor Howard in *Two Stars for Comfort*, by John Mortimer, the worst play I have ever seen.

March 23 Medical out-patients, 2.30 p.m. Poor Miss T. has died, aet 70, of 'pneumonia' [*an ex-patient and friend from his days in general practice*]. She was suffering from disseminated lupus erythematosus [*a slow, degenerative disease of the connective tissues*]. Her sister, aged 77, came to the Hospital to thank me. Her G.P. never sent for me; some doctors would rather see their patients die than do so.

March 24 [*Saturday*]   Today's *British Medical Journal* is sceptical about the use of anti-coagulants at all. The dangers of haemorrhage, subdural haematomas, haemopericardium, haematuria and rupture of the heart are reported. Rested until lunch. Afternoon, reading. To dinner at the Livingstones at 7.0 p.m. Emergency call to hospital for case of hypoglycaemic coma (possibly from insulin overdose). At hospital from 10.20 p.m. till 11.10 p.m., returned to Livingstones, and home at 1.35 a.m., new time. Clocks moved forward one hour tonight. Short walk with M., until 2.0 a.m. To bed at 2.30.

March 25   David in his dismal mood again. Very disturbing. Began 1st volume of D.H. Lawrence's *Letters*. To bed very late.

March 26   Phoned Gas Board yet again; rude and uncouth response. Ward rounds, 12, 15. Asked secretary to type list of Restoration Plays. St. John St., 4 cases. Finalized arrangements for USA and Canada.

March 27   Domiciliaries: left lobar pneumonia (aet 63, Stalybridge, admission arranged) and advanced tubercle [*tuberculosis*] (aet 63, Denton, admitted). St. John St., 2 cases.

3:0 p.m. [*Male, aged 55, postal and telegraphic clerical officer*] Five months ago he was knocked off his pedal cycle, suffering concussion, a cut on the back of his head and over his left eyebrow, and bruised calves. Today, he said that he did not 'feel with the day in the morning', that the morning was 'the worst part', and that he 'can't hurry in the mornings but only in the afternoons and evenings'. He was a healthy-looking man who looked younger than his years, with a normal and regular pulse and excellent blood pressure, 130/80. He also had varicose veins of both legs, with the left calf indurated, pigmented and discoloured. He told me that in the mornings his feet 'don't seem to touch the ground', and that he gets a 'mist over the eyes': he feels as if he wants to 'wipe something away', but cannot. His own doctor – whose name he could not remember – is giving him 'energy' tablets. He is suffering from a post-concussive neurosis, and will probably dawdle on in this way for another month or two, or perhaps longer. He had a 1″ scar over his left eyebrow.

March 28   Mrs Faulkner [*secretary*] asks me how I 'manage to go to all these places', referring to my planned visit to the USA: an envious question, characteristic of the local society. God protect me from my friends. St. John St., 4 cases.

2:30 p.m. [*Male, aged 16, apprentice patten-maker, Salford*] He was a healthy, muscular lad who has done some weight-lifting and plays football for his Works team. Six weeks ago, he was knocked off his bike and suffered abrasions which were dressed at the hospital. He was not asked to return, did not knock his head, was not unconscious, had no fractures, lacerations or any other injuries, yet he was off work for one complete month. When I asked him why he was off work for so long for such a trivial accident, he said it was because of pain in his left thigh. I regard his absence from work for a month as grossly in excess of the time needed; a few days would have sufficed.

4:0 p.m. [*Male, aged 46, works manager*] Six months ago, he had a coronary thrombosis and today says that he has a continuous feeling of discomfort at the upper part of his sternum. He called it 'a heaviness', and as if there was 'mucus' on his chest. He also said that he had no energy, and always felt tired. On the whole, I thought that he was too introspective and too anxious about his own condition. The lack of energy is entirely due to this anxiety state, and not to any organic condition. A holiday would do him good.

Dr L. called tonight. She has taken her MRCP London, and stands a good chance. She is very thin.

March 29   Flight to New York arranged, direct from Manchester, 27th April.

March 30   Rose at 4.30 a.m. with tinnitus [*ringing in the ears*]; very harassing, took Serpasil with some relief. Tidied books until 6.30 a.m. To Town Hall, to see Manager of Gas Board and to complain about leaking gas-stove. Ward 15, and emergency private visit (aet 77, Denton, cerebral haemorrhage, urgently admitted). Lunch 3/6d, and heavy Medical out-patients to 5.30 p.m. My BP, 170/100. Thereafter, four domiciliaries: congestive heart failure (aet 53, Droylsden); severe headaches (aet 61, Ashton, for diagnosis); rheumatic carditis (aet 14, Ashton, ECG arranged); coronary thrombosis (aet 58, Denton, ECG arranged). Very exhausting day, with insomnia and tinnitus.

March 31 [*Saturday*]   Sister G. phoned to say that Mrs. J. [*private patient*] had discharged herself, against advice, from the private patients' side Ward, 15. She objected to there being another patient in the same room. To Miss A. [*private patient*], Dukinfield, injection and tablets given: she was still asleep when I called at 10.15 a.m. Fruit purchased, 9/6d. Ward Round 12, in full, and Ward 15. My BP, 170/95; Reserpine 0.25 mgm, taken. St. John Street for letters, and home by 3.30 p.m. Not many days left before the USA.

April 1   Destroying old diaries most of the day. The most interesting one is for 1935 [*see Sept 4, 1960*] when I was still at Lewisham; a record of devotion and constant care of Mother. Phil P. [*contemporary, who died young*] was still alive, and we had many outings together, he with Marion Hutt and I with Rita Macmahon. On Good Friday, 1935, the four of us went to Marlow.

April 2   Arose at 3.30 a.m., tinnitus and insomnia. Went down to the Library and continued to read old diaries.

April 3   Saw Mr. F. [*consultant ENT surgeon*] about my tinnitus; he said it was nothing.

April 4   Domiciliary visits: advanced bronchogenic carcinoma and diabetes (aet 47, Audenshaw), and cor pulmonale (aet 72, Hyde, admitted). St. John St., no cases. Watched 'Tonight': on debutantes (a cattle market); a discussion of the Home Secretary's decision re Hanratty's Execution; latest film of the Royal Society's expedition to Tristan Da Cunha: and on the life of Charrington the Brewer, who turned to Temperance and gave up his fortune.

April 5   To Mrs. Faulkner [*secretary*]: her work has declined. Reports are not satisfactorily typed, however easy. Ward Rounds, 12 and 15, and thence to Medical Advisory Committee's luncheon-meeting. A boring affair as usual, with much heat generated for no particular reason. These people think they will live for ever. St. John St., no cases at all; Miss James a nightmare. A slack week, work deteriorating, but not worried really.

To W., the tailors: red velvet waistcoat purchased, £3.19s.6d. Then to Sherratt and Hughes: Mr. N. is an unsympathetic fellow, who gives no concessions and no proof copies. He has an ominous lump in his chest, attached to his ribs. He has seen Mr T., consultant; gumma(?), TB(?), sarcoma(?). Thereafter, to Walmsley's bookshop and the City Library, for tea in Colley's [*city librarian's*] office. 7.0 p.m.: Book Collectors' meeting, discussion on 'Old Booksellers of Manchester'; acted as chairman, meeting well-attended. Visited 'The Wyvern' afterwards with members. A row on getting home, M. complaining of my 'coming late' etc; 10.30 p.m., mark you ('marital bliss'). Entered this ledger at midnight. I am dyspnoeic [*short of breath*] and obviously overweight.

April 7 [*Saturday*]   Heavy rain and wind. Made breakfast for M. at 7.30 a.m. Set off for Southport with M., to see C.I. [*private patient*]. He had bilateral femoral herniae [*in the groin*], each one as large as an adult female breast. Photographs to be taken. Lunch at Prince of Wales Hotel, £1.12s.0d. Went for a walk along the promenade, cold and windy. Home by 3.45 p.m. Cambridge win boat race by many lengths, in very bad weather conditions.

April 8   Read *Sunday Times* and *Observer*, and all book reviews. It is impossible to read all the books recommended; life is too short. Budget day tomorrow. Canada facing economic difficulties, and appears to be in America's pocket. Tidied up books and found many plays, including Wm. Lower's *The Phoenix in Her Flames* (1639), May's *The Old Couple* and Davenant's *The Just Italian* (1630). Also found Roger Ascham's *Apologia* (1577), Thomas Cranmer's *Defence of the Truth of Catholic Doctrine* (1557) and Thomas Elyot: *The Castell Of Helth* (1541); and, later, Gay's *Beggar's Opera*, a mint first edition, and George Berkeley's *Philosophy*, 1710, first edition, published in Dublin. In the evening, read from Robert Boyle's *Origine of Formes and Qualities* [*1661*] and *The High Veneration Man's Intellect Owes to God* [*1685*]; also the interrogation of Prynne, Dr. Bastwicke and Burton by the Starre-Chamber, in June 1637. Their punishment was rigorous, painful and brutal, and Archbishop Laud behind it.

April 9   Supplementary out-patients at 10 a.m.: interesting cases, including C.B., a welder with phoeochromocytoma who has gone to work in Rotterdam, and earns £40 per week and expenses. He was a self-assured type, but appeared to be leading a riotous life. His BP was 190/110. My BP 150/90, took Guanethidine 5 mgm, and 1.5 mgm Marcoumar. To St. John St., 2 cases. Today's Budget News: 15% on sweets, ice cream and soft drinks; Schedule A Tax to be abolished in the not too distant future; and Capital Gains Tax to be levied on the 'wide boys' buying and selling stocks and shares. Otherwise, the mixture as before.

April 10   Literature obtained from N. [*hospital administrator*] for preparation of lecture in Virginia on the NHS [*see Oct 3 1960*]. No cases in St. John St., practice deteriorating. Six guests to dinner party at home, 8.0 p.m. to 11.30 p.m.

April 11   Did not attend Lodge meeting; getting tired of these futile ceremonies. More smallpox deaths in Wales.

April 12　From Henry Shaw, debt-collector, £2.18s.10d. Reports dictated, and collected Guanethidine, Marcoumar and Serpasil from Dispensary. Took 10 mgm Guanethidine, 1.5mgm Marcoumar and 0.1 mgm Serpasil, and thence to Benton's Cigar Shop, Manchester. Purchased cigars, £14.13s.0d; I am told at the shop that cigarette purchases are 'as bad as ever'. Prepared skeleton framework of speech for Virginia next month. Called out at 8 p.m. to private patient: A.W., aet 60, obesity, rheumatoid arthritis, cerebral vascular lesion, admitted *in extremis*. The residents, Drs. D. and F., gave her first aid treatment.

April 13　Rose at 3.30 a.m., made myself some tea, and spent some hours in the Library. Lunch at 'The Organ' with George W. and Tony T. Medical out-patients, from 2.30 p.m. Lengthy and heavy-going. There are many sick people, especially hypertensives, who are hard to control as out-patients, since they do not obey instructions. To bed early, at 9.30 p.m.; Pro-actidil tablet taken, a good soporific.

April 14 [*Saturday*]　To St. John St., for letters: work picking up again. Proceeded to Failsworth to M.L., a serious case combining lymphadenoma [*Hodgkin's Disease, cancer-like disorder of lymph nodes and spleen*] with fracture dislocation of cervical region in a car accident, causing complete Paraplegia. A cheerful patient, with a devoted wife, a hero in suffering. Home at 2 p.m., and phoned Dr. F. about a girl of 16 with drooping eyelids mistakenly taken to be myasthenia gravis: a case of hysteria.

April 15　Read papers: Death Sentence on Jouhaud, De Gaulle to decide; anti-semitism in Russia; Rainier of Monaco facing a crisis in his funk-hole of a Principality; trouble in Middle East, over Israel's diversion of Jordan Waters; aftermath of Selwyn Lloyd's miserable Budget; and Somerset Maugham's half million pounds from the sale of his Impressionist Paintings (£80,000 for a Picasso!). David's love for Hazel S. is intensified by his hostility towards us; he has gone to a performance at the Free Trade Hall of the St. Matthew Passion, conducted by Sir John Barbirolli. At

7.0 p.m., with M., to Indian and Pakistani residents' dinner: as usual, very tough curried chicken.

April 16   Disturbed night in spite of sedation. 560 dollars in travellers' cheques purchased for £200, with £1.10s.0d. commission. Ward 7, full round. Took one Apisate tablet to inhibit appetite. Lunch, 3/6d. Testimonial given to Dr. H., who is well-intentioned, but slow in the uptake. St. John St., 4 cases; Miss James refused to give me a cup of tea and said I could 'have a glass of water'. 'That's all that's free in this house', she stated. To Maurice G. [*friend and rabbi*] on the way home; smoked a cigar and had a double brandy.

April 17   Home early, intending to take it easy, but phone-call from City Librarian wanting me to come to Meeting of Book-collectors. Returned to town, and took the chair: Mrs. Beatrice Warde on her Reminiscences In the Field of Typography; not my field, but interesting.

April 18   To private patient, of Italian extraction: aet 69, Denton, with arteriosclerotic occlusion of the foot arteries. Incipient dry Gangrene, patient blind and difficult; admitted to private ward, paid £10.10s.0d. There has been a case of typhoid recently in the family, and they sell ice-cream! St. John St., one case only. To Manchester Medical Library, to see librarian: today slightly less sleepy. Passover; David silent. My BP 170/100. Feeling exhausted.

April 19   My new stethoscope lost (=stolen). St. John St., one case only. I am of the opinion that Miss James has ruined my practice, with her big mouth and lack of tact when making appointments. Watched Duke of Edinburgh describing his S. American trip: 54 days, 11 countries, 36,000 miles. (Note £507,000 cost of refitting 'Britannia'; original cost of Britannia £2,500,000. Figures quoted in *Daily Express* today. Compare poverty in S. American states). Anginal attack this evening, of some severity; BP 150/95, 10 mgm Guanethidine taken.

April 20 [*Good Friday*]   Dr. F. rang early about Mrs

C. [*private patient*], who died at 3.0 a.m.; strange that I dreamt about her last night, but I feel unmoved. She caused much unhappiness to people. To lumber-room; damp causing some damage. Brought downstairs Oliver Goldsmith, *Essays*, 1765, first edition, with engraved title; B. de Fontenelle, *Plurality of Worlds*, 1929, Nonesuch edition; D.H. Lawrence, *Reflections on the Death of a Porcupine*; and Herbert's *The Temple*, 1703, twelfth edition. (I have the 1st, 8th, 9th, 11th and 12th editions). Salan, the leader of the OAS, has been captured by the French. Bad weather lessens Exodus this Good Friday. Listened to 'Parsifal' Good Friday music from Winchester Cathedral.

April 21 [*Saturday*]   Awoke at 3.0 a.m.: insomnia without sedation. To bed again at 4.30. Purchased fruit, £1.16s.10d, and to hospital: Wards 11, 12, 15. Mrs. V. [*private patient*], an aberrant type, but better. My Prothrombin time 18 seconds, BP 160/100; 15 mgm Guanethidine. To St. John St., for letters; no merit award received. I note that seven have been awarded. Will see into the matter on my return from the States, but if Dr. X. has anything to do with them, I will never get one. Visited Maurice G. for tea, and heard about Majorca: now nothing but vulgarity, tourism, hotels and over-indulgence. Today, heavy cold has possessed me, due to indecent and boor-like sneezing in my face by an Arnfield's workman, on Wednesday last. The ill-manners of the masses have begun to appal me. Not limited to working classes.

April 22 [*Easter Day*]   Very bad cold; took anti-histamines. St. John St., for morning case (12.30 p.m.) After lunch, siesta, drowsy from anti-histamines. Judy is obsessed with Mahler, and this evening made a great deal of noise with records of his music. To bed at 2.0 a.m.

April 23 [*Easter Monday*]   Fine sunny day; the crowds are out motoring. Arranged US lecture in order of headings. These are happy days in spite of the ageing process, my BP and angina, the increased cost of living and the irritating bureaucracy of the Health Service.

April 24   Mrs. W. [*hospital employee*] comes to show me 'a rash'; it is herpes zoster, with chicken-pox and lymphadenoma [*Hodgkin's Disease*]. Lunch, 3/6d. To Dukinfield, to see U.T. [*see Feb 21 1962*]; the poor woman has the bone-pains of metastases. St. John St., 2 cases. Listened to Beethoven's Violin Concerto, with Menuhin and the London Symphony Orchestra, conducted by Colin Davis.

April 25   To hospital, and medical examination of 12 new trainee nurses, from Liberia, Barbados, Trinidad, Persia and Nigeria. The Liberian girl, who was 19 and very pretty, had a child of 3 (she had been raped, she said, when 15); the Persian girl had been to school with Queen Farah.

April 26   Awoke at 4.0 a.m., and read. Later to police, to notify them of our absence. Deposited cheques in bank, £75.9s.5d. To domiciliary: broncho-pneumonia and congestive heart failure (aet 75, Smallshaw). Ward round, 15: saw C.M. [*friend*], who has a perforated duodenal ulcer. Lunch, farewells, private patients seen, and instructions left with Dr. F. (His wife is a nag). Final touches to packing. Neville B. called with cinnamon balls, to be taken to Geoffrey[*son-in-law*] in New York.

*

[*This was his first visit to the United States, during which – as he wrote in his Diary on June 3 – 'I kept no journal and took no photographs'. Nevertheless, on June 3 he wrote up what follows 'from scraps, fairly successfully'.*]

*

April 27   Departure for America, 10.45 a.m. by Boeing 707, flight BA 537: 33 passengers, 32 Economy Class, one First Class. David had taken us to the airport; the night before he had spoken to M. of his infatuation, but he does not speak to me and I will not speak to him either. M. distressed by his folly. [*Her distress was that of a rabbi's daughter confronted by the prospect of her son's marriage to a 'gentile'.*]

April 28   Walk on the Broadwalk of Long Beach; weather cold, much litter on the sands and overhead noises from Jet aircraft. Jonathan [*grandson*] spoiled and difficult.

April 29   Visit to East Side, Brooklyn, in the afternoon; dirty. Delancy Street reminded me of Petticoat Lane and Whitechapel. Much hotter, 95°F or thereabouts, in New York. Walk through Central Park, and returned in the evening to Long Beach. Heavy, rapid and frightening traffic. Unsatisfactory initial impressions.

April 30   To Atlantic City, 180 miles: 75th Annual Meeting, or Convention, of the American Medical Association. Turnpike roads, to Teplitzky's Hotel, or Motel, 28 dollars a day for a couple, lunch not included. Excellent food and service, but American TV poor stuff, compared with the British: Westerns, old films, adverts, sponsored News etc. About six channels, each as bad as the other.

May 1   Listened to 'high-falutin'' medical papers: on marrow transplantation in Newborn Mice suffering from hereditary spherocytosis, and on some immunological aspects of the Evolution and Treatment of Leukaemia. Stayed up late listening to Mr. Teplitzky's life-story, while Jonathan ran up and down inclined floor, backwards and forwards.

May 2   Left Teplitzky's and proceeded to N.Y. in cold weather. In the evening, to Radio City, 50th Street, to see strange film-and-stage-show with grandiose tableaux, of a Walt Disney character, and a film of a spaceman with a woman on board (tosh). Then to Sardi's, 44th Street, where the theatrical folk go. Thereafter, to 'The Gas-Light Club' in 56th Street: aphrodisiac effect, with lightly-clad women in fishnet stockings exhibiting their mammary glands. Very satisfactory for the young, but frustrating for the aged and balding. New York is a wonderful place for the wealthy.

May 3   Michael Papantoniou took me to lunch at the Roosevelt Hotel: marinated herrings in Cream, Steak etc. Promises to call and see me in the Fall. Thence, with him to the United Nations building; a conducted tour, with much blather about the number of windows etc.

May 4   Travelled with Max S. [*brother-in-law*] in his Rolls Royce, via the Bowery district, to his factory. Inspected the manufacture of his bird-seed, etc, and saw his aviaries: canaries, budgerigars, toucans and small birds from West Africa with red underwings etc. His son made an objectionable impression.

May 5 [*Saturday*]   Much hypocritical solemnity in the S. family's religious observance; one of the sons highly repellent. Afternoon siesta. In the evening to Lower Manhattan East, and, thence to Reuben's, for apple pancakes.

May 6   In the evening to Idlewild airport, since Max S. was leaving for Dakar; a myriad of twinkling lights. Prior to his departure, he offered to phone David in Birmingham, who rebuffed him rudely.

May 7   A fine day; ascended the Empire State Building with M., and thence tc Fifth Avenue for lunch at '666 on the Roof'. Thereafter, to the Metropolitan Museum of Art on my own. The news of David's entanglement appears serious. We can find little peace at the prospect.

May 8   Went through Harlem in taxi, to La Guardia Airport: the taxi-driver was an educated, coloured young man. By propeller-driven Super-Constellation to Boston, one hour; fare can be paid on the plane, a 'shuttle-service'.

May 9   Crisp and sunny weather. To Christian Science Headquarters, and thence on a visit to Lexington and Concord. Saw the houses of Longfellow, Waldo Emerson, Russell Lowell, Louisa Alcott and Hawthorne's 'House of the Seven Gables'. In the afternoon, to the Bunker Hill Monument, Paul Revere's House, 'Old Ironsides' in Boston Dock and the Old North Church, where I spoke to the vicar.

May 10   Flight, by shuttle-service, from Boston to

Washington. Second rate hotel, $14.50 *nocte*, on the 7th floor, with air-conditioning and TV out of order. Thence, on foot to George Washington Monument, passing The White House. Weather rather chilly. Ascended to the top of the Monument by lift, and then repaired to an adjoining establishment for ices. There, talked to youth, the son of the kiosk owner; he was anti-President Kennedy and expressed strong pro-German leanings, perhaps a neo-Fascist. I was much impressed by the beauty of the Capital city and its buildings, and by the smart appearance of the coloured girls.

May 11   The queue outside the White House was very long; I barged my way in and was promptly reprimanded by two elderly ladies (Mrs. Charles W., widow, aet 68, from Brooklyn, and Miss Gertrude A., aet 64, Brooklyn 27). Great amity ensued when I discovered that they were both originally from Manchester, and had lived in the USA for 40 years; we went around the White House together. Disappointing, with much hustling and pushing. Thence, to George Washington's home in Mount Vernon, overwhelmed by large crowds of schoolchildren; a place to visit when all is quiet.

May 12 [*Saturday*]   Visited the Capitol, the Senate and House of Representatives in sunny weather. Thereafter, to National Gallery of Art; fine French Impressionists, also Braque and Picasso, together with the usual English, Dutch and Italian schools. Met a Mr. and Mrs. Joe S. from Milwaukee in the Gallery cafeteria: both zombies.

May 13   Wandered the streets with M., and looked into a crowded Roman Catholic Church on Rhode Island Avenue. Later, found ourselves outside the house where Lincoln died; visited it, and crossed the road to the Old Ford Theatre, now a Lincoln Museum with much detail of his Life and Death. To Smithsonian Institute of Natural History; the largest elephant seen. Cold and rainy evening, with nothing to do. A TV Boxing Match going on, and so to bed.

May 14   To Washington Union Station, for the Chesapeake and Ohio Railway. We had almost a two-hour wait; the nit-wits at the Hotel had no sense to tell us that the time of the departure given us was Eastern Standard Time. Thence to Covington in the Allegheny Mountains (a range of the Appalachians), where we were met by Harry W. Jr. [*a dairy farmer and bibliophile*]. Spent part of the evening looking at the books in his Library, which contained a large collection of Erotica.

May 15   Prepared for this evening's lecture. 7.30 p.m., address to the Alleghany-Bath Medical Society on the National Health Service; the Chairman's method of introduction left much to be desired.

*

Excerpt from report in the Daily Review, *Clifton Forge (Va), 'British Doctor Describes National Health Services', prefaced by an 'Editor's Note' declaring that the account was 'timely, in view of the controversy over President Kennedy's proposal for medical care financed by increased social security taxes'. The article continues:*

'Dr. Selbourne displayed a graphic chart of the administration of the National Health Service Act of 1946 . . . with authority over medical services filtering down through a vast government bureaucracy financed by taxation. Dr. Selbourne said that there were "rumblings" among the citizens – the patients – over the impersonalized medical services and delays, and the downward trend in the quality of medical service . . .

'He quoted J.H.F. Brotherston, professor of public health and social medicine at the University of Edinburgh, who has stated that "the general practitioner is in serious danger of becoming a subordinate medical auxiliary, rather than a key figure of the National Health Service" . . . Dr. Selbourne continued that after 16 years of "government medicine" in Britain, doctors have become increasingly involved in "squabbles" that divert them from the practice of medicine . . . while the rate of taxation stifles their enterprise, and the application of their best talents. Emigration of doctors from the British Isles is now running at the rate of 600 to 700 yearly. This medical system "is being carried on at a stupendous cost, which increases annually", Dr. Selbourne added . . .'

The 'stupendous' cost was in fact about £900 million in 1962–63, compared with £247 million in 1948–49 (the first year of the Health Service), and around £500 million per annum in the mid-1950s. At constant prices – that is, allowing for inflation – the increase was not that great. But the battle for reinstatement as a consultant, which my father had waged from 1948 to 1951 against the local administrators of the NHS – briefly referred to in the Introduction – had left its marks on him.

Chief among them was his constant objection to what he regarded as the operation of 'Parkinson's Law' in the Health Service, and to the 'bureaucratic indifference' which had 'blighted his career' and 'made so many medical men unhappy'. In his 1950 papers he even refers to the 'ruthless and bureaucratic absurdities of the Regional Hospital Board', and earlier in this volume describes some of its members as 'half-literates'. Indeed, he was continuously critical of the powers over doctors given by the NHS to unqualified laymen and local worthies, such as those who served on hospital management committees, his own included.

That health services had at last been made available to all in 1948, irrespective of ability to pay, he clearly (and naturally) welcomed, provided always that the doctors themselves were given the means to 'satisfy the demands of the public', as he put it. 'This poor man', he said in 1952 of a 'poverty-stricken' and 'thin' hawker of donkey-stones with carious teeth, 'is in need of some dental treatment, which he could easily have now under the Health Service . . . He is a debilitated type, and needs the care and attention which it can provide him.'

Yet his criticisms of some patients' – and doctors' – abuse of the system are also frequent in his papers, and do not diminish as time passes. (By 1966, he regarded abuse as 'very common in our Welfare State'.) There are the familiar criticisms of 'futile calls', when he was still in general practice; criticisms of practitioners who were ready to provide patients with certificates of incapacity for work 'until Doomsday'; then, increasingly, criticisms of the 'well-off' who used the NHS but could afford to pay for treatment. In other words, like many (most?) doctors, he was ambivalent about the Health Service, while firm in his support for the principle of it.

He also strongly objected to the system of 'Merit Awards', often very large supplementary annual payments made in conditions of considerable privacy, even secrecy, to some medical consultants. He believed that the system of awards was 'corrupt', said so openly, and, unsurprisingly, never received one.

*

In the days after his talk on the National Health Service, my father spent time 'looking at Harry W.'s library' – some items in which had originally come from the collection of Oscar Wilde's son, Vyvyan Holland – and talking to 'local citizens' in and around Covington, Virginia. He then returned, with my mother, to New York and Long Beach, where he 'inspected' various bookshops. In one, 'void of customers', he saw a 'delightful book of translations of Chinese poetry, with fine illustrations. It was too heavy to take with me, so I left it reluctantly in the shop, which was deserted.' On May 25, they boarded the Canadian Pacific's 'Empress of Britain' in Montreal. 'The ship', he reported, was 'overrun by Canadian youth, with blaring transistor sets in their hands, and going everywhere with them.' He found the voyage home 'dreary'; a 'lengthy film about a psychiatrist marrying a wealthy patient', which he watched in the ship's cinema, 'relieved one form of boredom with another'. However, the journey was redeemed for him, four days out, by the discovery on board of 'one of my old pupils at Lewisham Hospital, who turned out to have accompanied me on Ward Rounds twenty-eight years ago', and with whom my father sat up talking 'until the early hours'.

*

May 30   Cold wind and sunshine. Nil of note until a conversation with a steward, who told me how a Captain under whom he had served – who 'logged' crew members for the slightest infringement – had been beaten up by his own crew when in mufti, and off duty. Weather improving as we enter the Firth of Clyde and pass Arran.

May 31   Approaching the end of the journey; packing, and getting restive. Stopped at Greenock, to put off 175 passengers by tender, 'The Maid of Ashton' (!!). Admired the beauty of the Scots mountains, the Clyde, Dunoon, Holy Loch and Rothesay. Today, the stewards and waiters became particularly obsequious; £5.0s.0d. to the Restaurant Supervisor, 7 dollars (£2.9s.0d.) to the table waiter, and £2.0s.0d. to the cabin steward. Passed very close to Elsa Craig in the Firth of Clyde this afternoon. Thereafter, rubbishy passport formalities, with superfluous officials engaged in much stamping and tearing of pieces of paper.

June 1   Awoke at 3.0 a.m., and went on deck: the ship had dropped anchor and was waiting for the tide. Docked at Liverpool at 6.0 a.m.; 2/6d porterage to customs, a relief after the American cut-purses. Rail tickets to Manchester, 2 x 11/-. Home, to open many letters; flowers from Dr. F. ever thoughtful. Also a phone call from Miss James; she gives me the shocking news of the death of Dr. O. ten days ago [*the Manchester Royal Infirmary pathologist who had been helping to treat him*], confirmed by immediate phone call. Eichmann, the most evil of men, hanged last night, unrepentant.

June 2 [*Saturday*]   Rose at 10 a.m. Letter of condolence to Mrs. O. Began to read accumulated Sunday papers, beginning with *Observer* profile of Macmillan (29.4.62); 'Who Killed Webern?'; and other interesting matter. Golda S. [*friend*] for lunch; siesta. David appeared this evening. Lengthy conversation. He intends to marry Hazel after all. One could sympathise, but M. felt it acutely. He left after a few hours. I tried to dissuade him, but he appears to have made up his mind.

June 3   Phoned Dr. F. He tells me that Mr. C. [*consultant surgeon*] has been up to his old tricks again. In my absence he discharged one of my private patients, and put one of his in the vacant bed without consultation with the Registrar; an unethical fellow.

June 4   Air France Boeing 707 crash, at Orly Airport,

soon after take-off; 131 dead (American). A charter flight, probably overloaded. Two air hostesses were thrown clear. Copy of the *Daily Review* [*see May 15*] received from Harry W. in Virginia. To Bank to remove Will, and instruct solicitors. Credit balance, £737. To hospital: transferred one of Mr. C.'s private patients into General Ward, and did Ward round, 15. St. John St., 4 cases.

3:0 p.m. [*Female, aged 50, school-cleaner, Salford*] Sixteen weeks ago, she tripped over some broken flagstones in Salford and severely lacerated her right wrist. In addition her denture fell out and was fractured ('right across the middle of it'). One tooth was also 'knocked out' of the bottom set. First aid was applied in an adjoining warehouse, where she was taken by passers-by; from there she went by taxi to hospital, where ten stitches were inserted in her wrist. She has not worked since, because her 'nerves' are 'bad'; she said she 'hoped to go in tomorrow, on trial'. Her hands, she explained, 'are in water' (i.e. at work), and though she wears gloves 'they are a nuisance for wringing cloths'. She was a healthy looking woman, whose pulse was regular and blood pressure normal (140/80). There was a vertical scar, ½" long, on the front of her right wrist and a smaller one – a little less than ½" long – radiating therefrom in an inward direction. I found a slight limitation of flexion of the right little finger into the palm, the right-hand grip was slightly weaker than the left, but flexion of the wrist-joint was normal. Her disability is minimal; nevertheless she had a fortunate escape, since a laceration in that region of the wrist could easily have involved one of the main nerves, and caused some muscular palsy in the hand. She looked younger than her years, and was accompanied by her married daughter.

Watched 'Panorama': the Dalai Lama interviewed by Ludovic Kennedy. Much exhausting book-keeping tonight, and irritability of temper.

June 5 David's wedding-day. [*The marriage actually took place three months later*]. Disinherited, in accordance with yesterday's instructions. To Mrs. K., p.v., ring reintroduced, £1.0.0. To Anti-coagulant clinic: my Prothrombin time 19 seconds, 36%. Talked to Mr. C. about transfer of his patient yesterday. St. John St., 3 cases.

4:15 p.m. [*Female, aged 57, housewife, Salford*] She was a worried-looking woman, whose body was thin and emaciated. She had a malar flush [*flushed cheeks*] and the characteristic features of cardiac disease; she had rheumatic fever in adolescence, and suffers from mitral stenosis [*valvular disease of the heart*] of some severity. There was a marked presystolic and late diastolic murmur at the apex, followed by a low first sound. Her blood pressure was 130/80. She has no children. When she weighed herself on my scales, she said 'I have lost seven pounds'. What struck me was her intense depression, and her sickly appearance. She said that she felt 'very tired'.

Home early to comfort M., who is inconsolable. The moral of today's event is that we must not spoil our children and give them too much. For they take all, and give nothing in return. Walk with M., and thereafter watched football match, Italy v Chile; disgraceful behaviour by Italy, fist-fights etc. Italy 0, Chile 2.

June 6   To Arnfields. Thereafter, to Mrs. Faulkner [*secretary*]; gave her American gift and told her about David. She wept.

June 7   To domiciliaries: rigors [*violent attacks of shivering*], malaria(?), brucellosis(?) (aet 46, Ashton, for investigations); senility (aet 80, Denton, admitted). Deposited cheques at bank, £59. 14s. 0d. Ward round, 12. Afterwards, walked with Dr. F. round the hospital grounds. To St. John St., 3 cases, including bronchogenic carcinoma(?).

3:30 p.m. [*Male, aged 26, single, bricklayer*] He was a healthy young man of good physique, whose hobby is riding a motorcycle. Six months ago, in a storm of sleet, he ran into the back of an unlit, stationary lorry. He fractured his nose, broke a molar in his lower left jaw, and lacerated his lip, the bridge of his nose and his forehead. He had 12 stitches in the facial lacerations, his nose was straightened under anaesthesia, and since the molar tooth was cutting his tongue at the back of his jaw, it was extracted. He said today that he feels fit, but his facial scars were somewhat jagged, thickened and conspicuous; one of them extended obliquely from the right nostril to the margin of the upper lip, and another, 1″ long, was vertically disposed across his forehead.

R.G. [*acquaintance*] called, with his wife and son, aet 5. He took up much time showing me his drawings and poetry etc. Home at 6.15 p.m. Aidan Crawley gets in as Conservative in West Derby by-election, majority only 1,200; Liberals second. Also, report on stolen Goya published; inadequate safeguards. Watched Fyffe Robertson at Fingal's Cave, Staffa; and, thereafter, for a walk with M. down Ford Bank, to the river. It was a fine evening. Met a sub-leader of the Hallé, out walking with a woman not his wife.

June 8   Fruit purchased, 10/-. Follow-up clinic, heavy-going. To Shaw's [*solicitors*], to collect new Will. Thereafter, Medical out-patients; very large crowd. Home at 6.0 p.m. To the Fays [*neighbours*]; my new Will witnessed by them.

June 9 [*Saturday*]   M. telephones David telling him not to bring Hazel tomorrow. Bright sunshine for Whit-holiday. To Judy, 10/-. Ward rounds, 14 and 15. To Opera House, 8 p.m.: 'Irma La Douce', with Mary Preston, mildly entertaining. Streets deserted, because of Whit Holiday.

June 10   Quiet day. The D.'s [*friends*] wanted us to call. Mrs. D., a neurotic, has gallstones, so did not go, to avoid kerbside consultation. Instead, to the Harrises for supper, and home by 11 p.m., approximately. Pleasant evening.

June 11   Ward round, 14; and to see Mr. G. [*private patient*] in Ward 15; improving, but BP going up. My BP (160/90) taken by Dr. F., a good fellow, very loyal. After lunch, 3/6d, called at Dr. J.'s. He and his wife asked about David in a searching sort of way, I thought. Home early.

Watched Nureyev and Margot Fonteyn in *Giselle*. Thereafter, to the Josephs [*friends*] for cigar and brandy = vaso-dilatation [*widening of the blood vessels*].

June 12   Ordered Bio-Bibliography of Florence Nightingale. Letter from bank trust-department, recommending Lloyds Bank rights issue. Purchased toothpaste and razor blades, 8/-. Thence to solicitors, and surrendered Will, with due alterations. Phoned Superintendent Registrar for Edgbaston district of Birmingham; informed that David cancelled the marriage last Tuesday [*June 5*], but is getting married tomorrow at 10 a.m. Great sorrow in my heart.

June 13   Arnfields; received 1961 payment, £750. Ward 15, round; saw Mrs. C. [*patient*] whose son, now aet 21, I once delivered. St. John St., 3 cases, including a very strong and active young plasterer, aged 22, some of whose teeth were knocked out in a street accident 5 months ago. He has had false teeth fitted to replace them. The GP who removed the stitches from his various lacerations, Dr. T., has since died, so he told me.

4:15 p.m. [*Male, aged 23, single, butcher*] He is a butcher, unmarried and 'not courting', who indicated that for 2 or 3 years he has had an erratic heart beat, with synchronous attacks, or paroxysms, of anxiety. He does not smoke or drink, eats well, and has a fresh complexion; 'I work hard, but I enjoy it', he told me. His pulse was regular, his blood pressure was normal, (he weighed 13 stone 6lbs), and his heart was sound. He said that he recently got up in the night and woke his mother to tell her that his heart was missing beats, and that he felt frightened and anxious. After this attack, and his conversation with his mother, he passed 'a lot of water'.

On examination, his response to effort was normal: after touching his toes 10 times his pulse rate only went up 90, which is quite a reasonable figure, and returned to 66 after 3 mins. It was when I began asking him about his hobbies that I got the first clue about the nature of his condition. He rears prize bantams – he said that he pays as much as £20 for a hen – and when he goes to work each morning he feels anxious about leaving his poultry. 'His poultry are his life', said his mother, who came with him; indeed, I gathered from our conversation that he has no girl-friends, never goes to dances, is not interested in TV, and essentially has no real intimates, apart from his mother and his bantams. Indeed, he registered some emotion whenever he mentioned the subject of bantams, said that they had recently been doing badly in competitions, and finally told me that when he is at work 'children throw stones at them', which presumably interferes with their development. When I suggested that his heart-beat could be regulated with a sedative, which would stop the paroxysms, he said somewhat sharply, 'You are giving me tablets for my heart, but I would rather fight it'. The diagnosis here must be that of an anxiety state, or cardiac neurosis, associated with an obsession with bantams; passing a large amount of urine, in the circumstances he described, is also consistent with histories obtained from obsessional people with anxiety neuroses. If he goes on this way, and ordinary sedatives do not help him, I told him and his mother that he will end up with a psychiatrist on his tail. A strange case, my dear Watson!

Gave the monster, Miss James, a lift to her friends. At 8 p.m. L.S. came from Chorley, for a long private consultation about his impotence. Walk with M. thereafter.

June 14   St. John St., 3 cases.

3:30 p.m. [*Male, aged 46, bus driver*] He was walking home shortly before midnight from the bus depot, where he had left his bus for the night, when a motor cyclist travelling at great speed towards him lost control at the bend in the road where he was walking, and crashed into a wall. The motor cycle, he said, then bounced across the pavement into a lamp-standard close by him – the lad on the motor cycle was knocked unconscious – but a mudguard of the cycle flew off into the air striking him across the back; he had 'run up some steps off the pavement' to avoid direct impact and had at that moment turned his back on the proceedings. He was able to walk home (a short distance away), though it took him '25 minutes' to do

so because of the pain in his back. He was thereafter off work
for seven weeks, for most of the time with his ribs strapped
up, and with 'terrific' pains in his stomach; they were 'like a
vice squeezing the wind out of me', he said, so that he had to
'fight' for his breath. He added that he had to 'climb on the
couch' because of the pain in his stomach; the only relief he
got was from peppermints. During these seven weeks, which
at one point he called a 'nervous breakdown', he also used to
have 'cold sweats and go grey in the face'. On examination, he
was of slenderish build, spectacled, and of good colour, with
a slight tremor of his outstretched hands and a normal blood
pressure. He was always a bit of a neurotic; I have known him
for years. He was once the rodent exterminator for the local
Town Hall, and I first met him in that capacity. I was not
much impressed today with his account of his symptoms, nor
with his claim to have continuing tenderness, one year after
being struck by the mudguard at the back of his right loin.
In fact, there was nothing wrong with him. His only ailment
was a compensation neurosis.

Miss James spilled ink over my desk and BP apparatus.
Alas, how I suffer from that nit-wit!

June 15   Restful day at home, no shave, no bath.
Conservatives suffer heavy defeat at West Lothian; Labour
in, with large majority, 11,000. The OAS have blown up a
large hospital in Algiers. Read *BMJ*, *Lancet*, *Guardian*, and
last week's *Observer*, etc.; including review of Samuel Butler's
Letters, Toynbee on a *Life of Braque* and Harold Nicolson on
Norman Douglas' *Old Calabria*.

June 16 [*Saturday*]   To St. John Street, for letters;
today, all of them medical adverts. A scandalous increase
in them of late. Proceeded to Colam; salmon and plaice, £2.
To the hospital, Ward 15. Flowers from P.M. room, 5/-. It
appears that my stethoscope was stolen either by Dr. X. or
by Dr. Y., both Indian house physicians. Proceeded to Woods
Hospital, for Ward Rounds. Toffees, 2/-. Home for lunch, and
siesta. To the Carlebachs [*friends*], for tea. There I saw some
German stamps, with the British crown on them, printed

in anticipation of the wartime occupation of Britain. Some hopes!

June 18   Phoned Registrar of Marriages, Birmingham; found that no fresh date has been fixed for the marriage. Mrs. P. [*private patient*] died during the night, at Woods Hospital; left ventricular failure. Arnfields, and Wards 14 and 15. My blood test: 20 seconds, 33%. St. John St., 3 cases, including woman, aet 26, who needed medical defence for shop-lifting. Canadian election today, Diefenbaker or Lester Pearson. Read *BMJ* on hypertension; also an obituary of Dr. E.R., but no mention of his lechery and gluttony.

June 19   Rose at 5.15 a.m. Went down for a snack, made myself a cup of tea, and read a well-written piece in last week's *Sunday Times* on Ibiza, by Laurie Lee. David does not write or make contact. St. John St., 3 cases.

3:45 p.m. [*Male, aged 60, labourer*] He had to stop work last November, (after 17 years as a labourer with the same firm since his demobilization, in 1945, from the Royal Navy), because of increasing shortness of breath and emphysema. He thinks 'the fog started it', but his bronchitis is of long standing, and until last Christmas, when he says that he stopped smoking, he had for years smoked 30 to 40 cigarettes a day, and drunk '6 pints a week'. He has also been attending the Chest Clinic, where his sputum was examined, but no TB found. Today, he said that he coughs 'mostly in the mornings', sleeps propped up with 2 large pillows, and that his dyspnoea is 'getting gradually worse'. He has very little sputum, like most of these cases. He was a man of slender build, with slight clubbing of his fingers, who wheezed on breathing. Chest examination showed all the features char-acteristic of chronic bronchitis with emphysema: prolonged expiration, wide sub-costal angle, adventitious sounds, and hyper-resonance. His blood pressure was normal, but his pulse was irregular due to extra-systoles. Two weeks ago, he resumed work with his firm: during the first week he 'sat down', but is 'dumping cartons of fat now'. He said that he likes work. 'I will keep going until I have to give up', he added. He still has some residual elasticity in his lungs, and is not totally disabled. But his condition is steadily progressive. Within the next three years, at most, he will not be able to continue.

Walked with M. this evening. Long discussion about David. Very tiresome problem.

June 20   M. could not resist telephoning David. She therefore did so, and got a dusty reply; she was crestfallen and hurt after the conversation. I told her not to grovel to him.

June 21   Longest Day today. Letter to trustee department, re taking up Lloyds share offer. Visited Dr. T.; he is getting ready for his departure from general practice. Not a bad fellow. To travel agency: preliminary enquiries re West Indies, long talk with bearded employee. St. John St., 2 cases; practice seems to be picking up a little. Intake of food much less today; BP reading, 165/95. Washed dishes after supper. For a short walk with M. and Judy, in the light rain; a pleasant smell of grass and leaves. Began to read *South Wind*, by Norman Douglas.

June 22   Medical out-patients hectic, including patient with recurrent laryngeal palsy. Dr. W. tells me of his troubles with his colleagues. Boeing 707 disaster at Guadeloupe, the second Air France Boeing this month, the fourth this year: 112 dead. Last year, 1,000 were killed in air crashes. Chinese concentration of troops opposite the off-shore islands of Quemoy and Matsu, and £126,000,000 loss on Railways, announced by Dr. Beeching. The Establishment is enjoying Ascot, while all this goes on. M. to bed early; long walk with Judy, who tells me about her examinations.

June 24 [*Sunday*]   Leisurely day, dressed at 6.0 p.m., no walks. Severe gales today, Midsummer Day, in some places; strong gusts on Tyneside. Many fires, also, in various parts of the country. Today, suffered from postural hypotension [*fall of blood pressure on standing*], with nausea. Took 1.5 mgm

Marcoumar and one Salupres; also 500 mgms of Tetracyclene, because of ulcer on my tongue. Am taking too many pills; must resist the tendency.

June 25 Destruction of sentimental documents of no interest to the children, 6 a.m. to 7.10 a.m.

June 26 Cold wind, rain and sleet. Anti-coagulant clinic, 34 patients: my test, 22 seconds. BP, 165/95; 10 mgm Guanethidine and 3 mgm Marcoumar taken. Ward round, 15. Thence, to domiciliary: viral influenza (aet 36, Ashton, consultation). Heard of the death of poor A., the income tax man. St. John St., no cases. Proceeded to Shaw's Bookshop. Purchased the Pickering Edition of Herbert's *Temple* (1857); *The Works of Dr. Sydenham*, 9th edition (1729), a nice clean copy, with cracked hinges, £2; Peter Shaw, a 'Physician at Scarborough', *A New Practice of Physic* (1735), £3.10s.od.; and *The Rationalist Annual*, with articles by J.B.S. Haldane, Maugham and Bertrand Russell. Thence, to Sherratt and Hughes, where I bought *The Letters of Oscar Wilde*, edited by Rupert Hart-Davis, £4.4s.od. The weather eased up in the evening. Discovered that *South Wind* has an autograph letter, by Douglas to Sir Lees Knowles, Bt., pasted in at the back of the volume. It is dated 1917, from Paris.

June 27 Letter from D.B. and Co [*solicitors*]: writ issued re my accident [*see Sept 11 1960*]. To hospital: my BP, 155/90, have diarrhoea from Guanethidine, but my onslaught on my hypertension is justified by results. Dr. F. tells me about Dr. X's misdemeanours with a nurse, who accuses him of the paternity of her pregnancy and is blackmailing him for money. After lunch, I spoke to Dr. X about the dangerous situation he finds himself in. St. John St., 2 cases. Dr. F. phoned this evening, to say that the Matron agrees that Dr. X is being blackmailed.

June 28 To Shaw's [*solicitors*]: will signed and witnessed, paid £5.5s.od. Thence to hospital, and brought Dr. X back to Shaw's. But, under cross-examination, and after I spoke to the Matron later, it became obvious that Dr. X. is the guilty party. St. John St., 3 cases. Much ado today about the Pilkington Report on TV, and its recommendations. The *Manchester Guardian* and *The Times* are in favour; most papers with vested interests in ITV shares are against it. Money is the main motive of the dissenters, as always.

[*The Report contained some severe criticisms of Independent Television, which was held to 'fall well short of what a good public service of broadcasting should be'. Its programmes were 'frequently lacking in real substance', and they 'tended to portray a world in which moral standards were either ignored or flouted'. There was also 'excessive violence'. The Committee recommended that the BBC should continue to be 'the main instrument of broadcasting in the United Kingdom' and awarded it a second television channel. The Chairman of ATV described the Pilkington Report as a 'sorry document', and declared that the 'lethargic standards' of the BBC had been raised by ITV's 'energetic competition'.*]

M. is desolated at the continued silence of her son, and my satisfaction at his disinheritance increases daily. As Geoffrey [*son-in-law*] says, his attitude is a mixture of *Times Literary Supplement* and undergraduate beatnik.

June 29   A lovely afternoon; visited Mottram Church and Churchyard with Dr. F., and saw the tomb of a boy, aet 15, whose body was snatched by 'Resurrectionists'. Thence, to Medical out-patients; talked at length to Dr. V. [*consultant physician*] who had an enlightened attitude about Dr. X., and placed much of the blame on him. Churchill brought to England from Monte-Carlo, after fracturing the neck of his femur. Watched rare film, made by a personal secretary, of the Dalai Lama undergoing his religious trial, before his installation in Lhasa.

June 30 [*Saturday*]   Reading my diary for 1935. *May 31st, 1935*: 'Pay-day at Lewisham Hospital, £33.3s.0d. received for the month. Returned £5 loan from Brown [*medical colleague*], and gave Mother £10.10s.0d. Applied for post as Medical Registrar at Southend General Hospital [*a post he obtained*]. Saw 'Reckless', with Franchot Tone, Wm. Powell and Jean Harlow, at the Empire, Leicester Square, accompanied by

Rita McMahon'. *June 1st, 1935* [*Saturday*]: 'Bad earthquake in Quetta, India. Saunders under the influence. Chatted to Reuvid till 2.0 a.m. Did Night-round for 3 other doctors, in addition to my own'. *June 2nd, 1935*: 'Weather frightful, rain and wind. Took Mother to Bow, to visit her obese friend, Esther'. *June 3rd, 1935*: 'Purchased blazer, light hat and sandals for £2.2s.0d. at Davis's'. *June 4th, 1935*: '"The Normandie" wins the Blue Riband of the Atlantic'. *June 5th, 1935*: 'Derby Day today, weather atrocious. Bought 50 State Express (Astorias), 4/-. Bathing costume, 15/-. Went out drinking with Brown at the "Swan and Mitre", Bromley.'

Urgent call at 8.45 p.m.: cerebral haemorrhage, (aet 55, Audenshaw, admitted). Thereafter, to hospital until 10.45 p.m., Mrs. K. *in extremis*.

July 1 Mrs. K. died this morning. Read articles in the *Observer* on 'Fascism in England', and editorial on the Pilkington Report. To wedding luncheon at The Midland: Mrs. Horwich [*friend*] with extraordinary hat.

July 3 In Ward 14, unpleasant patient reprimanded. Also noted Dr. F.'s bad habit of coughing in one's face. St. John St., 4 cases. Continued to read in my 1935 Diary from May 8th. The earlier part unfortunately destroyed [*see Sept 4, 1960*]. *May 10th, 1935*: 'My Mother's 52nd Birthday'. *May 12th, 1935*: 'Visited the tombs of my father and grandmother [*in Edmonton cemetery*], and offered up a Prayer'. The same evening I visited the abode of Rita McMahon. *May 15th, 1935*: 'To the Dinner of the Socialist Medical Association at the Cafe Royal, with Miss O'Brien [*Matron of the Grove Hospital*]. Met Mr. and Mrs. Somerville Hastings, Lord Kinnoul, Edith Summerskill, Ellen Wilkinson and Major Clement Attlee.' *May 20th, 1935*: 'Saw film of "Les Miserables" with Mother, at the Tivoli: Sir Cedric Hardwicke, Fdk. March and Chas. Laughton'. *May 21st, 1935*: 'Phil P. [*student contemporary*] bought a Renault car for £150. Purchased a cruise ticket for myself on the "Doric" for £18 (Deck A, Cabin 18), to depart on June 15th'. These events are likely to be forgotten, if the Diary is destroyed.

July 4   Rose at 2.15 a.m., and sat in my room reading the entries in my 1935 Diary. The names which appear frequently are Phil P., Rita McMahon, Brownlee and Dr. Saunders, Ambrose and his orchestra, my Mother, Marion Hutt, Eunice Jones, Beatrice and Esme, Brownlee's future wife. *May 6th, 1935*: 'King George Vth's Silver Jubilee. Wonderful weather. Amazing Jubilee scenes in the Mall, Trafalgar Square and Piccadilly Circus. Buckingham Palace floodlit. The King spoke at 8.0 p.m. Much C_2H_5OH consumed by all and sundry'. Further extracts are to be written up in this Journal, until 1935 Diary is destroyed.

To Arnfields, and Ward Rounds. My mac has disappeared. Lunch at Masonic Temple, with Professor D.; he told me of the love-affair of A.S. [*former Matron of a hospital in Nigeria*] with a Syrian, and her loss of £1,000 which she loaned him. St. John St., 5 cases, including L.S. [*see June 13*], who said that the treatment [*for his impotence*] had been successful; paid £5. Gave Miss James £2, for her holidays; her gratitude was inaudible.

July 5   Refused invitation from solicitors to submit independent report on negligence alleged against two doctors and a chemist. Ward rounds, 14 and 15; Ward 7 filling up. Mac lost, or stolen from car. St. John Street, 2 cases. Maurice G. called this evening; opened and sampled 1924 brandy. Beautiful stuff. Watched film on Algeria, interrupted by phone-call from Dr. F. telling me that a provisional diagnosis of 'acute rheumatism' (aet 28, Audenshaw) is an acute leukaemia.

July 6   Weather cold and bad. 8.45 a.m., domiciliary visit: cerebral thrombosis (aet 78, M/c 20, admitted). Did Anti-coagulant clinic, and thereafter spoke to P. [*hospital administrator*]. Parkinson's Law is in operation throughout the Health Service. From 2.30 p.m., heavy Medical out-patients, with increasingly exacting patients, tiresome to a degree. A largeish waiting list has also developed; to attend on Friday mornings, until it is clear. Civil War in Algeria; Morocco sends in troops too. Chichester, the 'lone yachtsman', arrives in New York. A masterly achievement.

July 7 [*Saturday*]   Bank credit balance, £1,282. To Woods Hospital, to see 3 patients. Home for lunch, and siesta. Watched Wimbledon women's finals: Mrs. Susman the winner. An Alitalia DC8 has crashed outside Bombay; 94 dead. Heavy cold. Took Piriton, 1 tab; Veganin, 1 tab.; 10 mgm Guanethidine; 2.5 mgm Pempidine; 3 mgm Marcoumar; 1 large Brandy and 1 Havana Cigar. Albert J. [*friend*] has had a coronary; his condition fair only.

July 9   Heavy cold continues. Ward Round, 12; too many patients who need not be there. Watched very interesting 'Panorama': the New Friendship between De Gaulle and Adenauer; the poor craftsmanship in house-building in Britain; explosion of Rainbow Bomb in the Pacific and the disruption of Radio Communications; discussion between Canon Collins and an acidly hostile Labourite on Collins' attitude to unilateral disarmament.

July 10   To bed at 6.30 p.m., with continuing heavy cold. Got up at 9.35 p.m. to see first transatlantic TV picture direct from Andover, Maine, by rebound from satellite. Richard Dimbleby gave description of proceedings, but anticipated picture did not materialize. Went to bed to read my 1935 Diary. *May 24, 1935*: 'To Royal Society of Medicine, to see demonstration of case of gallstones in a girl of 8. Listened to Harry Roy and his band in my room at Lewisham Hospital, with Brownlee'. *May 25, 1935*: 'Listened to George Robey on the wireless, and Mattheson Long in 'Mr. Wu'. Saunders in my room, depressed'. *May 26, 1935* [*Sunday*]: 'Visited Mother, and then went for a walk on Box Hill with Phil P.' *May 27, 1935*: 'Introduced to a Mr. Fishman, in order to meet his daughter, with a view. Afterwards heavy alcoholic session with Brownlee'.

July 11   St. John St., 4 cases.

4:15 p.m. [*Male, aged 40, licensee*] He was a thick-set, large man who weighed 15st.7lbs, and whose pulse and blood pressure (130/80) were normal. He said that he could not lift barrels or crates of beer, was 'getting worse', and had pain over the upper part of his right buttock. In addition, when he crosses his right leg over his left, he gets pain in the back; 'I notice the pain', he stated. Yet he was able to stoop fully, rotate laterally, his reflexes were all normal, and there was no muscular wasting. His doctor has got him a surgical corset, but he was not wearing it. Because of this alleged pain in his right buttock, he has an extra Barman in, three or four times a week, to help him; when Barmen are not available he 'brings up' the bottles 'separately, or in baskets'.

If he had what he claims – a severe strain in the sacro-iliac region, which has 'weakened the muscles' – he would have presented with more physical signs, and would have been unable to stoop with such facility. All X-Rays have been negative. Moreover, he said he was worse yet he was not wearing his surgical corset. (When I asked him why not, he said he had come in his car to see me and could not wear it while he was driving.) I could find nothing at all the matter with him.

Sent a copy of Herbert's *The Temple* (1857 edition) to Robert S. [*recently met*] in Washington; the binding is somewhat Gothic. [*In his accompanying letter he wrote: 'I shall send you some further information about George Herbert so that you may know what kind of man he was. But if you look up page 158 of the book I am forwarding to you, and read poem 121, you will see a sympathetic and kindly attitude towards the Jews'.*] Visited Albert J. [*see July 7*] at Manchester Royal Infirmary after supper. He is in the same bed as I was. I found him very groggy, with a poor pulse and in a dangerous condition. Later, the Goldings [*friends*] came and stayed much too long. To bed exhausted.

July 13   To Mrs. Faulkner [*secretary*] for stationery: kept in a sorry mess, dirtied by carbon papers. Did follow-up clinic; my BP, 160/100, 10 mgm Guanethidine taken. Domiciliary visit: dermato-myositis(?) [*a virus-related disorder affecting the skin and muscles*] (aet 66, Tintwistle, admitted). Thereafter, Medical out-patients. Large Cabinet Re-shuffle announced. Seven cabinet ministers sacked, including Selwyn

Lloyd, Lord Kilmuir, Charles Hill, Sir David Eccles etc.

July 15 [*Sunday*]   Reading my 1935 Diary. Twenty-seven years ago today, I met M. at 2.10 p.m. in Oman Avenue and took her to Whipsnade Zoo. [*They had met for the first time two weeks earlier on June 30th, 1935.*] It was a pleasant run, the day was very warm, and we had tea together in a cool lounge at the Zoo. I took her Belgian address, and returned to Lewisham at 10.30 p.m.

Phone-call from Dr. F., re Friday's domiciliary in Tintwistle [*see July 13*]. She has dullness in her left upper lobe, a growth; blood urea, 400 mgms%. To three small boys, for cleaning M.'s car, 3/6d. Miss Lambert [*Arnfields secretary*] to tea; gave her a book about Byron. Mrs. J. telephones for kerbside consultation about Albert; some friends are very good at this, but in an emergency will often send for other doctors.

July 16   Letter to Brentano's, New York, offering them my Sussex Edition of Kipling. Domiciliary, at 9.30 a.m.: respiratory infection, with congestive heart failure (aet 74, Hr. Openshaw, admitted; transferred to private patients' Ward 15 after admission). Ward Rounds, 7, 12, 15. St. John Street, 3 cases.

3:45 p.m. [*Female, aged 55, widow*] Her husband was killed in a road accident on Christmas night 1960. After his death her health rapidly deteriorated – she has had bronchitis for many years – with worsening breathlessness, even without exertion; she would 'get up in the night panting for breath'. Four months ago, she developed a weakness on the left side of her face after a slight stroke. Today, her blood pressure was still very high, 240/120 sitting, and 190/115 standing. She is thick-set, not keeping to a diet, her speech was slurred, her heart was enlarged, and she said she 'stammers and goes dizzy'. There was an advanced degree of changes in her optical discs, compatible with serious high blood pressure. Nevertheless, nearly every few months a new and better drug becomes available for the treatment of hypertension; rapid progress is being made. Within a year or so greater strides will be made, and the longevity of hypertensives further extended. She has been taking Guanethidine, but I shall have to reorganize her treatment in the follow-up clinic, since her blood pressure is rising again, and try her with Methyldopa. At the moment, her expectation of life is only five or six years, at the maximum. But her life could also end suddenly tomorrow, with a further cerebral haemorrhage.

July 18　Heavy rain today. Foul weather for July. Received *Revue d'Histoire de la Médecine Hébraique*, from Paris. Domiciliary visit with Dr. J.: congestive heart failure (aet 54, M/c 18, admitted). Invited Dr. and Mrs. J. to dinner on Saturday at The Midland. Ward rounds, 14 and 15; a boy of 15 with leukaemia died last night. My BP 165/95; am taking 20 mgm of Guanethidine daily now. St. John St., 4 cases, including L.S. [*see June 13 1962*], further injection given, paid £5. Passed serious accident on way home: a Rank Flour lorry and a motor-cyclist, aet 17, killed. Watched entertaining ITV programme on Women, with Anna Quayle, Malcolm Muggeridge, Kingsley Amis and Bernard Levin.

July 19　Medical examination of 10 cadet nurses, 3 from Uganda, and Ward Rounds, 7 and 12. To Manchester, at 12 noon: presented with new mac by the E.'s, [*private patients*], 'Gents Special length 42, with S.B., Fly-Front', fits well. Lunch at Masonic Temple. St. John St., 3 cases.

3:30 p.m. [*Female, aged 47, nurse*] Four months ago, she was knocked down by a light van as she was crossing the road, was rendered unconscious – she kept 'going off and coming to' in Casualty – and sustained various bruises and lacerations, but no fractures. She rested in hospital for 6 hours, and was offered admission, but refused, since she has three small children whom she had to go home and look after; she is separated from her husband, who is a chronic alcoholic. (She said that he had been violent with her once, and split her lip, but otherwise her life had been a 'very happy' one.) She was off work for 10 weeks, during which time a bald patch developed on her scalp, at the site of the laceration. She is an intelligent woman of good type, who said she was 'not quite as well' as she was before the accident, and feels 'very tired'. Her reflexes were brisk, because of her nervous state, and her blood pressure (170/100) was slightly raised. She works very hard at the hospital, including on night duty, has domestic anxieties, and must make special arrangements for the children. She has no leisure at all. She could do with a good holiday and a rest. The hair over the bald patch will grow again, in due course.

Home to read my diary for 1935, as follows (excerpts). *June 8th, 1935*: 'Listened to Grace Moore as Mimi in Act III of "La Bohème", relayed on the radio from Covent Garden'. *June 9th, 1935* [*Sunday*]: 'Disturbed 3 times during the night with piffling casualties. Outing with Phil P. Travelled in his Renault, with Marion and Rita, to Slough, Maidenhead and Henley. Rowing boat at Henley, and tea at the Angel Hotel. Invited to a Garden Party by his parents, on June 30th' (where I met M.) *June 10th, 1935*: 'Permission to go to Southend for interview. Will take Mother with me. "Chance makes relations, but choice makes friends" ' (Delille). *June 11th, 1935*: 'Phoned Mother, to tell her that I was taking her to Southend tomorrow, and for a trip to Hayling Island.'

No letters, no cards, or communications from David.

July 21 [*Saturday*]   Woke up at 2.30 a.m. to read, worried about my blood urea of 57 mgm. Nocturia twice. Took Methyldopa, 250 mgm. Later, to St. John St. for letters, and called on C.B. [*patient who had radio and TV shop*] in Clayton, to order new Murphy TV set of modern design. Flowers from post-mortem room, 2/6d. Home for lunch; took another Methyldopa, 250 mgm, and siesta. Methyldopa acts as a soporific. No Guanethidine today. To bed, and read about medicine at the Court of Louis XIV; Madam de Montespan had seven bastard sons of the King. [*The more common version is that she had four illegitimate children, two sons and two daughters.*]

July 22   Repercussions of Cabinet sackings in today's papers. Feel better with Methyldopa, but hospital pathological reports are so unreliable that progress can only be estimated. Note frequent errors in spelling of late, my memory not as good as it used to be. I cannot remember names, places, or recent events = cerebral vascular changes. Serious fighting this afternoon with Mosley's gangsters in Trafalgar Square; a large crowd of 8,000 people, 300 police, 50 arrests. Psychopaths, preaching hatred to the neurotically unstable masses, should be taken into custody and given ECT [*electro-convulsion therapy*] to rehabilitate them.

July 23   Saw 18-minute direct TV transmission from America to Europe: baseball match in Chicago, President Kennedy's 3.0 p.m. Press Conference, South Dakota National Park, New York Skyline, San Francisco and Quebec. Tinnitus in right ear at midnight.

July 24   Anti-coagulant clinic, 10.30 a.m., muddle and confusion, and Ward round, 12. Mrs. E. [*private patient*], in Ward 15, suffering from Senile Dementia. St. John St., 3 cases. Thinking of taking it easy tonight, but the Goodmans [*friends*] called at 9.0 p.m; I walked them home at 11. Feel much better on Methyldopa; my nocturia has diminished. No one will read this diary anyway. Purely kept for self-edification and interest, and essentially a mental exercise.

July 28 [*Saturday*]   Ted Heath, dealing with Common Market, gets into difficulties over Commonwealth Trade Preferences. 125 miles of motor-car traffic, nose to tail, from Gloucester to Exeter; the people are enjoying themselves. My nocturia still present, but urgency diminished, possibly due to water retention. Note Methyldopa causes increase in weight. Also, some haemoptysis [*blood spitting*] this morning. Letter from David, but am partially indifferent to his verbiage. Dinner at The Midland, 9 p.m., £6.6s.0d., and 10/- tip. M.'s desire to be constantly going out irritates me, in my state of indifferent health.

July 29   Up at 5 a.m. Back to bed at 6.20 a.m. and wakened at 10.15 by Miss James, phoning about U.T. [*see Feb 21 1962*]. I had intended to stay in bed today, but went out to Dukinfield to see her, after hearing a magnificent sermon from a Bolton church, on morning TV, by Rev. Glyn Jones. Wrote to congratulate him. Got U.T. admitted to an amenity bed. Visited Wards 11 and 12. My BP, 160/90. To St. John St., to collect letters; gave Miss James a lift to an address in Nelson Street, where she had to feed a cat. Home at 1 p.m. Have increased my dose of Methyldopa to 250 mgm, 4 times a day. Makes me very sleepy, but BP must be kept down. Fighting in Manchester this afternoon, at a Mosley Fascist meeting. Why is Racial Incitement not banned by law?

July 30   News from hospital, that poor U.T. died at 8.20 p.m. 'Panorama' direct from USA by Telstar; amazingly clear pictures of 5th Avenue, N.Y. and the Rockefeller Center, with Richard Dimbleby and James Mossman in a Drug-Store.

July 31   Anti-coagulant clinic, very busy indeed; much help rendered by Dr. B. My Prothrombin time 25 seconds, 26% activity; my blood urea 54 mgm %, alarming reading! Made appointment to see Dr. W.F. [*his heart physician*] on August 9th.

Aug 1   Received account from my solicitors, a dishonest charge. St. John St., 1 case; another life insurance case. Some of these insurance companies try to sweat consultants for small fees; unfortunately, there are so many doctors willing to submit. Home early. Watched TV, on 'How to Meet Death'. The question was not really answered, although many customary points, all gone over before, were raised about Euthanasia, life hereafter etc. B.A. [*friend*] died suddenly in hospital yesterday, during convalescence from a coronary thrombosis which he had three weeks ago. I have had no anti-coagulants for 4 days now; my BP rising without hypotensive drugs.

Aug 3   Cloudy and overcast. Received *Reader's Digest*, first subscription issue; my resistance was worn down by repeated importuning.

Aug 4 [*Saturday*]   Bad weather, cold and cloudy. A

restful day, did not dress. Read *BMJ*, *Lancet*, *Guardian*, and began *The Blue Nile* by Alan Moorhead. Note anti-semitism in the Argentine; well-established in Germany, Egypt, Russia, and Arab States, and rearing its head in England. It is fairly universally distributed, despite the murder of 6 million in the recent war. M. and Judy have gone to the Palace Theatre, to hear Adam Faith singing his rubbishy songs.

In their absence, I read 80 delightful pages of *The Blue Nile*, and thereafter my 1935 Diary. The house was peaceful, while I was reading.

Aug 5   Jamaica gains her Independence, after 300 years of Colonial Rule. But there is not a building in the whole of Jamaica worthy of note, or of historical interest; it was much exploited by Britain in the slave-days. Princess Margaret, a poor hardworking girl, represented the Queen at the celebrations. Death of Marylin, or Marilyn, Monroe announced; found dead in bedroom, with door bolted on the inside and many sleeping tablets (barbiturates) lying about. Very sad at the news. Thereafter, George N. [*friend*] came to tea with his wife, a horrible woman. After a gluttonous tea and no thanks for it, she rammed herself into her car, without saying 'goodbye', or 'come and see us sometime'; a beast. Never again.

Aug 6 [*Bank Holiday*]   No letters today, coldest and wettest bank holiday this century: rain, cloud, gloom and depression. Ward round, 12, in full; wards 14 and 15 visited too. Home by 3.0 p.m. All the newspapers are full of Marilyn Monroe's death. The *Guardian* had the best articles on it, by W.J. Weatherby and Alistair Cooke. Common Market talks break down over commonwealth agricultural exports; France proving difficult. National Socialist rally in Norfolk: Nazi thugs. I have a low opinion of human nature, which is easily roused to prejudice and hatred. More Russian atom tests in the atmosphere. On 'Panorama', some parts of Marilyn Monroe's films were shown, and Dame Sybil Thorndike said a few words about her. Also Edward Heath interview on the Common Market, James Mossman report on Jamaican Independence, the Archbishop of Canterbury on his Moscow visit, and debate on Free Speech between Ronald Bell M.P. and Tom Driberg. The former is a nasty piece of work, Conservative of course, who is in favour of Fascists.

Aug 7   Heavy downpours, rain incessant, and cold as a November day; the worst August for 60 years. Most of my letters macerated by the rain; visited GPO (local branch), to complain. To Boots, Droylsden; assistant refuses to give discount, but I stood firm and she had to do so, 7/7d. Home by 6 p.m., and to bed early. My health is not all that could be desired.

Aug 8   Request from *The Times* to subscribe to the *Times Literary Supplement*: will consider it. St. John St., 2 cases, including M.J., who when I asked him for a urine sample asked me if I wanted him to defaecate as well!!

Aug 9   Special interim dividend from Leyland Motors Ltd., £3.16s.7d. To Manchester Royal Infirmary to see Dr. W.F. for consultation. Prothrombin time, $20\frac{1}{2}$ seconds = 30%; blood urea, 43 mgm; BP 190/110. An ECG done, and screening. He advised me to stick to H-Chlorothiazide K. (Esidrex), one daily, and take no hypotensives for 3 weeks. I am somewhat reluctant to abandon my own therapy, with BP of moderate severity; however, I will try. He states my heart is not enlarged, on screening, and ECG much improved. Gave him 18th century oblong quarto with navigational maps of Mediterranean Ports, fine copy, c.1727–1730.

Aug 11 [*Saturday*]   Restful day in bed; M. also has a day off in bed. Russia sends up Vostok 3, with space man Nikolaev in orbit; to stay up a long time. David arrived this evening, complete with beard. Read a play he has written; great ability demonstrated, obviously self-revealing. His approach to us much more filial.

Aug 12   Taking things easy. There is no point in self-destruction for the Manchester Regional Hospital Board, which is indifferent to my effort.

Aug 13   Beginning of Wakes holiday; most people absent at Arnfields. St. John St., 4 cases, and home by 6 p.m. Two Russian astronauts are circling round the Earth in the same circuit, separated from each other by only 72 miles.

Aug 14   St. John St., 3 cases, including a woman who is back from Montreal after two years' emigration. She states that she 'did not like it'.

Aug 15   Southern Rhodesia stock to be sold, in exchange for Charringtons United Breweries Ltd., at 14/6d. 3 gallons of petrol in Reddish; suspected attendant of cheating ½ gallon. St. John St., no cases. This evening, briefly visited Albert J., who is pretty groggy [*see July 7 1962*]. His coronary has shaken his self-confidence, and given him an anxiety state about the curtailment of his money-making. Watched CBS TV programme, 'Eisenhower on the Presidency'. He gave the impression of illiteracy; partisan without reason or calculation, golf-mad, indolent and stubborn, and mentally incapable of having held so high an office. He also exhibited a self-hypnotic approach to religion.

Aug 16   A pugnacious little squirt, Dr. H. of C., wakes me from my sleep after midnight, to bellyache about the admission of a lad who has run berserk; Dr. E. has refused, quite rightly, to admit him. To hospital, and talk with R. [*hospital catering officer*] about larceny and food thefts by staff; 3 sacked last week. Called at Bank, and purchased 100 Marks and Spencer A Shares, and 500 Charrington Breweries Ltd., cost may be in region of £800. Returned to hospital and saw Dr. H. of C. in Ward 15: an unpleasant and dangerous little fellow. Phoned Jack; he tells me that cousin Marie [*in Montmartre*] is dying of cancer, aged 59.

Aug 17   Ordered a new Morris 1100, delivery in 6 weeks. At Anti-coagulant clinic, saw slides of erythro-blastoma. Proceeded to Ward 4, to see Mrs G. [*private patient*]; elephantiasis of leg, amputated. Saw other patients of mine, including woman with avulsion of Brachial Plexus [*network of nerves at root of neck, torn away*]. She had necrotic trophic changes at her finger-tips; looking at them, it reminded me that I delivered her once. Yesterday's private patient extremely ill. Medical out-patients; Sister H., a bitch, would not let me use her office to talk to a patient's relatives. Absurd. Also saw Miss N., Dukinfield bank cashier, aet 32; neurosis, man required. Home early by 5.0 p.m., or thereabouts. Judy has gone to Spain with the Tweedles [*friends*]. We two alone for Dinner. Beethoven's Eroica Symphony on the Third Programme suddenly interrupted by a Pop-Singer; apologies, thereafter, for a 'technical hitch'.

Aug 18 [*Saturday*]   Awoke at 3.40 a.m. and read James Morris on Adelaide. He deplores Australia's allegiance to the Crown, and will probably receive abusive letters. Received a patronising letter from Brentano's, New York, about my Kipling set; will reply in equal measure.

Aug 19   Woke at 7.0 a.m., one hour's work, then made breakfast for M. Read in Sunday papers on Lord Harewood (his life story by one of his friends); comments on Soviet jubilation about their 'heavenly twins'; Indonesia's annexation of Dutch West New Guinea; *Observer* article by Colin Legum on Nkrumah. Will he leave the Commonwealth? (Tendencies that way). U2 aeroplanes arrive in England; rising tensions in Berlin about The Wall. Dr. F. phones, to say that Mr. G. [*private patient*] has died. To bed early, and read about Ezra Pound's obsession with usury.

Aug 20   Woke at 6.30 a.m., and arranged work for the day. Trip to Greek islands in October contemplated. Account sent re late U.T., 25 guineas. Domiciliary visit: congestive heart failure, oedema of legs (aet 70, Dukinfield). Ward round. Spoke to Matron, re visiting hours for patients. St. John St., 3 cases.

3:0 p.m. [*Female, aged 30, part-time cleaner*] She was a pleasant, obese young woman with a rapid pulse and a tremor of her outstretched hands. Whilst cleaning the inside of a window she lost her balance and fell backwards on to some stairs, striking her back and twisting her neck. She told me that she remained lying on the floor for half an hour after the fall, as there was no one about to help her; 'steam came off my body', she added. (I presume she meant she was sweating from the shock.) She eventually got up, went to see the lady next door — for whom she also worked — and then walked home. She told me today that her left leg drags when she walks: 'it has not bucked up at all', she said. On examination, I found some tenderness over the left sacro-iliac joint, but she was able to stoop fully; her difficulty was due more to her obesity than her injury. I found her general health sound, but she is exhausted by her three young children. She said that she 'snaps' at them and that when she stands at the sink, her knees 'buckle' under her; 'I cant wring my washing', she added.

'Tonight' programme has restarted at 6.50 p.m.: Alan Whicker in Alaska, man with tame owl, new book on Mao Tse-Tung by Hungarian, and Miss Sarah Miles (girl from Roedean) has achieved film fame.

Aug 21   Good night's sleep, without sedation. Anti-coagulant clinic, and domiciliary visit: congestive heart failure (aet 73, Ashton, admitted). Wards 12, 15. Lunch: new salad diet, no meat, no added salt, no yoghurt, no cheeses. No tablets of any kind today, no **BP** readings or clinical tests undertaken.

Aug 22   St. John St., 4 cases.

3:40 p.m. [*Male, aged 39, ex-lorry driver, see Oct 2 1961*] Since last October, apart from a few weeks' work as a bar-tender and 'steward' in a Conservative Club — from which he was sacked 'after a row with the president' — he has not worked since April, has been 'signing on' at the Labour Exchange, and has been awarded a 15 per cent disability allowance. (He said that his wife was 'keeping an eye open' to find a job for him as a porter, at the hospital where she works as a cleaner). I asked him what his day consisted of. He replied that he gets up at 8.0 a.m., makes the breakfast for the three children at school, 'cooks the meals and does the shopping', and goes to bed 'at about 11.30 p.m.' In addition, a month ago he had a 'terrible pain' in the back of his neck. On examination, his weight had risen another half a stone, his pulse was rapid (96), and his blood pressure was 190/110 (a considerable rise for his age); he had a soft systolic murmur at the apex, and a loud second sound over the aortic area. He attends his doctor only spasmodically, for treatment for his blood pressure – his last attendance was four months ago – and he has increased his intake of fluid. He is now drinking '6 to 8 pints on Saturdays and Sundays, and 4 pints on other days', and his smoking has increased to '20 to 30' cigarettes a day. His wife and two working children are bringing in their wages, so that he has no particular incentive to work; 'I do not think I will drive lorries again', he added. He strikes me as a layabout.

Attempted assassination of General de Gaulle, 4th attempt this year. Watched film of D-Day, June 6th, 1944, and tragic deaths of our soldiers; young lives wasted, because of one accursed man's hatreds and ambitions. A peaceful and quiet evening, reading. Complete change of diet for last 2 days.

Aug 23   Obscene telephone calls this morning; went to police station to ask for M.'s protection from bandits. In heavy rain to domiciliaries: cerebral thrombosis (aet 60, Denton, admitted), and haematemesis (aet 78, Denton, admitted). Ward 11, round. Mrs. L. [*private patient*] in Ward 11 has ascites, and undoubted metastases from carcinoma of the breast. St. John St., 2 cases; rain incessant. On getting home found David, with hair growing down and beard massive. Watched Armand Denis film on expedition to Nepal looking for the Yeti, and then out to dinner with the Livingstones for our anniversary [*see Aug 25*]; half share, £3.3s.0d. On return listened to Luigi Alva singing aria from Donizetti's *L'Elisir d'Amore*, and to bed thereafter.

Aug 24   Follow-up clinic, including Miss O., with fits. Ward 11, round. Met Sir Charles Lythgoe going round the hospital with D. and N. [*hospital administrators*]. Phoned M., and heard disturbing news about David: he had told her he was 'going out for a short time', and had not returned. After-noon clinic cancelled, and hurried back home at top speed; M. hysterical over David's absence. Phoned police and Maurice G. [*rabbi and friend*]. He came immediately and we went together to Hazel S.'s parents. It appears that David called there this morning, and has gone out with her. His conduct is that of a 'beatnik'; he returned at 7.30 p.m. To North Western Gas Board, £5.11s.10d. Much distress at David's intentions.

Aug 25 [*Saturday*]   Our 26th Wedding Anniversary; M. is tearful, and is not used to David's verbosity. I wish he would marry that woman and have done with it.

Aug 26   Heavy rain and wind. Read Brendan Behan in the *Observer* on his early days in Dublin, and another instalment on Lord Harewood and his marriage. Cuba 'shelled' from two boats manned by anti-Castro students, based in Florida. Holidays in Elba recommended. Interesting review by Raymond Mortimer of a new book on architecture by Jacobs, which recommends continuation and maintenance of old architectural styles, instead of today's box-like structures, etc. Afterwards felt depressed and tired, with sore throat. Must be checked up next week; have had no anti-coagulants, no hypotensive drugs, no sedatives, no diuretics. Took Ledermycin, 150 mgm (for sore throat). Maurice G. came. He has spoken to David and Hazel. He likes her; thinks she is clever and will make David happy. He recommends that we approve of her. We have no option.

Aug 27   Visited Ward 11; B.T. [*father of private patient*] disgruntled, and Mrs. L. a pain in the neck. On my rounds, caught sight of her son E., who had been visiting her; I delivered him 21 years ago. Gave Dr. F. red peppers. St. John St., 2 cases. A distinctly uncharitable attack on Sam Goldwyn by Alistair Cooke in today's *Guardian*, for his 80th birthday.

Aug 29   Domiciliary visit: congestive heart failure, auricular fibrillation (aet 62, Openshaw, admitted). Swab taken from my throat by Dr. F. Ward Round, 7; felt lousy and weak. St. John St., 4 cases including lead poisoning and L.S. for his injection, £3.0.0. On return home, felt very weak and could not concentrate. Read James Morris's tenth excellent article on Australia (Perth). Felt so bad had to go to bed. Heard David come back, at 1.0 a.m.

Aug 30   Up intermittently during the night taking Penicillin, Aspirin and sucking lozenges. My oral cavity always vulnerable. Stayed in bed till 12 noon. Long talk with David, who left for North Wales [*via marriage in Birmingham, on Sept 1*]. Lunch at home; Dr. F. and Sister G. telephoned to inquire about my health. St. John St., 3 cases; twelve cases this week. To bed early, but could not sleep because of throat pain.

Aug 31   To Anti-coagulant clinic; swab taken from throat for culture. My blood cholesterol 207 mgm%. Lunch, 3/6d; swallowing much better. Medical out-patients, and thence to domiciliary: cerebral thrombosis, auricular fibrillation (aet 58, Ashton, admitted). Feel better working.

Sept 1 [*Saturday*]   Received catalogue of Exhibition of Notable Books on Science and Medicine, from University Medical Librarian. The diagnosis of my oral lesion must be Erythema Multiforme, without cutaneous affection. Judy came back from Spain today looking well, and returned £10 in travellers' cheques. M. still depressed about David; she finds it hard to take. Read some letters of D. H. Lawrence.

Sept 2   Severe earthquake in Persia; area involved the size of Wales. At least 4,000 killed, and thousands injured. Fascist speeches in Ridley Road, with evil slogans. Article on Lord Harewood (part 3) concluded, and review of Harold Nicholson biography of Mrs. Browning. David telephoned this morning; 'We are going to Wales', he said. Spoke to Dr. F., and criticised him for not informing me more quickly about Mr. T.'s [*private patient*] blood urea of 90. To Judy, £1.0.0. = a total of £4.10s.0d. saved. (I act as custodian). Walk with M. after supper. Mounting death toll of Persian earthquake, and fighting between Fascist and anti-Fascist (Yellow Star) groups in the East End.

Sept 3   Visited Mrs. Faulkner [*secretary*]; she never offers a cup of tea. Phoned S.F. [*travel agent*], re visit to Greece in October. At hospital, saw Dr. H. [*ENT specialist*] about my throat; he said it was naught. Blood count done on me in Haematology [*Dept*]: hb.++, differential not very significant, 5,800 w.c.c. Ward rounds, 12, 14 and 15, outstanding problems dealt with satisfactorily, including lad of 19 with Crohn's disease [*inflammation of intestine*]. Saw Mrs. L. in Ward 11; the poor woman is garrulous, and has much ascites. To domiciliary visit: bilateral chest signs, loss of weight, icterus [*jaundice*] and clubbing of fingers (aet 46, Denton, admitted). St. John St., 3 cases. Quiet evening, reading.

Sept 4   Car ran out of petrol in Stockport; took bus to Reddish garage, 3d. Because of incompetent cleaning of carburettor, trouble and waste ensured for the rest of the day. Morris 1100 to be obtained on Friday [*Sept 7*]. To domiciliary: congestive heart failure *in extremis*, (aet 59, Droylsdon, admitted). In Ward 12, post-partum suicide attempt, lesbian.

3:0 p.m. [*Male, 41, electrical fitter*] He was on his way to work on a motor scooter at 7.15 a.m., and on the crest of a hill, when the door handle of an overtaking car, 'driven by a woman', caught his right elbow, lacerating it (7 stitches) and knocking him off the scooter. (He said he was 'brushed off' his vehicle). He also suffered abrasions to his face and forehead, and a fractured bone in his left hand. He had six weeks off work, for all this, four months ago. He was a thick-set man and pleasant, with no children, who told me that his left hand felt a 'little weak' and his right arm ached when he had to 'tighten up things with a screw-driver'; otherwise, he was 'feeling better all the time'. I tried his left hand grip and thought it was quite good; any residual weakness in it will eventually clear up. He said that after the accident he had had pains 'all over the body'. His pulse was regular, and his blood pressure normal (130/80).

Gave lino to Miss James [*receptionist*]. Magistrates release

Colin Jordan; it is impossible to eradicate his kind of hatred. Men are evil. To bed early.

*

Sept 5   Rose at 7.20 a.m.; nocturia twice. Made breakfast for M. Arranged night-flights to and from Greece, so as not to waste days. Ward 15 visited. St. John St., 2 cases, including a man who said he would 'get me seats at Glyndbourne'. At 5.0 p.m. to Dr. A.J., for medical examination re accident on Sept 11th 1960. He appeared to have a sympathetic approach to my problems.

*

Excerpt from Medical Report by Dr. A.J., on Dr. Hugh Selbourne, aged 56 years, Consulting Physician:

'Prior to the accident, he had a whole collection of illnesses. In 1941, he was found to have a duodenal ulcer and hiatus hernia, and could not enter the Forces. In 1953, he had angina of effort, which was said to have been caused or aggravated by overweight and overwork. Six months later, he had a frank coronary thrombosis, was in Hospital, and was off work for eight months. Since then, he has been taking various tablets for his heart condition. He tells me he was "on an even keel" at the time of the accident on Sept 11th 1960, when his car was "struck amidships", and sustained bruises to the forehead, left shoulder and right hip, and fractured the base of the end phalanx of his left middle finger. His blood pressure, which shortly before the accident was 180/110, rose to 210/120, his anginal pains increased in severity almost at once, and he was taking up to 15 tablets daily for several months. In December 1960, he developed a further coronary thrombosis, and at one time was desperately ill, although back at work in April. Since these various attacks he has cut down his activity considerably.

'On examination, he was alert, still considerably overweight, and very frank in recounting his disabilities. He was somewhat short of breath even at rest, and I did not feel justified in getting him to do any exertion. The heart sounds were tic-tac but regular, and he had an occasional moist sound at both lung bases. There was no oedema of ankles or sacrum. His blood pressure was 180/115, and his optic fundi were normal. There was no tremor or undue sweating. His pulse rate was 60. The urine contained no phosphates or albumen, though he said that it had done in the past. My opinion is that the physical injuries he sustained in the accident were not severe, and that the rise in blood pressure he reports was no more than may occur from time to time in any hypertensive. The further coronary thrombosis that followed the accident would in all probability have occurred without it. His general health is such that he will be wise to restrict his activities in future.'

*

Sept 6   David was married on September 1st, in a Birmingham Registry Office, to Hazel S.; all over bar the shouting. To St. John St., in heavy rain and thunderstorms; 4 cases.

3:0 p.m. [*Female, aged 16, case-maker*] She was a healthy-looking girl, but with facial acne, and was accompanied by a married sister. She was run into by a motor-scooter (nearly a year ago) while she was crossing the road with a friend. She had abrasions to the legs and knees, and was concussed; she said that after the accident she was 'laid down' on the pavement. She was detained in hospital for 5 days but no fractures were found, and she required no stitches. She was off work for 6 weeks thereafter, because she had 'bruised a muscle' in the back of her left leg; during this time she also 'broke it off' with her boyfriend. Today, she said that she got headaches 'once a week', which 'disappear' when she takes an Aspro, and that she 'keeps knocking' her legs at work. She has just come back from three weeks holiday in the Isle of Man. When I asked her what she had done there, she replied smilingly 'everything', at which her sister laughed. In addition to this, she had spent time 'sunbathing and doing the Twist'. 'It had me going', she added. There was damn all the matter with her.

Decided not to accept C.B.'s invitation to his Lodge meeting: nonsensical ceremonial, gourmandizing, and empty speechifying. Home at 6.30 p.m. Maurice G. called to discuss

David's prospects with Hazel. He was reassuring, and said he thought highly of her.

Sept 7   Purchased new Morris 1100, 4-door de luxe tartan red, heater, seat belts, road tax to Aug 63, total £747.15s.3d. New registration Number WJA 508. To Anti-coagulant clinic. Will go on low-protein, salt-free diet, with fruit juices, for next two weeks. Lunch, 3/6d. Medical out-patients; spoke to Cretan doctor, and told him we would visit Crete in mid-October and hope to visit his father. Eventful week: Judy returned from Spain, David married, serious earthquake in Persia.

Sept 8 [*Saturday*]   Weather cold and cloudy. Morning case at St. John St.: aet 59, Droylsden, with left hemiparesis, subdural haemorrhage possibly, to be investigated. Paid 6 guineas. Home by 11.30 a.m. in new Morris 1100. Siesta after lunch, and pleasant walk with M. Peaceful evening at home reading through my Diary for 1958. In May of that year, Dr. W. found my BP to be 180/120, and I went temporarily on a low calorie diet; in June, David took his Finals at Balliol, and Ruth [*daughter*] was busy with her suitors. We were also entertaining fairly frequently, with little reciprocity.

Sept 9   To Midland Hotel, for wedding reception; parking in railway station, 2/-. On return, read Somerset Maugham, 'The Judgment Seat', and Bertrand Russell, 'Are the World's Troubles Due to Decay of Faith?' [*Two essays in the Rationalist Annual; see June 26 1962*]. David telephoned; I am sad at heart about him.

Sept 10   Virulent attack on David and Hazel, in letter from Ruth and Geoffrey, caused me much distress. John Ogdon played Chopin Concerto at the Proms. My albumen less.

Sept 11   Appointments committee for new house phy-sician: Dr. L., MD (Peking), born in Hong Kong, appointed. Two domiciliary visits: broncho-pneumonia (aet 46, Ashton, admitted), and generalized carcinoma, carcinoma of pancreas (aet 64, Ashton, admitted). At St. John St., 3 cases, including a young woman of 20, who most unconcernedly raised the question of her sexual intercourse with her fiancé.

Sept 12   Domiciliary visits: abdominal pain (Mrs. N.Y., aet 17, Hyde, admitted); coronary or cholecystitis (aet 74, Stalybridge, ECG arranged, case for diagnosis). St. John Street, 2 cases, including Miss J.B., a charming person on oestrogens who had a castration operation twelve years ago at St. Thomas' and has good female development, though still somewhat masculinized. Not mixed up psychologically. Thereafter, to Walmsley's bookshop, and home.

Sept 13   Breakfasted at hospital. Full ward rounds, 12 and 15; finished by noon. To St. John St., one case, and thereafter Hazel and David visited me. Guarded optimism, and mixed impressions. Took them to the Kardomah for coffee, 5/-. David at home for supper. Listened to Haydn's Horn Concerto and saw film of recovery of amphorae from Roman wreck in 200 feet of water, off the coast of Sicily. I felt sad throughout the film at David's struggles, and will give him washing machine and savings certificates.

Sept 14   Geoffrey and Ruth have set sail for England. To hospital, where I saw E.E. [*patient and freemason*] in follow-up clinic. He told me that I would be promoted in Provincial Lodge this year; Warden(?). Ward rounds, interesting cases in medical out-patients, and domiciliary visit: coronary thrombosis (aet 73, Ashton, admitted). St. John St., no cases. In the evening visited Mr. T. [*private patient*], *in extremis.*

Sept 15 [*Saturday*]   Wet, cold and unsavoury weather. Made lunch for M., who remained in bed. Judy went to Old Trafford: Manchester United 2, Manchester City 3. Short walk in the evening, and so to bed. M. refuses to meet Hazel.

Sept 16   Very drowsy. Leader of the OAS attack on De Gaulle last month [*see Aug 22*] hangs himself in his prison cell. In Sunday papers read reviews of new biography of Harold Macmillan, Lord Boothby on Sir Thomas Beecham, and Rees-Mogg on the Commonwealth and the Common Market (pro-Common Market). Visited by T.'s son [*see Sept 14*]; a tiresome interview. He has a monotonous voice. Lunch burned, owing to his visit. M. phones Maurice G. who advises her not to meet Hazel as yet; letter to David cancelling Wednesday's [*Sept 18*] meeting between M. and Hazel.

Sept 17   Bad night, nocturia twice, awake for many hours. Fine sunny morning, but cold. Letter from Hazel thanking me for receiving her kindly at St. John St. Ward round 12, in full. Returned home to get my spectacles and thence to St. John St., 4 cases. Pleasant letter from Miss J.B. [*see Sept 12*], re my understanding of her condition and sex changes. David phones this evening. I told him that M. wont meet his wife, unless Hazel tries to adopt Judaism. I feel sorry for the lad, and will have lunch with them next week and give him some Savings Certificates.

Sept 18   Cold and bleak day, as usual. Anti-coagulant clinic, 62 patients. Returned nurses' examination papers, marked, to Deputy Matron; 6 failed out of 18. St. John St., 3 cases, including mitral disease with asthma. Home early, passing a wedding.

Sept 19   Full ward round, 15. St. John St., 3 cases, including L.S., injection for impotence, £5.0.0. Two letters from Hazel rejecting conversion; M. has a good cry.

Sept 20   Sifted through applications for Senior House Officer in Medicine, and selected short list. St. John St., 4 cases.

4:40 p.m. [*Male, aged 54, inspecting engineer*] His work mainly entails the inspecting of cranes. The average height at which he has to work, climbing up the structure of the crane, is 120 feet; he said that he had been up to 300 feet twice in his life. Eleven years ago he began to develop giddiness and headaches, and Menière's Disease was diagnosed. Thereafter, for ten years, he gave himself injections three times a week for it. Last year, he was 'up 30 feet on a tower crane', 'went round', and had great difficulty getting down again. He consulted another doctor, an ENT surgeon, who said that he had never had Menière's Disease, but that something was wrong with the labyrinth in his right ear; the whole of his inner ear was then removed eleven months ago, after which he said that he felt a 'new man'. He was a thick-set individual of florid complexion, with a raised blood pressure (200/120) and a deaf-aid in his left ear, the result of a past punctured left ear-drum.

Today, he reported that he hears a high-pitched hum or buzzing in his right ear (tinnitus) when he is tired, and that if he gets up suddenly from a seated position and has to turn quickly, he feels off balance and unsteady; and, sometimes, as if his head was 'going to come off'. When 'sitting, talking, reading or watching TV', he is 'all right', as also when he gets up 'quietly' and stands perfectly erect. Despite his claim that the operation has made a 'new man' of him, what has happened is that the removal of his inner ear has deprived him of his uncontrolled or reflex balance; he can, however, control his voluntary balance reasonably well, though everything depends upon the speed of his movements. (His relatively high blood pressure does not help him.) He is trying to go on with his work at heights, but is really unable to do so, since he has lost his sense of balance.

Saw 'Adventure' film on Ionides, 'The Man Who Loves Snakes'. Rail strike all set for October 3rd. Fell asleep during speech by Macmillan on the Common Market.

Sept 21   During clinic car cleaned by mental patient. Home at 6 p.m.: Ruth and Geoffrey have returned from the USA. A happy reunion.

Sept 22 [*Saturday*]   No peace at all, Jonathan [*grandson*] spoilt and noisy. Spiritual, physical and mental fatigue, with much praecordial pain. Looking forward to holiday, and to retirement. Taking stock of the situation as a whole, I may add a codicil to my will in due course, reinstating David.

No sleep this afternoon; disturbed by Jonathan's rantings. The meanness of Geoffrey is manifest; he has bought himself transistors, cameras etc., but came to us empty-handed. Food for thought. To reconsider my attitude. Retired to bed at 10.45 p.m., but unable to sleep owing to loud continual conversations in the Hall, without thought for others. Had to get up, stood at the top of the stairs, and told them to keep quiet. An important day for me in making decisions.

Sept 23   Restful day. To Mr. T. [*private patient, see Sept 14 1962*]; ascites still present, condition deteriorating steadily. Yesterday, my eyes were opened suddenly, as if I had made a great discovery, and the truth has dawned upon me about those who, without dignity or charity themselves, grasp what they can from others. I must change my will again before it is too late; I cannot disinherit my son in such circumstances.

Sept 24   Awoke at 4.20 a.m. I thank the Almighty for my sudden realization, and that He has given me the vision to perceive it, before it was too late. To Betty Shaw [*solicitor*], for alteration of will: David included as executor and beneficiary. The new will to be ready on Friday morning [*Sept 28*], at 9.30 a.m. To hospital, and talk with Dr. V. [*consultant physician*]; he complained angrily about the dumping of cases on us by certain GPs. Ward Round 15, in full. St. John St., 4 cases. The Friedlands [*friends*] called this evening at 9.30 p.m.; while they were here F.B. [*ENT consultant*] phoned, re case of malingering. After they had gone, helped M. to wash up, as Geoffrey and Ruth, who lose their tempers easily (in nonsensical outbursts of extreme bad taste), had gone off to bed without saying good-night. What a life!

Sept 26   New Morris 1100 mass-produced rubbish. To domiciliary visit in Rover: coronary thrombosis (aet 60, Smallshaw, ECG arranged, not yet admitted). Ward round, 12. David and Hazel for lunch. They appear quite happy; David showed me a letter from Nevill Coghill, professor of English Literature at Oxford, about one of his plays. To St. John St., one case only, very slack week. Weather getting worse in Europe; heavy storms in Barcelona area, with many missing, after period of long drought. Remarkable rescue of 48 people from ditched Super-Constellation in Mid-Atlantic. Clerical work, with domiciliary forms etc, etc., until midnight.

Sept 27   Made breakfast for M., who does not feel well. To *Manchester Guardian* office, to purchase James Morris booklet on South America, 2/-. Lunch at Masonic Temple; ordered 200 shares of Smith and Nephew at 14/1½. Thence to Shaw's Bookshop, and St. John St., 2 cases. Watched TV film on Jordan, 'In the Footsteps of Lawrence of Arabia'; not very good. Storms in Spain have damaged the textile trade. 700 dead. Faint trace of albumen in my urine.

Sept 28   The cruel Imam of Yemen assassinated after 8 days' rule. To bank, and withdrew old will of June 28th 1962, to be destroyed. Thence to Shaw's [*solicitors*], to sign fresh will; feel better as a result. The change has been made exactly three months after the one in June. Medical out-patients; very busy indeed. Lunch and, thereafter, domiciliary visit: myocardial ischaemia (aet 68, Ashton, to attend anti-coagulant clinic). Second Medical out-patients clinic, heavy going, but interesting cases. Two further domiciliaries: pneumonia, *in extremis* (aet 78, Droylsden, admitted); and Pakistani neurotic (aet 60, Ardwick Green, will not admit him). Long sleep in chair, after excellent dinner. Entered this Journal at 11.30 p.m.; a full day.

Sept 29 [*Saturday*]   Intensely sore throat, chiefly right pharyngeal region near internal meatus of Eustachian Tube. I have very little resistance, but I hope to battle on to enjoy some years of retirement, after having worked hard all my life. I shall therefore leave St. John St. at the end of March 1963, and refrain from Court Attendances. The main thing is to maintain my health, and relax from irksome duties. Bad faith and evil, false friends and ingrates, all flourish; the rest go to the wall. A storm this evening, wind and rain. Oh, my throat! Very exhausted.

Sept 30   Up at 1.20 a.m., with violent sore throat, probably viral in origin, and identical with the one of some weeks ago; localized to right superior constrictor muscle of pharynx, without ulceration. Did some useful clearing in my room, and returned to bed at 4.0 a.m. Severe gale in the early hours. Constantly disturbed in morning by loud voices. Some relief from the strain when Geoffrey, Ruth and Jonathan left, although I love them. The pain in my throat may be apthous ulceration, but essentially it is a psychosomatic manifestation. I have had enough tensions, strains and fears of late – David's marriage, Geoffrey's selfishness, M.'s sadness, my increasing fatigue and high blood urea – to do for a lifetime.

Oct 1   'Panorama' with Ernest Marples and Sidney Greene on Wednesday's [*Oct 3*] rail strike; Nkrumah and Ghana, with Robin Day; near Civil War in Oxford, Mississippi, over John Meredith, negro student for enrolment, with Federal and State troops involved; and on the career of Hugh Gaitskell. Interviews with his sister Lady Ashton, Shinwell, Attlee (gaga, nearly finished), Earl Longford and Betjeman.

Oct 2   Disturbed night, painful throat. Awoke frequently to relieve anguish on swallowing. To domiciliary visit: thrombo-phlebitis of leg (aet 79, Audenshaw, to be admitted as private patient). Anti-coagulant clinic; my BP taken by Dr. F., 165/95. Trace of albumen today. Saw F.B. in ENT Dept, re throat: nothing abnormal discovered, 'probably a virus'. Local analgesic recommended. To Masonic Temple, for meeting of Past Masters. Waiting list for Menorah Lodge [*his own*] approximately 5 years.

Oct 3   Awake from 3.0 a.m. to 5.0 a.m. Went down to Library. Insomnia well marked, but throat possibly slightly better. Letters slightly earlier than usual this morning, despite 24 hours railway strike. Put £1,000 from share windfall in Leeds Permanent Building Society. To garage; minor jobs attended to by man in oily dungerees, which transferred themselves to my clothes and hands thereafter. To Arnfields; Miss Lambert [*secretary*] has resigned, and tells me about her love life, etc. She will manage a hotel in North Wales. Ward Round, 15; a paper round. To St. John St., 4 cases, including the aunt of the D. girls. One of them, unmarried, lives in sin and has a child; the other – who had hairy legs and was always violent and psychopathic – committed suicide by drowning in a Reservoir. Paid rent for rooms, £64.5s.0d. and thereafter to Black's for a sandwich with M., 10/-. 7 p.m., first concert of new Hallé Season, with Barbirolli: Berlioz' *Carnaval Romain*, Brahms' Second Piano Concerto in B Flat, played by Gina Bachauer (Greek), and Beethoven's 7th. Dead tired, will take sedative.

Oct 4   Sunny and crisp morning. Ward Round, 15. After lunch, to domiciliary visit: congenital muscular dystrophy (aet 16, Hr. Openshaw, for wheelchair). Friendly reception from Dr. G., who called me. Thence to St. John St., one case only.

3:0 p.m. [*Female, aged 57, cook at 'hand-bag works'*] Eight weeks ago she was waiting on the doorstep of her house, which is on a main road, looking out for her husband to get off the bus on his return from work. (She has been doing this for years; as soon as she sees him, she 'gets his tea ready'). But on this particular day a lorry mounted the pavement and crashed into the front of her house, 'hurling' her 'behind the front door', and – from what I could gather – compressing her between the front door, where she had been waiting, and a glass vestibule door behind her. She said that the front door, on the other side of which was the lorry, was 'on top of' her, though she was still standing; 'I couldn't turn round to get the other door open', she stated.

Eventually the police came, the lorry was backed out, and she was retrieved, suffering from shock and bruises to both shoulders, brought about by the pressure of the door on them. She said that she was 'put to bed' by her doctor, who gave her 'an injection' and 'tablets'; she has been unable to go to work since and has consulted solicitors. Her present situation is that she is able to do her own cooking, cleaning and washing, but she has 'a girl who does the shopping'. Today, she told me that her 'inside' was 'all of a work'; that she goes 'all dizzy'; and that her face goes 'funny'. She also goes 'all shaky' when she gets 'to the edge of the pavement', etc. However, she has recently been to Morecambe for a two-week holiday in her caravan, driven by her 35-year-old married daughter, who owns a car. This improved her, but her 'nerves have gone bad again' because of the 'noisy street' she lives in; since the accident she has slept in her 'back bedroom'. She was a thick-set woman with a very anxious demeanour, an appreciably raised blood pressure (190/130) – with accentuated second sound – and a marked tremor of her outstretched hands, in particular the right one. She has obviously had a severe shaking from her frightening experience, and her description of things was genuine. What is clear is that she will not improve until the case has been disposed of, and she receives a satisfactory lump sum settlement, so that she can then revel in telling the tale of the accident for the rest of her life. She said that her face 'goes red about twice a day'; 'a bit of excitement brings it on'. 'It goes as red as your carpet', she told me.

Home early. M. had gone to a Mannequin Parade at The Midland. Successful space-flight recorded from America: over 9 hours and 6 orbits, with 80% fuel still left in machine. Sir John Barbirolli's mother, aet 91, died 2 days ago, yet he conducted the concert yesterday nevertheless (!). Geoffrey and Ruth called after we had gone to bed. Atmosphere not very cordial, and no enquiries made about my health. Happy, however, at my recent revelation.

Oct 5   Throat very sore today, but on left side instead of right. Ward round, 7; spoke to E.E. [*patient and mason*] who told me that Lord Derby was not proving a very good Provincial Grand Master, upsetting many people. David and Hazel arrive from Birmingham; lunch with them in the mess. Domiciliary visit, thereafter: ischaemic heart disease (aet 66, Ashton, ECG arranged). Interesting cases seen in Medical out-patients. To second domiciliary on way home: chronic bronchitis and emphysema, congestive heart failure (aet 53, Denton, to be admitted). De Gaulle's Government defeated. Judy meets Hazel for the first time; likes her.

Oct 6 [*Saturday*]   To St. John St. for letters; bookings looking up. Thereafter met D.V. [*Pakistani businessman*] with Dr. Z. [*Pakistani doctor*], at hospital. Invited to Karachi by the former, to his son's wedding. M. agrees to go. Forgot my spectacles at the hospital. Home, and siesta.

Oct 7   Bright sunny day. Beginning to pack necessary trifles and reading matter. Roland S. [*friend*] calls to tell me about his recent visit to Greece; it was less widespread and intense than mine will be. Today is the eve of the Day of Atonement. As I get older, whatever savours of self-flagellation seems to me of nuisance value only, and devoid of real religious connotation. It merely serves to make life more unpleasant, in a world already made unhappy by selfishness, hatred, lust, love, and money-madness.

Oct 8   M. fasting devotedly; Jonathan uncontrolled and damaging furniture; Ruth cannot keep a confidence, a malign and frightful gossip. Watched 'Panorama' on The Mafia in Palermo.

Oct 9   Purchased £50 in travellers' cheques from Cook's, and 400 drachmas (82.50 to the pound). To police station, informing them of my absence, and postal sorting office, complaining about state of letters on delivery. Anti-coagulant clinic, Ward rounds, and thence to St. John St., 4 cases. BOAC total deficit of £64,000,000 announced, including depreciation of planes. Heard that Maurice G. is reading Ethiopian, for an M.A. or Ph.D. Full day, hectic before departure.

Oct 10   To Arnfields; Miss Lambert, who is resigning, lachrymose. Called on Dr. J., and told him to look after Arnfields in my absence. To Mrs. K., Dukinfield; ring inserted, £1.11s.6d., and G.D. [*private patient*] complaining of uterine haemorrhage. P.V. examination, long cervix, no retroversion, uterus bulky. Will wait till I return. To hospital; farewell to Dr. D., whose father I will see in Crete. Ward round, 15; asked Dr. V. to see my cases in an emergency. He was in good mood. Hurried lunch, and to St. John St., one case only.

Cheque received from Henry Shaw, debt-collector, £6.10s.9d. M. does not look well; I hope the rest will do her good. Gave Judy [*daughter*] £15, for shopping during our absence.

Oct 11   Disturbed night, unable to sleep because of mounting anger at the two-facedness, double-dealing, hypocrisy and greed around me. The total indifference of others to my health is characteristic. Received two books from Harry W. Jr. [*see May 14 1962*] in Covington, Virginia: one on Chinese eroticism and the other on Eroticism in Hindu Sculptures. Proceeded to Wards 7, 14 and 15; Pakistani house-cap presented to me by Dr. Z. St. John St., 2 cases. Home early. D.V. [*Pakistani businessman*] came to the house at 6 p.m. to take us to the airport. I gave him liberal potions of whisky. Left London at 11.0 p.m., by Comet. 2 glasses of lemon-squash on plane, 1/-.

*

During his visit, with M., to Rhodes, Crete and Athens, he kept a detailed record, and observed (among other things) that the goats and bulls in the Rhodian countryside 'looked hungry and dehydrated'. He thought that Rhodes was 'spoiled by too much group travel and corrupted hoteliers, who as a result could not care less about individual and personal service'; inspected a Rhodian garden 'with its hibiscus, oleander, fig trees, oranges, lemons, peppers, thyme and orchidaceous leaves', after having struck up a conversation with its owner in the street; enjoyed 'the cool breeze from the sea and the sound of the waves upon the beach'; and read Lawrence Durrell as he travelled the island.

In Crete, he met Dr. D.'s father ('aet 78, deaf, glaucoma, senility and Parkinsonian tremor, a hospitable old gentleman'). He noted the 'kindliness shown by Cretans towards one another'; and had a 'kerbside consultation' – 'thrust upon me' – with an army officer's wife 'said to be suffering from osteoporosis'. She had had, he wrote, 'hundreds of useless investigations and multiple forms of treatment'; a 'mixture of massive doses of steroids, androgens and aspirin together', which he calls 'blunderbuss poly-pharmacy, dangerous and dreadful'. At Knossos, he noted the 'elliptical and rectangular sarcophagi, with burial in the crouched position'; and at 'enchanting Hierapatra, facing the Libyan Sea', where the air was 'soft and balmy', he ate 'Soupa Trachana which tasted like a linseed-oil poultice'.

From Crete, they flew to Athens ('the Greek passengers rushed for seats in the aircraft as if they were fleeing collapsing masonry in an earthquake'); and visited Corinth 'where thieves' dens lined the streets selling "refreshments", including lukewarm Nescafe at dishonest prices'. In the sanctuary of Aesculapius at Epidaurus he noted that 'snakes used to be kept in the subterranean passages for therapeutic purposes; compare shock treatment for mental patients'. On his last day in Athens at the Hotel Grande Bretagne – where 'everyone, chambermaids, porters and lavatory attendants, was waiting, ghoul-like, for tips' – he 'bought trinkets for friends, 70 drachmas, and a lamp for Miss James, 30 drachmas'.

*

Oct 26   Return from holiday in Greece. We left the Plaka [*Athens*] at 2.0 a.m., and at 4.15 a.m. took the bus to the airport. Felt broken and exhausted by two hours' late departure of aircraft. Home by 2.30 p.m., to find flowers from David and Hazel, and Judy in good spirits. Broke the back of two weeks' correspondence, and listened to Greek music on gramophone records, purchased in Athens yesterday. Getting things straight.

Oct 27 [*Saturday*]   Woke at 7.30 a.m. and made breakfast for M. Serious news from USA and Cuba; the *Guardian* devoted the major part of the newspaper to the Crisis. Phoned Drs. L. and F., Sister G. and Dr. V., who sounded fairly dispirited. Other news: India invaded by the Chinese in the North, and Rabbi of ultra-orthodox sect, aet 55, murdered in New York and another stabbed by youth, aet 16. Siesta, making up for loss of sleep. Phoned Miss James; she has a varicose ulcer on the ankle, and is in much pain. Perused recent book catalogues; book prices maintained at satisfactory level. Preparing for next week's work.

Oct 28   World crisis over Cuba still on, though it appears slightly easier. Mattei, Italian industrialist, killed in plane-crash. Phoned S.F. [*travel agent*] to complain about hotel incompetence, cold water etc. Ruth, Geoffrey and Jonathan called this afternoon; altercations avoided, though they accuse me of irreligion. Dr. F. also came round with hospital news:

191

Dr. X's nurse-friend [*see June 27 1962*] has had twins; Dr. C. refuses to cooperate with Dr. V. [*both consultant physicians*]; P. [*hospital administrator*] has haematemesis, and is a surgical in-patient. Better news tonight from Cuba; Khruschev decides to pull out his bases.

Oct 29   Gave Dr. J. reproduction of Mycaenean cup. Breakfast at hospital; gave Dr. D. a gift from his parents. Full Ward round in 12; spoke to Drs. C. and V., Sisters G. and F., and new Sister K. on Ward 12. Visited P. [*hospital administrator*], in Ward 14. St. John St., 3 cases, and large number of letters; many appointments coming along. Gave Miss James some Grecian pottery, which she appeared to appreciate. Thereafter, briefly to Freemasons' Club; encountered P.E. [*masonic official*], a hard-bitten and uncharitable fellow, who disguises himself as an upright Christian. 'Panorama' on Cuba, with discussion *ad nauseam*, and conjecture upon conjecture, as to what Khruschev thinks.

Oct 30   Cold. To Anti-coagulant clinic. Ward rounds, 7 and 15, and dreadful lunch. St. John St., one case only, who was trying it on good and proper.

3:0 p.m   [*Male, aged 45, branch manager, yeast and baker's sundries*] He was a healthy looking man, whose general condition was perfectly sound, with nothing the matter. Eight weeks ago in Rochdale, he swerved into a wall in his van after a collision with a Ford Anglia driven by a woman; he says he 'jerked' his back against the seat. He continued at work, but a week later went to the local hospital complaining of back pain. Since then he has consulted solicitors, has been attending an osteopath for massage, has purchased a Philips infra-red lamp, has seen an orthopaedic surgeon at the hospital, has received heat treatment to the small of his back in the Physiotherapy Department, and claims that the hospital Casualty Officer – whom he called 'a coloured gentleman' – told him that if his back were 'not attended to', he would be 'an old man in 10 years' time'. Today, he complained of a 'gnawing pain' over the sacral region, and said that when he lies on his stomach

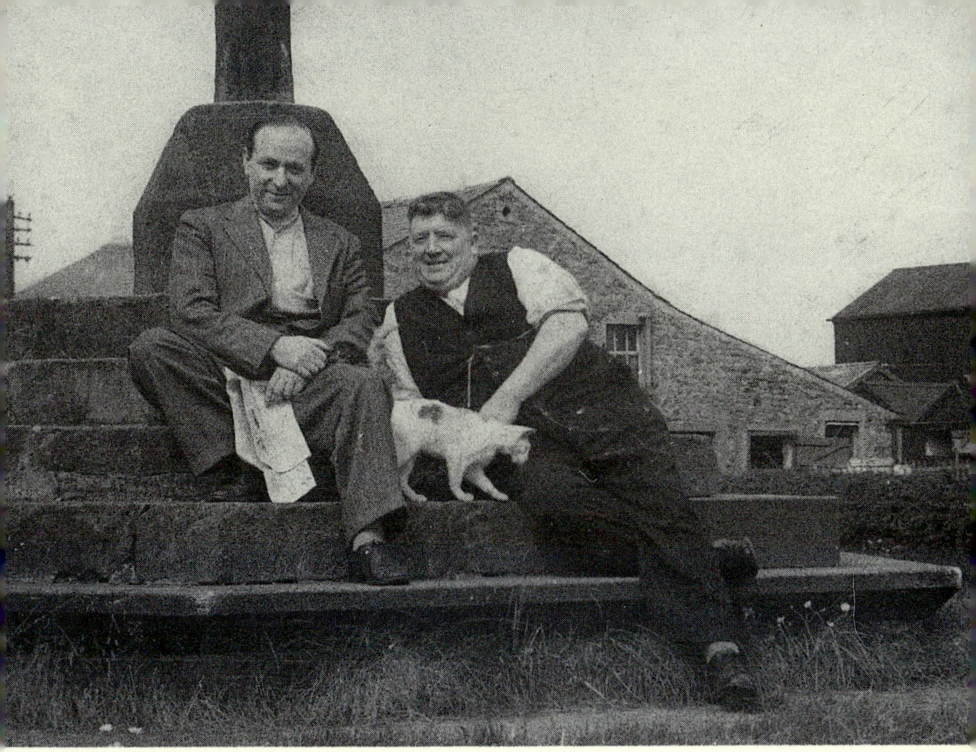

Hugh Selbourne with a Lancashire farmer patient

The Selbourne family in Dukinfield, 1949

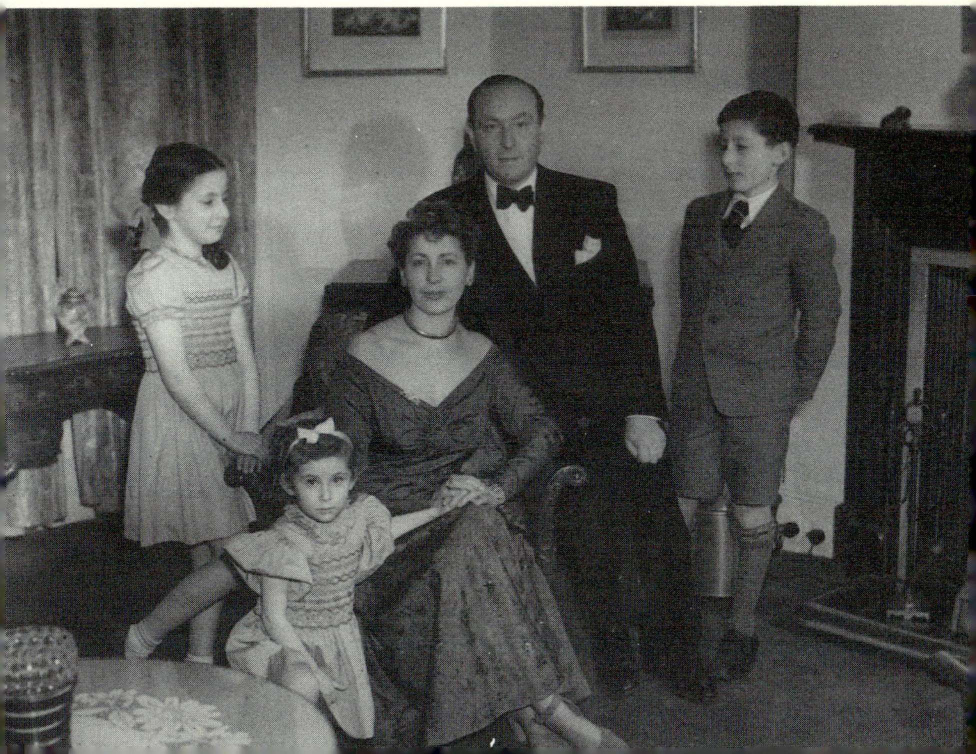

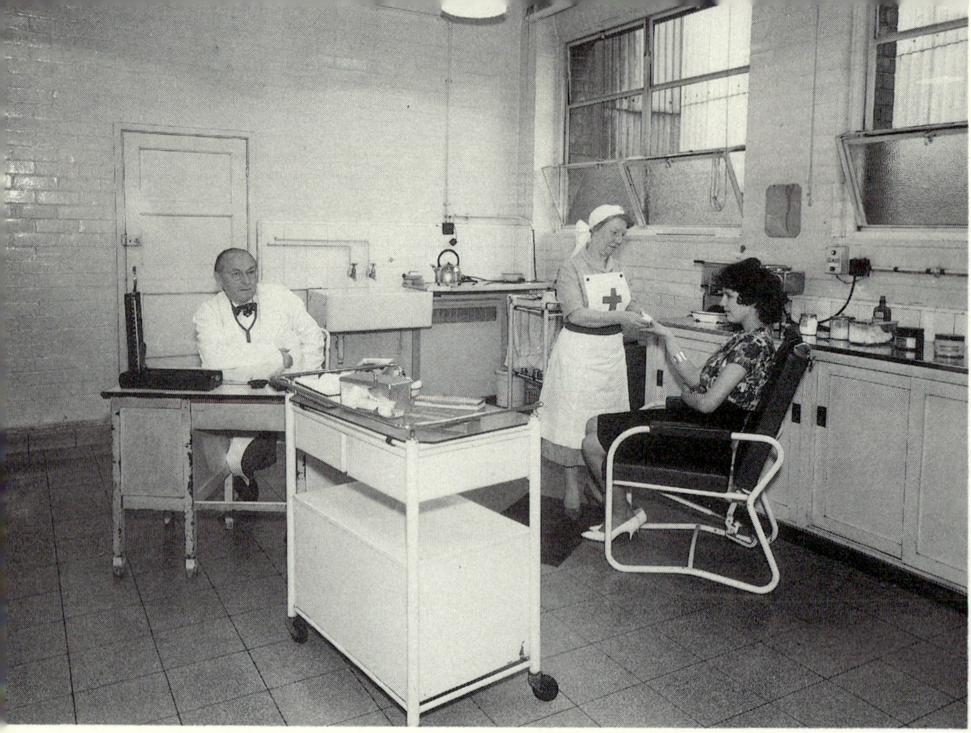

Works Doctor, Arnfield's, Audenshaw, near Manchester

With Sir Michael Bruce at Sherratt & Hughes, the Manchester
booksellers

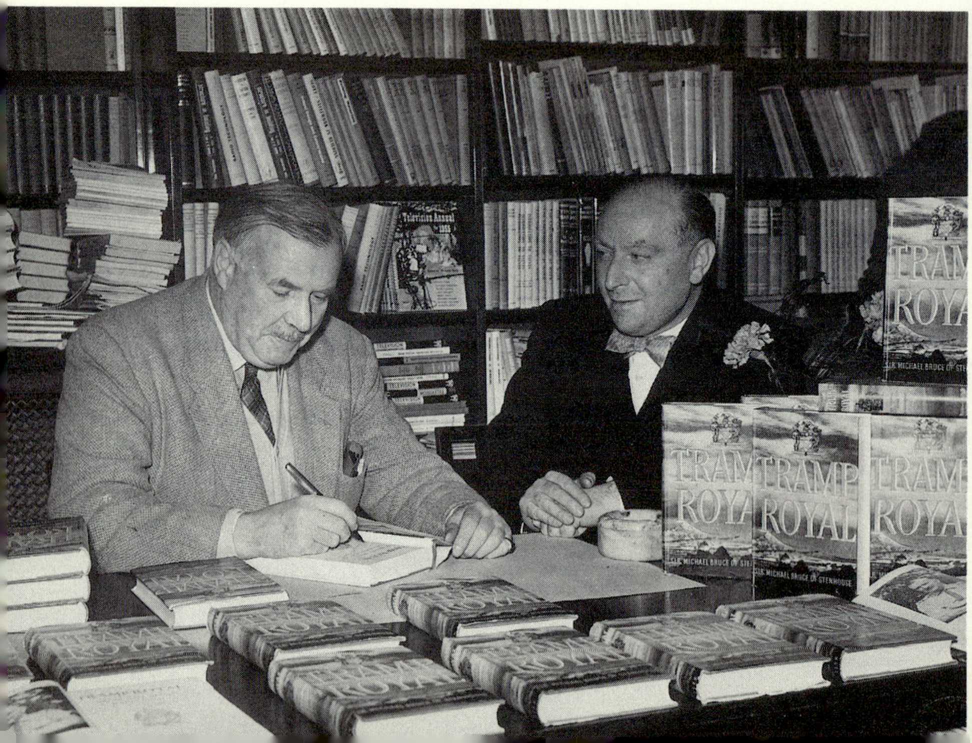

or 'in a draught' the pain 'creases' him. Despite these dire symptoms his appetite is sound, and he sleeps well. When I asked him how long it would take him to get well, he replied 'It is entirely in the hands of the doctors'. This situation has dangerous potentialities; he is revelling in an imaginary disability, and most of his symptoms are poppycock. He was able to stoop fully and rotate his spine in every direction necessary. When he was leaving he told me that he had 'always been an athlete', was 'a bit of a crank in health matters', and a 'firm believer in Epsom Salt-baths'. There was bugger all wrong with him.

It gets dark early. Wrote and posted letter to the D.'s in Crete, thanking them for their hospitality. Quiet evening and early to bed, to read the papers, catalogues etc. Heavy rain tonight, and very cold.

Oct 31   To Arnfields and domiciliary visits: hypertension (aet 57, Ashton, to be dealt with in out-patients); chronic bronchitis (aet 60, Ashton, for out-patients). St. John St., 3 cases. Thereafter, to supper at Black's with M., £1.2s.0d, and proceeded to Hallé concert, excellently conducted by Bernard Haitink, aet 33: Haydn, Brahms, Prokofiev. Programme and beer, 5/-. On return, watched 'Panorama Special' about Indo-Chinese frontier war.

Nov 1   Received 'Proceedings of the M/c Literary and Philosophical Society' Vol 104, 1961–2. Renewed TV and Wireless Licence, £4.0.0. Bought Wilkinson's razor blades, hard to get for past 3 months. To hospital and learned that Dr. T. of Oldham collapsed and died during administrative appeal to the Regional Hospital Board about the number of hospital sessions allotted to him. What a circus of evil men constitute the Regional Board and its bureaucratic ringleaders! Also, heard of difficulties in getting Dr. X.'s twins adopted. Visited Dr. A.; in-patient, Ward 14. He had a left lobectomy in 1953 for adenoma of lung (heavy smoker); he now has laryngeal palsy, and rheumatoid arthritis. St. John St., 3 cases, including woman with 13 children, one with hydrocephalus.

2:30 [*Female, aged 61*] She lives alone and is a registered blind person, suffering from glaucoma in both eyes. (Her husband left her in 1939 with three daughters to bring up, one of whom is now a hospital cleaner.) She has also suffered for the last six years from Parkinson's disease. Four weeks ago she was dragged along by a bus for about 130 yards, was very badly shaken and frightened, and sustained abrasions to her ankle and foot, which were dressed in the hospital, but she was not detained. After the accident her Parkinsonian tremor, which is limited to the right arm, worsened and she kept having nightmares, in which she saw herself 'holding on to the bus' with her foot dragging in the roadway. She wept bitterly while telling me this. She herself thinks she is 'getting over it', and is 'certain' she will get better. (It is well known that accidents can temporarily aggravate Parkinson's disease and other neurological disorders; in another month or so, she may have returned to her pre-accident state.) She added that she does not go to her doctor very much; 'I dont believe in it', she said. She was a pleasant woman of great courage, of good colour but very thin, and with a marked tremor of her right arm. There was also some associated muscle wasting, but she was so thin that it was not easy to assess the extent of it. She made light of her disabilities, had a sense of humour, and said that she did her own cooking and shopping.

Poor weather all day. Rain, cold, misty, unpleasant.

Nov 2   A week since return from Greece. Sotheby's want 15% commission for any sale of books, and all the books at once; will think it over. Medical out-patients lengthy, with the unpleasant Sister H. assisting. Spoke to E.E. [*see Sept 14 1962*]; am angry at not being promoted this year, will resign from the Club for a start. M. met Hazel for the first time, her impression the same as mine after first meeting. They both strike me with pity; David is bearded and devoid of ambition. Gave them the Flatley clothes-drier. I hope their marriage will turn out all right.

Nov 3 [*Saturday*]   A sunny, cold morning. To St. John St., for letters. Thence to Middleton, for medico-legal examination, aet 23, a very sad case of crash fracture at C5 [*the* *spine*], with complete quadriplegia [*paralysis of all four limbs*]; wife 20, and infant daughter of 15 months. Home, and studied Sotheby's auction results. Book prices appreciating very markedly, Newton's *Optics*, £90 (cf. £24, when I bought it in 1953); Laennec [*L'Auscultation Médiate*], £250 (cf. £22 in 1948); Audubon's *Birds*, Vol 1, £4,100, when all 4 vols used to bring £3,000 a few years ago.

Nov 4 Rose early for a Sunday, 7.40 a.m. Left house at 10 a.m. to domiciliary visit: scurvy and coronary thrombosis (aet 63, Ashton, admitted). Thereafter, called in at Wards 12 and 15. Poor lunch at home today; thinking of siesta, when the Horwichs [*friends*] appeared, Bill H. very drunk from a party, ebullient and noisy. Tried again to rest, but interrupted by the arrival of Drs. F. and L. for tea. To bed early, exhausted.

Nov 5 Excellent map of Central and East Africa arrived with *Geographical Magazine*. Ward rounds, 12, 14 and 15; Mrs. L. [*private patient*] is struggling on bravely, yet remains exclusively interested in money, a negation of understanding and reason. What a type! She is near to death, yet spends her time in the Ward looking constantly at the *Financial Times*, without seeming to contemplate the unknown for a moment. 'Panorama' on Havana during the crisis (secret film), James Mossman reporting from Nepal, and Robin Day at Harvard, speaking to Professors of History on Kennedy's achievements so far as President.

Nov 7 A letter from David, reassuring in tone. Successes in mid-term elections for Kennedy, Rockefeller gets in as Governor of New York, and Nixon faces political extinction. St. John St., 2 cases, including a toyshop assistant, aet 55, with anxiety state and marital unhappiness. Paid £6.0.0d. This evening, inclined to go to bed, but many phone calls, including kerbside consultations.

Nov 8 Bad cold, bronchitis, difficult to get up. Made breakfast for M. however. Left at 10 a.m., feeling very groggy. Domiciliary visit: chronic bronchitis and byssinosis [*a form of pneumoconiosis from cotton dust*], TB(?) (aet 61, Ashton, admitted). St. John St., 2 cases, including a man who came 75 minutes late, but was very casual about it. He said he 'fell asleep in front of the fire'!! He failed to attend last week altogether.

Nov 9   12 cases, including C.B. [*see April 9 1962*], phoeochromocytoma, who said that he had been suspended for three months from his job for striking the foreman and knocking out six of his teeth. His BP 150/100; my BP 180/100. During clinic, Dr. D. rang me to say that his father had been taken acutely ill in Crete, and that he had been summoned to the bedside; a Professor of Medicine has also been summoned from Athens. I am deeply grieved, and hope that D. senior survives and gets decent treatment. Medical out-patients in afternoon; interesting cases, but badly afflicted with headache, coryza [*cold*], conjunctivitis, depression, and anxiety about my BP. Heavy traffic on way home; it gets worse and worse.

Nov 11 [*Sunday*]   Moving obituary by Dennis Brogan on Mrs. Eleanor Roosevelt, who died a few days ago. Also articles on Cuba and Russia, India and China, and the tangled international situation. Remembrance Day article in *Sunday Times* by Lady Violet Bonham Carter. Sorted out some old Valentines, rare prints, water-colour drawings and autograph letters from upstairs room.

Nov 12   Restless night, nocturia three times. I need sedation. Judy oversleeps and misses school. Additional morning clinic, new patients, including poor woman of 50, bleeding p.r. [*per rectum*] for three years (!!), with a large carcinoma of rectum; her GP is Dr. X of Hyde. There were also two cases of recent 'coronary attacks' sent up as out-patients! What is medicine coming to in this country? St. John St., one case, and home early. Sent telegram to Crete, to inquire about Mr. D.'s health. I do hope he gets better. 'Tonight': reactions to Thalidomide verdict; and views of zombified teenagers about their parents. 'Panorama': discussion between Lady Longford and Barbara Wootton on Thalidomide babies and artificial limbs. Further income tax demand today for £2,500 (1962–3).

There is no incentive for work in this country; but some people make it fairly easily.

Nov 13   Twelve student nurses examined; a brighter lot than usual. Mrs. N. [*private patient*] gave me 2 packets of Wilkinson's Sword Edge Blades. No lunch today; one egg and one cup of coffee in Dr. F.'s room. St. John St., 3 cases, including a splenectomy, a schoolgirl, and a solicitor's clerk. Geoffrey [*son-in-law*] called to see me, advising me to 'sell the Library' and enjoy myself. He says that I will 'live another 30 or 40 years' etc, etc.

Nov 14   To two domiciliaries: glycosuria and blackouts (aet 73, Denton, admitted); hypertension and congestive heart failure (aet 63, Ashton). St. John St., 5 cases, and thence to Black's with M., pre-concert. At the table, met a Mr. Francis of the 'Friendship' Lodge; told him that it was a misnomer. At 7.0 p.m., to Hallé: conducted by Laurence Leonard, Paul Badura Skoda playing Tschaikovsky's B Minor Piano concerto. We left at the interval. I am not required in court tomorrow for the R. [*medico-legal*] case; he has pleaded guilty to manslaughter.

Nov 15   To St. John St., 3 cases.

4:15 p.m. [*Male, aged 63, despatch clerk*] He worked until 12 months ago as a bleacher, spending many years exposed to chemical fumes, and now has marked emphysema and chronic bronchitis. Today, he complained of cough, shortness of breath – he sleeps with four pillows – sputum, and occasional ankle-swelling. He said that he had been given a Franol spray to assist his breathing, but that otherwise his GP 'never listened'. He had double pneumonia fourteen years ago, and his brother, aet 50, also suffers from bronchitis. He has no children. On examination, his chest expansion was only ¾", he had sonorous rales [*abnormal sound from the lungs, higher pitched than a wheeze*] and rhonchi [*wheezes*], with prolonged expiration and other typical features of emphysema. His peripheral blood pressure, as expected, was normal (140/90). His general condition was bad, and I could not hold out any promise of recovery. However, I told him that we could at least try to prevent an aggravation of his symptoms in the coming winter, and he agreed to come into hospital. The rest itself will do him good. Despite his worsening chest condition, and incipient right-sided heart failure, he continues to smoke '12 to 13' cigarettes a day. He is a very sick man indeed; he said to me himself that he was 'steadily deteriorating'.

To Shaw's Bookshop, and thereafter to meeting of Manchester Society of Book Collectors; met a Mrs. Dobbin who collects children's books, and a Miss Wadsworth who collects books about roads. Spoke today about Harry W. Jr. of Virginia, his farming and his collection; will speak on Dec 13th about Thirty Years of Collecting.

Nov 16   Examination of 14 trainee nurses, some from Uganda, Kenya, Jamaica. A mixed bunch, including one obese, of 18 stones. Sister X., who has lesbian tendencies, fondled the girls' breasts during the examination, a needless procedure.

Nov 17 [*Saturday*]   Restful day. David and Hazel came to tea; relations with M. improving. M. gave Hazel a bracelet, and I gave them a 17th century Dutch print of singers and merrymakers, which I have had in my study for many years.

Nov 18   Very cold. Malcolm Macdonald made Governor of Kenya, Tshombe ignores U.N. re integration into Congo, China captures Walong in India in a heavy offensive. Trouble in Cuba not yet over, Sino-Soviet relations worse than ever, Adenauer senile and anti-British in the matter of entry into the Common Market. Listened to Goossens and Menuhin in the Bach D Minor Concerto, for oboe and violin. Gales and heavy snow in Scotland.

Nov 19   Received telegram from Crete, announcing the death of poor Mr. D. on Sunday, Nov 11th. Sent letter of condolence to family. St. John St., 2 cases.

4:0 p.m. [*Female, aged 41, telephone operator*] She had stood up, preparing to get off a bus on her way to work, when it pulled up suddenly and she fell backwards, striking her head against the back seat and twisting her left side as she fell. To make matters worse, she had just started menstruating, the conductor fell on top of her, and his ticket machine struck her on her right ankle. She felt shocked, was bruised 'along her legs' and at the back of her neck, and had a swollen ankle. She was off work for a month, and today – four and a half months after the event - complained of headaches 'at any time' (which 'last two or three days' and 'start at the back and go over the top'), and a pain over the kidney region which 'stays in one place, like toothache'. She also does not know when she will have her period next, as she has been irregular since the accident; the pain in her side is more severe 'when it happens'.

She was a woman who looked much younger than her years, is divorced, has two teenage daughters, and has lived with her mother for some years. On examination, there was deep tenderness in the left iliac fossa, low down in the pelvis and over the left kidney region, with a fair amount of muscle-guarding; together with marked tenderness in the left fornix and in the region of the left Fallopian tube. It may well be that when she 'twisted' her 'side' and the bus conductor fell on her, she suffered some inner strain – perhaps some abnormal rotation of her Fallopian tubes or uterus – which has produced a gynaecological or renal disorder; her urine sometimes 'runs away' when she coughs or sneezes. (There was also no doubt about the abdominal tenderness, which she registered every time I returned to the same spot.) She needs a renal and abdominal X-Ray, though a neurotic element cannot be excluded, as she has had a fair amount of domestic trouble.

Called on Mr. T. [*private patient; see Sept 23 1962*] on my way home; his condition has deteriorated sharply. Chinese invasion of India more extensive and serious.

Nov 20   Anti-coagulant clinic, and Ward rounds, 7 and 12; spoke to Miss S. about her dying father, and posted chilblain ointment to Hazel. St. John St., 2 cases, including

13st. 4lb., 5′11½″, football-playing chartered accountant, aet 24, who is a regular blood donor. Home early. China invades Assam, grave news from India. Late night announcement: ceasefire suddenly ordered, by Chou or Mao.

Nov 21   Domiciliary visit: praecordial pain, auricular flutter (aet 50, Hr. Openshaw, ECG arranged). To Arnfields; talk with E.G.T. [*managing director*], re giving annual check-up to Higher Executives (25 for £250), thus pushing up my salary. Ward Rounds, 14 and 15. St. John St., 2 cases, including emergency consultation with drunken man who was brought to me by Harry K. [*friend*]. Waited in vain for L.S. from Chorley; Miss James (varicose ulcer) gave me a pain in the neck, with her long face and sour manner.

Nov 22   Letter from Hazel, thanking me for ointment; replied immediately. Heavy fog this morning; unable to go to Ashton. Maurice G. advised me to cancel St. John St. appointments and stay at home. I wish I had listened to him. To St. John St., fog deepening, and apprehensive. On arrival, emergency call to private case in Ashton: aet 51, coronary thrombosis, admitted. Returned to St. John St., 2 cases, including news editor, aet 31, humourless fellow, obese and slightly hypertensive. Left for home at 4.30 p.m., in the worst fog ever experienced; arrived at 7.10 p.m. [*a distance of about 5 miles*]. To bed at 8.30 p.m.; exhausted by strain of driving.

Nov 23   Awoke at 2.30 a.m., either insomnia or by then adequately rested. Read *Radio Times*, made tea, tidied room etc. till morning. Follow-up clinic, assisted by Nurse R., highly efficient. Thence, to two domiciliaries: cerebral embolism (aet 60, Ashton, admitted), and broncho-pneumonia, almost dead, death-rattle (aet 61, Hyde); a 'quickie', as Dr. H. [*the G.P. who called him*] described it. Wards 12 and 15, urgent cases seen, and Medical out-patients. Thereafter, a further domiciliary: pernicious anaemia (aet 69, Ashton, for investigation). Home by 6.30 p.m; Dr. N. [*GP, friend*] phoned about B.A. [*private patient*], carcinoma of cervix, or body of uterus. Row with M. and Judy over their interruptions whilst listening to News

Bulletin. Went off to bed early in a temper, wondering why there is so much selfishness on their part, when so much affection is showered on them.

Nov 24 [*Saturday*]   Disturbed night, sleeping in fits and starts. Rose at 9.0 a.m., insufficiently rested, weather cold and damp. Quarterly telephone account, £11.7s.0d; wrote letter of complaint to Telephone Manager about rotten service. Read *Manchester Guardian*: death of James Bone C.H., aet 90. Further rudeness from Judy at lunch-time. To dinner at the Freedmans [*friends*] at 7.30 p.m., 6 other guests and large amounts of food. Returned home at midnight. Thereafter, walk with M. and Judy, damp and misty; a light burning upstairs at Mr. T.'s [*see Nov 19 1962*], *in extremis*.

Nov 25   A moderate fog. D.V. [*private patient*] telephones from London. His wife has 'hiatus hernia' according to yet another doctor, a Pakistani in practice near the Cumberland Hotel (phoned him, sounded a bit shady). Read article on Churchill, who is 88 on Friday [*Nov 30*]. It described his disappointment at being defeated at the 1945 elections, and the doleful reactions of his entourage. Thereafter, emergency call to poor Mr. T. I dressed, and called on him, a good man who is on his way out. It is sad that he will not see his daughter married; Mrs. T. a noble woman.

Nov 26   Called first thing at Mr. T.'s, but could not make myself heard. Thereafter to garage, for attention to car-horn (rather hoarse). To hospital, phoned R.H. [*broker*] to order 100 Elliott Automation Shares at 47/6d, and Mrs. T., re her husband: I.S.Q. [*in statu quo, no change*]. Medical out-patients, additional session; Dr. C. off-duty for next two weeks with 'slipped disc' (very dubious affair), and Dr. V. on holiday. Had to cope alone. Ward Round 15, in full, and umpteen phone calls. Wanted at Assizes immediately, but unable to go; case settled. To domiciliary visit: senile dementia (aet 70, Denton, admitted). St. John St., 6 cases, including C.D., aet 77, hypertension and loneliness, to be admitted.

Nov 28   Patchy fog. To Arnfields; Miss Lambert

wants me to buy her a *History of the Opera* as a parting gift, before she goes off to run her hotel. Full ward round, 15; parts of 14 and 12. Thence to domiciliary visit: pregnancy with thrombo-phlebitis of leg (aet 41, Denton, consultation). St. John St., 2 cases; L.S. from Chorley, and G.H., aet 65, Miss James's spinster friend (carcinoma?). Did not go to rubbishy Provincial Grand Lodge meeting: a racket, in which a few people at the helm prance about like demigods in a schizophrenic world they have created, and then claim kudos for it.

Nov 29   Phoned G.H.'s doctor [*see Nov 28*] and Miss James, to reassure her. To domiciliary: J.K., cerebral thrombosis (aet 72, Stalybridge, admitted to private ward). No cases in St. John St., and home by 3.30 p.m. M. exasperatingly slow about getting ready to go out to dinner tonight. Dr. E. [*house-physician*] rang, grateful for my testimonial.

Nov 30   Ward round, 12; yesterday's cerebral thrombosis, J.K., moribund. Medical out-patients heavy; R.B. [*see Nov 8 1961*] came to see me, with anxiety state. David and Hazel to dinner; they are staying the night. Showed Hazel the library. Dr. F. phoned very late, to say J.K. had died earlier this evening.

Dec 1 [*Saturday*]   M. did not wish me to go to Hospital today. David and Hazel came down to breakfast at 10.30 a.m.; I wonder if the marriage is a success? I feel sorry for them. They took away sundry items for their home. Very tired today, afternoon siesta, Golda S. [*neighbour*] to tea. At 7.0 p.m., we went to the Livingstones for dinner. Poor Judy is always left at home, but she does not seem to mind. She can study, listen to radio, watch TV as she pleases.

Dec 2   Made breakfast for M., and then to hospital to Dr. V.'s [*consultant colleague*] lecture-demonstration, on psychosomatic aspects of medicine, to post-graduate students. The demonstration was quite interesting, but the audience was comatose, mostly coloured students, mostly dull. My three cases turned up for demonstration: phoeochromyctoma, chronic lymphatic leukaemia and aneurysm of left ventricle, following myocardial infarction. Ward 7 visited, before leaving.

Dec 3   Disturbed night, severe frost this morning. Hot water needed to thaw out car-doors and windows. Home in patchy freezing fog. Admission to hospital arranged for G.H., Miss James's friend [*see Nov 28*]. Large explosion of Olympus engine (secret Hawker Siddeley aviation project); loss said to be £1,000,000.

Dec 4   Fog, frost, cold, misery and damp. All but five displaced by the Tristan da Cunha earthquake [*see Oct 11 1961*] wish to return to the desolate isle. Full ward rounds; saw F.B. [*ENT surgeon*] about my throat. Left for St. John St. in heavy fog. Rang Dr. G. [*psychiatric physician*] about Jamaican psychopath, with accident neurosis.

Dec 5   Patchy fog, but London has the worst of it. Domiciliary visit: chronic bronchitis and emphysema (aet 62, Ashton, for investigations). Saw poor E.F. [*private patient*] in Ward 15. Telephoned his adopted son, and told him about the cancer. Restful morning at hospital for the first time in many years.

2:15 p.m. [*Male, aged 56, steeplejack and chimneyjack*] He was a thick-set man, with a tremor of his hands, slightly raised BP (160/95) and irregular pulse, who wore a leather splint on his right wrist, which he said he 'got off an ambulance chap'. Three months ago, he was thrown off his seat ('three rows from the back') on the upper deck of a bus, when an 18-ton lorry collided with it; he put out his right hand to stop himself falling and fractured the small scaphoid bone, known as the 'anatomical snuff-box', which connects to the wrist-joint. His glasses fell off, and broke; his upper denture was also fractured when his mouth 'snapped', as he put it, in the impact. (His mouth must have been partly open at the time). He was then assisted downstairs by the conductor, and went home on another bus, sitting on the lower deck. He is self-employed, with a partner, had only one day off after his mishap, and has since been doing 'one-handed jobs', with 'no climbing or steeplejacking'. (Their main work is renewing lightning conductors, and they have had to employ a 'mate' to replace him.)

Today, he complained that he was a 'bag of nerves' and that if he picked anything up his hands trembled. 'I cant keep them still', he said, declaring that his wife would not let him pour the tea because it went 'all over the place'. He also said that he had pain in the wrist; 'I cant sleep for it'. On examination, his right grip was weaker than the left, there was some tenderness over the scaphoid bone, but nothing much wrong with his wrist movements. The fracture he sustained is very common, and often arises in the way he described – falling with hand outstretched. It is a fracture which can take a long time to heal, and in many cases arthritic changes take place in the wrist-joint after such an accident. Moreover, X-ray pictures are not necessarily a guide to prognosis in particular cases: an X-ray may show only a thin fracture and yet the person be unable to move the wrist; conversely, a worse fracture with marked arthritic changes may not be an impediment to hard manual work. In this case I doubted whether he had as much pain as he made out, and told him that if he discarded the splint he would get on much better, and in due course be able to get back to steeplejacking. Rehabilitation even in bone-fractures depends a great deal on the personality of the individual.

K.D. [*friend*] phoned, distraught about his son, aet 7½, who has had a tracheostomy. Phoned pediatric registrar for information. A fairly clear road home. Heavy smog in London, and many deaths. Mortality rises eight-fold in London in smog-outbreaks. Sunbathing today in Folkestone.

Dec 6   Started sending out Christmas cards in earnest.

Dec 7   Laryngitis this morning. Ward rounds, 12 and 15; nothing can be done for E.F. Toffees, 4/9d. Quiet evening, reading on the History of Mathematics, 'from Euclid to Einstein'.

Dec 8 [*Saturday*]   Rain in torrents, but fog washed away. Mrs. K.S. [*private patient*] sends me a felt hat for Xmas. Letter from L.F. [*solicitors*] re my accident: derisory offer, £100 for M., £275 for me, liability admitted by the other side, offers to be rejected. News: Abu Simbel Temples in Egypt to be submerged by Aswan Dam; 30 million dollars required to lift them 200 feet above floodwaters, but UNESCO cannot raise the money. Egyptians angry. To St. John St. for letters, and to give Miss James lift to hospital, to see her friend in Ward 12. Sister F., another bitch (I will deal differently with her in future), would not give Miss James lunch; Dr. F. provided it for her in his room. It is fortunate that there are as many decent people in the world as shits [*seven names follow, three of them those of hospital administrators*] to equalize things. To bed after lunch, to read the *BMJ* and the *Guardian*. Prepared outline of talk for Book Collectors' Society next Thursday [*Dec 13*], and watched 'That Was The Week That Was', BBC TV satirical programme, 10.45 p.m. Excellent, I thought.

Dec 9   No rest today, with the comings and goings, too much food as usual, Ruth, Geoffrey and Jonathan etc, etc. Time only for a short siesta, and heard Schubert's Fifth Symphony on radio. Among others today, spoke to Dr. G. [*consultant physician*], who is deeply interested, to the point of obsession, in trains and trams; and a Mr. R., Johannesburg surgeon, whose wife has a recurring tumour at the upper end of her femur, and who said that he earned £60,000 a year in South Africa. But what does it avail him?

Dec 10   Criticism in papers of Saturday's 'That Was the Week That Was'. Distressed to hear of the death of Dr. W. [*friend and local GP*]. He was brought in dead yesterday afternoon. (He died of a coronary thrombosis after Sunday lunch.) Went to P.M. room to view his body, and found place like a shambles. Woman of 33 and boy of 20, killed in motor accident, were lying dead, still on stretchers. What a sight! And B. [*secretary*] sitting there typing, quite unconcernedly. St. John St., 3 cases.

4:0 p.m. [*Female, aged 65, pointer of bolts*] She has six children, all married, and told me that she had been 'brought up in the workhouse'. She was well-built, verbose and very depressed in appearance, and came with her husband. Twelve months ago, a heavy steel handle struck her on top of the head 'at about 11.30 a.m.', as she was bending down 'into the sud trough' – she said that she fell to the ground, but was not unconscious, and was assisted to the works rest-room where the nurse 'rubbed some stuff' on her head. (She added that she felt sick, and had a 'bump as big as a duck egg'.) After resting on the 'sofa', she was accompanied home on the bus by a 'young lady from work'. However, she returned to her job the same afternoon and struggled on for three months, since she was in need of the money, despite headaches and 'blackouts twice a week', until she 'could not last out' any longer. She has been off work since, that is for the last 9 months.

Today, she said that she had pain and 'swelling' at the back of her head; a 'crack' which 'goes across' her forehead and temple; and her eyes are 'plaguing' her, 'running all the time'. She also said that she was 'not the same woman', since the knock on her head – in which her husband concurred – goes 'funny' when sitting in her chair, and 'fell on the floor last Friday'. During these 'blackouts', of which she had two last week, she is incontinent. Her symptoms can be attributed to an accident neurosis, brought on by the trauma to her head (the site which most frequently arouses such responses); the fact that she had seldom been away from work previously has added to her feelings of anxiety. She and her husband were both simple folks who struck me as honest. She said, 'I have had a hard life, and been a good worker'.

Watched 'Panorama' on blind Chinese refugees in Macao, a battle in Brunei (north of Sarawak), and increasing armed hold-ups in London. Also Malcolm Muggeridge interviewing Maurice Cornforth, a Marxist, who made a complete fool of himself.

Dec 12   Received Xmas card from Senator Randolph Collier, encountered at the theatre in Epidaurus. Visited

Dr. K. [*see June 21 1960*], who is fed up with the practice; he kept calling the patients 'filthy' and 'dirty' and all manner of obscene terms. He has lost over 300 cards [*i.e. patients*] and said he was 'almost bankrupt'; gave him £1. To Ward 15; N.H. dying. Mrs. H. thanks me for what we have tried to do. St. John St., 5 cases.

3:0 p.m. [*Male, aged 45, textile traveller; see June 5 1961*] He was slightly less miserable than on his previous visit, has no more 'bangs and flashes' before his eyes, and was not limping. However, 21 months after fracturing his kneecap, he is still only working part-time (on half-pay) 'cant carry anything' – he has 'tried and tried', he told me – and has difficulty 'walking up and down', not only with rolls of cloth but even without them.

The orthopaedic surgeon has told him that there is 'nothing further he can do', and from what I could gather he is being advised by his G.P. to see a psychiatrist; his GP has avoided telling him outright, by referring to a 'neurologist'. On examination, however, I found an enormous amount of grating in his right knee on movement, with the features of post-fracture osteo-arthritis. He was able to kneel on the floor of my room, but had a great deal of pain in doing it. What we have here is compensation-neurosis, superimposed on real arthritic changes. He needs mental rehabilitation; substantial physical rehabilitation will then follow.

To Hallé Concert: Henry Szeryng, stupendous in Brahms' Violin Concerto, and Vaughan Williams' Sixth Symphony conducted by Barbirolli; coffees 1/2d, programme 1/-. My BP, 180/105; have increased dose of Methyldopa to 250 mgm, three times a day. Albumen++.

Dec 13   To Friths, with M., to select carpets for house. Thence, to Jackson's the Tailor; measured for lounge suit, dinnersuit and overcoat, and purchased 2 pairs of shoes at Dolcis, £7.10s.4d. St. John St., 4 cases. Afterwards, swotted up parts of talk for tonight, and so to Central Library at 7.0 p.m. for talk (by me) on 'Some Recollections of Thirty Years of Book-Collecting'.

[*On hereditary predisposition*] '. . . There might have been a hereditary predisposition in me to make me want to collect things; one of my grandmothers collected old silver, my brother collected stamps and still does, an uncle collected rugs and old china, and one of my favourite cousins collected match-boxes . . .'

[*On his purposes*] '. . . But I also realised when I qualified as a doctor, at the early age of 21, that there was a danger of becoming too preoccupied with my work; that unlike doctors of the past, who lived in a more leisurely age, our generation of medical men mistakenly tended to be unappreciative of literature, the arts, travel and conversation. I set out from the start to broaden my outlook and to learn as much as I could about the beautiful world we live in, and the way in which people have expressed themselves, not only scientifically, but spiritually, through literature and the fine arts. I wanted to occupy my mind, and in my earliest days would forego a meal to afford a book . . .'

[*On dukes, plebeians*] '. . . One hundred years ago, if every book-collector was neither a duke nor a prince, no duke or prince worthy of his name was not a book-collector. As P.H. Muir says, Debrett was almost a ready-made address-list for the antiquarian bookseller. Now, we plebeians have come into the arena . . .'

I told them of mistakes booksellers have made, and mistakes I have made – like passing up Newton's *Principia* for £100; described booksellers I have known, like J.D. Hughes [*original partner in Sherratt and Hughes*], who, when I was ill with a coronary, gave me a first edition of Boswell's *Life of Johnson*; and showed them my Laennec, a Spanish mediaeval manuscript with faked pages, and the *Book of Revelation*. At the end, I said that if bibliophiles are an "idiotic class", as A.E. Housman put it – and we are usually harmless – some of the visitors to my Library are no less so. Some will say, "Have you read all these books?", and others, looking at my shelves, will suddenly declare "You collect old books". "No, old boots", I tell them. Vote of thanks, and adjourned to 'The Wyvern' for alcoholic session.

Dec 15 [*Saturday*]   Read Sacheverell Sitwell article on Paris, and in *BMJ* on 'Emergency Resuscitation' by

Professor Gordon Wyant; he was once my house physician (and married a nurse). Discussion in press on 'Why did the Allies refuse to bomb Auschwitz?'. The answer, to me, is obvious. Talks in Paris between Macmillan and de Gaulle, the latter's moment of triumph. Severe gales today, with winds of up to 90 miles an hour; much havoc wrought to Xmas decorations and trees in London, and other towns. Watched the fourth edition of 'That Was The Week That Was'; much watered down in the face of critics.

Dec 16　　Charles Laughton, aet 63, died in Hollywood. John Steinbeck, aet 60, gives interview about himself in today's papers. Ignominious political situation in Britain, Macmillan greatly discredited and Conservative Party in the doldrums; 'Edwardian posturings on ancestral grouse moors', Harold Wilson's description of him. Listened to Bayreuth recording of *Götterdämmerung* on radio, and began to read *King Lear* for the first time.

Dec 17　　Letter of apology to Matron for not coming to Annual Ball, £3 to Dr. C. for Nurses' Party, £5.5s.od. to Dr. V. for Residents' Xmas Gifts. Ward 7, round, and Boots' gift token to Sister A., £1.1s.od; Wards 14 and 15. Purchased gin, sherry and orange juice, £3.3s.od. St. John St., one case, two failed to attend. Party at home, 8.30 p.m., eleven guests. Stupid invasion of Library, instigated by Bill H., to see books; chaos and confusion. David rang. He has no friends, and nowhere to turn except to us, whom he has spurned for so many years. Continued to read *King Lear*, when everyone had gone.

Dec 18　　To St. John St.; 2 cases, one of whom gave me a bottle of whisky and Coty perfume. Posted a further 20 cards this evening, approaching one hundred; Xmas a racket.

Dec 19　　To Arnfields; received box of 25 Havanas (Romeo and Juliet, Corona Size), from E.G.T. [*managing director*]. Whilst at the factory examined a girl who said 'my nose was scraped for cyanide trouble'. Went to Woods Hospital, Glossop with Dr. F. and did full ward rounds; saw Mrs. W., who preferred to stay in Hospital over Xmas, since she is not wanted by her daughter. St. John St., 3 cases. M. phoned, God bless and protect her. This evening went over some pictures: probably a Gainsborough sketch, and perhaps a Dutch old master drawing. Also a manuscript in contemporary Elizabethan hand describing the Globe Theatre, with a careful drawing. Must explore its value.

Dec 20   Mrs. L. [*see Nov 5*] died yesterday, aged 64. Incoherent letter from Max S. [*brother-in-law, N.Y.*]. It was in reply to mine, and my criticism of his hostile remarks about David. A spirit of amity, however, persists. Purchased further Boots' tokens for Xmas gifts, and deposited £115.10s.0d. in cheques. Saw Dr. D., and gave him a photograph I took of his father in Crete: the last that was taken of him. Thence, to two domiciliaries: uncontrolled diabetic, with diarrhoea (aet 68, Hyde, admitted into private ward, paid 10 guineas); broncho-pneumonia, *in extremis* (aet 68, Denton, unfit to move). Thence to St. John St., 2 cases.

3:30 p.m. [*Male, aged 56, nursery representative*] He was having a week's holiday with his wife in Bournemouth – where he had gone by coach – in late September/early October this year. Coming down the stairs of the hotel on the last morning, at 7.0 a.m., he had reached the top stair of the second flight when he caught his right shoe in the 'loop of a loose rubber thread' at the edge of the stair, and 'somersaulted down 12 stairs to the landing below'; he said that he 'finished up' with his feet against the wall, and his arms 'up in the air in a U-shape'. He said that he lay 'winded' on the floor for 'about ten minutes', with people afraid to lift him, according to his account, for fear that he had 'broken something'. (He hadn't). However, he was eventually 'helped up to a chair' and a doctor summoned, who pronounced him fit for the return coach journey. When he got back home at 6.0 p.m., 'I felt sore', he said, 'got undressed, and my wife checked me over', though nothing was visible at this examination. In the morning, he visited his doctor, whom he claims told him that 'the shock had not come out' and advised a few days rest. Two days later, he 'started with' a painful attack of shingles round the waist and into the left groin, and was off work for a month. (He also claimed to have had 'angina two years ago', to have had no symptoms since, but to be taking Peritrate tablets – for the angina which he does not have – twice a day.) During this time he consulted solicitors and issued a claim for damages against the hotel. He was a healthy-looking, well-built man with satisfactory blood pressure (150/100), a regular pulse, no abnormalities in his back and shoulders, a sound heart and half a dozen spots on the lower lumbar region and over the left thigh, which were the residuum of the attack of shingles. In fact, I could find nothing at all the matter with him, nor could I attribute the shingles, painful as may be, to his unfortunate somersault down a staircase. The two events were fortuitous, and cannot be medically connected for the purpose of litigation. The claim is idiotic.

£3.3s.0d. to Miss James, as Xmas gift. Her friend, Miss G.H., had bought me an azalea. A further 16 cards dispatched. Listened to very fine *Carmen* on television, produced by Rudolph Cartier, with Rosalind Elias (aet 28, from the Lebanon) as Carmen, Raymond Nillson (Australian) as Don Jose, and John Shirley-Quirk as Escamillo. Macmillan and Kennedy meet in the Bahamas; Skybolt scrapped.

Dec 21   Destructive criticism of yesterday's 'Carmen', by Philip Hope-Wallace in the *Guardian*. An avalanche of cards received. After lunch, called to Dr. Y. [*house physician*] in her room; vomiting. Medical out-patients sheer chaos, including case of chronic lymphatic leukaemia. Thereafter, very dreary Xmas party in Out-patients dept., and home at 6.20. Drs. C. and E. [*house physicians*] to dinner. Mrs. L.'s funeral [*see Dec 20*] took place today. Read *King Lear* again tonight.

Dec 22 [*Saturday*]   Xmas cards still coming in. Unable to get to hospital, because of dense fog. Twenty-four football matches cancelled or abandoned. Read in bed, including newspaper article on the persecution of Bahai's in Morocco; three sentenced to death because of their religion. Watched

'That Was The Week That Was', sometimes tedious.

Dec 23   More cards. The second restful day in succession without dressing, shaving or going out; M. sympathetic. Read *Observer* and *Sunday Times*; but it all escapes almost immediately unless written down *statim*. Editorials on Kennedy–Macmillan meeting at Nassau; discontent in Conservative Party; must get Alison Lurie, *Love and Friendship*, first novel, recommended by Atticus. Phoned David; it was Hazel's birthday yesterday. Began Swift's *Gulliver's Travels*, in the unexpurgated Nonesuch Press edition.

Dec 24   News: the return of 1100 American prisoners from Cuba for a ransom of 17 million dollars' worth of food and medicines, and very large Xmas turkeys on sale at Smithfield for 45/-.

Dec 25 [*Christmas Day*]   Dressing-gown day like Sunday [*Dec 23*], did not go out, much too frosty and cold. Expected in hospital for party, but thought better of it; will leave the residents to their own joys and devices. 25 road-deaths last night, higher than last year, heavy drinking doubtless a cause in many cases. Read *Bart's Hospital Journal* for Nov 1962, Dr. Robert Pitt's *Letters to John Locke* (revealing the quackery of the times), and an appreciation of Gerard Manley Hopkins, priest and poet. Also a useful review of a new book by W.B. Jennett on *Epilepsy after Head Injuries*, which establishes that the likelihood of developing late epilepsy, and *status epilepticus*, is four times as great with those who suffer a first fit within 24 hours of the trauma, than those whose fit occurs after a longer interval. Dr. F. phoned this evening about the day's events in hospital: 6 admissions, one diabetic coma, three private patients better, and Dr. M. dead drunk.

Dec 26   Snow and icy roads; a white Boxing Day. Must get away, if possible, next year. Did morning shopping for M., and proceeded to hospital on slippery roads, with car trouble from no anti-freeze; overheating, with hell of a smell. Repairs carried out at garage by a fellow-customer, who spent 1½ hours removing my dynamo, banging in loose core, and filling with anti-freeze. Proceeded on my way to Ward rounds. Saw Dr. D.; the 40 mourning days for his father are over. Gifts to Sisters will be cut down next year, and Xmas cards to fellow-consultants who never reply. Drs. M., S. and F. have bought me some lousy cigars, which I hope to turn in at the cigar merchants, for fewer but better ones. Drove home in descending fog on glassy roads, like the end of the world. To the Goldings [*friends*] for tea; they were discussing the Marquis de Sade's *Justine*, not worth reading or even handling. Thence to Ruth and Geoffrey; he gave me two packets of sword-edge razor blades. Railway accident north of Crewe: 17 killed and 60 injured, so far as is known. Watched film on the life of Henri de Toulouse-Lautrec.

Dec 27 Woke up late; frosty. Ward round and domiciliary: cerebral thrombosis (aet 62, Denton, admitted). St. John St., 4 cases, including blimp with obesity and hypertension. To Lodge meeting, proposed health of Worshipful Master – my speech called a 'masterpiece' – and home by 10 p.m. A hard frost tonight.

Dec 28 Misery, no let up in the weather, but proceeded to four domiciliaries: right lobar pneumonia (aet 67, Audenshaw, admitted); congestive heart failure, mitral stenosis, had to get in through back of house when no one answered (aet 56, Audenshaw, for investigation); chronic emphysema, bronchitis and angina pectoris (aet 62, Ashton, to be admitted), and cerebral thrombosis (aet 49, Ashton, to be admitted in a few days). Ward 12, round in full; Mr. W.E. has active senile TB, to be transferred. Medical out-patients, including post-traumatic epilepsy. My BP, 155/95. News tonight included revelations of secret despatches between Edward VIII and Duke of Coburg, revealing Nazi sympathies of the Royal Scoundrel; admired Cassandra's attack on the wretch in the *Daily Mirror*.

Dec 29 [*Saturday*] Rested as much as possible; appalling weather. Read *BMJ* on Senile Tubercle. Went through some of my books, etc: *Ballad of Reading Gaol* by 'C.33' (1898), original letters by Harrison Ainsworth, a photograph of Charles Dickens with letter by his son attesting the true likeness thereof, a Charles the First binding, some juvenilia of interest, and an original sketch by Thackeray illustrating *Vanity Fair*. Thrilling stuff. Judy has gone out for the evening; M. and I feel very much alone in the large house. Watched 'That Was The Year That Was'; Millicent Martin fascinating, but the sting seems to have gone out of the satire.

Dec 30　　Bitterly cold, with snow; drifts 20 feet deep in Devon and Cornwall. To domiciliary, in icy conditions: bronchogenic carcinoma (aet 66, Stalybridge, admitted). Have done 50 domiciliaries this Quarter, in spite of absence in October. Proceeded to very good sherry party at hospital, Dr. F. the host: spoke to Drs. C. and G. and sundry Sisters. Heard that Dr. A. [*neuro-surgeon*] is giving up medicine and going to the Bar. Thereafter, visited the Wards; have four Private patients simultaneously for the first time ever. Home at 3.30 p.m.; Judy has tantrums and in an aggressive mood, on hearing that Bessie G. has got a place at the University of London. She lacks confidence in herself, but I have faith in my little Judy. She should do well, but is immature and intimidated easily by extraneous factors. Watched a lot of rubbish about pop singers on ITV. Have taken four Methyl-dopas today; cannot resist desire to lower my BP to reasonable figures. Have had a full and hectic year, full of interest but with many distressing features, including David's marriage, which has hurt us, and the realization of others' mercenary motives. God bless M. and protect her; her health and vigour have deteriorated as a result of David's action. Insomnia.

Dec 31　　Horribly cold and gloomy. Ward round, 7, and Wards 12, 14, 15 completed; saw R.D. [*private patient*], holding on. To Uppermill, near Oldham, for private call: cerebral thrombosis (aet 76, admitted unconscious). Thence, to St. John St., one case only, aet 51, a bad neurotic. Blizzard unabated, the country snowbound. M. and Judy went to bed early. Watched old film of the Marx Brothers, 'A Night in Casablanca', and read book catalogues into the New Year.

1963

Jan 1   David, snowbound, telephoned. Has been celebrating the New Year with Hazel; M. took over phone with altercations etc. Proceeded in biting cold wind to Hyde, and called on the Livingstones. They have their problems with their daughters; their youngest, aet 16, returned at 3.30 a.m. Called on Mary S. [*friend*]; observation of varicose veins of great severity. Thence to St. John St., snow falling, place deserted. Watched discussion on TV about the Honours System with Lord Boothby. He loves this poppycock; they should be totally abolished.

Jan 2   Still snowing, but worse in Scotland and the South of England. In blizzard to domiciliary visits: bronchial pneumonia, cor pulmonale (aet 72, Lower Openshaw, admitted); diabetic coma, cerebral vascular lesion (aet 80, Ashton, too ill to move). Two cases in St. John St., and home by 4.30 p.m. Sam D. [*friend*] has got an OBE. He deserves it.

Jan 3   Winter worsening. M., restless, woke me at 3.20 a.m. To domiciliary visit: damned neurotic (aet 64, Hyde); trailed to see her in heavy snow, but nothing the matter.

Jan 4   Will restrict protein intake. Medical outpatients, and thence to domiciliary visit: congenital syphilis, nose absent, cor pulmonale with intense cyanosis, *in extremis* (aet 63, Denton, admitted). Home in heavy traffic, slush and squalor.

Jan 5 [*Saturday*]   Day of rest. Read a great deal,

including 'Reflections on Ageing and Death', by Sir Robert Platt in today's *Lancet*, and *The Dream of the Red Chamber* by Tsao Hsueh Chin, a Chinese novel of the Early Ching period, first published in 1791. The narrative covers the period 1729–1737. Interrupted by arrival of washing-machine service-mechanic, who appeared after ten days of phone-calls; his manner lazy and casual, his appearance unprepossessing. Examples of this kind of British workman are multiplying, indifferent to threats of loss of custom. Imagine the wail of lamentation which would go up from the darling public if a doctor had to be called three times, without avail, in an emergency. In the train disaster on Boxing Day, the driver had ignored the danger signal, and telephone messages for help were not transmitted! The Welfare State is to blame for this decadence in the will and spirit of the people.

Jan 6   Have very bad cold. Made breakfast for M. and rested through the morning. Ruth, Geoffrey and Jonathan came for tea; Geoffrey asked me how I was, for the first time since his return from the USA. Thence to the Sassoons' [*friends*] engagement party at the Steele Hall: I consumed too much food and had too much alcohol for my complaint. Chatted to many people whom I did not know, but who claimed friendship with me. Home very exhausted. News: 2,300 passengers from P. and O. vessel 'Canberra' stranded in Malta because of electrical defect, giant airlift attempted; shocking conditions on St. Helena exposed, poverty, dirt, maladministration and poor medical services; Hugh Gaitskell ill, and in the Middlesex Hospital.

Jan 7   Very bad cold. Hesitated as to whether I should set out for the hospital, but decided to go because of pressure of work. Called en route on R.J.T. [*managing director of small local engineering firm*]; he will make a profit this year, but has had to sack 100 of 200 employees. St. John St., 2 cases.

3:0 p.m. [*Male, aged 58, bachelor, labourer*] He was a pleasant and friendly Irishman, tall and of slender build, who walked with a slight stoop. Three and a half years ago he was about to climb out of a trench 5 feet deep, when he was caught between the rear of an excavator, which struck him forcibly in the back, and the steel piles of the trench. He was not kept in hospital, suffered no fractures (he says), but spent a month 'in bed' at home with 'chest and back' pains, and was off work for a further eight months thereafter. (During this time he commenced proceedings against his former employers, but he was very hazy about everything concerning dates, times, names and other details). When he resumed work, he got a light labouring job 'pointing kerbs' with a firm of builders, but was 'paid off' on Dec 28 last. Today, he complained that he has had 'constipation of the bowels' since his accident 3½ years ago, and that his 'water' was 'not as free as it used to be'. He also has pains in his chest, has to sleep on his right side, his 'nerves' are 'bad', etc. etc. He told me that he smokes 20 cigarettes a day, and has 'an occasional pint of beer'.

I could not find much wrong with him, though he was thin-chested and had a few bronchitic sounds in his lungs, as one would expect at his age and given his heavy smoking. Forward movement of his spine was of full range, but backward movement was not quite complete. His pulse was normal, and his BP (140/90) excellent. He must have had a fright at the time of the accident, but his alleged constipation and urinary difficulties – the latter not unusual in men of his age – cannot be attributed to it.

His real problem is that at his age and with the present degree of unemployment it may be difficult for him to find a job. There was also an element of post-accident neurosis in his performance. When he is 'near an excavator', he said today, he goes 'all of a tremble'. As he was leaving, he announced that he was going off tonight for a 5-week holiday in County Mayo.

Jan 8 Bad cold still and nocturia. Did not want to go to Hospital today; phoned Dr. F. and cancelled morning visit. Called at travel agents for information on Pakistan, and purchased 'James Morris in Australia' [*see Sept 27 1962*], a *Guardian* pamphlet, 2/-. To Masonic Temple, for lodge committee meeting, and thereafter to St. John St., 2 cases.

3:0 p.m. [*Female, aged 21, single, secretary*] She was a healthy-looking, athletic girl, alert and intelligent, who was knocked off her Vespa by a passing car three and a half months ago, while she was on her way to work. She was thrown into the roadway, and was assisted into a nearby shop by a passer-by and the car-driver; she rested there for ten minutes and was then taken to hospital by the man who had knocked her down. She was X-rayed, not told the findings, and taken home by ambulance. Her own doctor told her to rest, gave her vitamins for a week, and allegedly advised her to 'warm her back in front of the electric fire tor ten minutes before going to bed'. She has not worked since the accident. Today, she said she had a constant pain over a wide area of the small of the back, and especially in 'the groove of the buttocks, at the top'. She also said that she 'cannot sit on a hard seat for long', and has had some tingling and numbness of the legs. On examination, the main tenderness was over the sacrum, especially over the right sacro-iliac region. She showed many features of a strain of the aponeurosis, or the muscle sheaths and ligaments over the right sacro-iliac joint, and I was inclined to the view that her pain was genuine. That is, she fell on her backside and has coccydinia.

Summoned urgently to two domiciliaries: congestive heart failure, auricular fibrillation (aet 71, Ashton, admitted), and broncho-pneumonia (aet 66, Ashton, admitted). Magnificent account of the History of Nice, Monaco and the Riviera on BBC TV, with Baroness Agnes de Stakhel.

Jan 10   Second breakfast at hospital, with Dr. A. Full Ward rounds 7, 14, 15; there are eighteen medical cases of mine in Ward 15. Sister N. collapses in Orthopaedic Dept. I was summoned to see her; nil abnormal found. Thence to Woods Hospital, Glossop, for Ward round: a lovely place in the snow. I would like to live in Glossop. Proceeded to St. John St. in dark, cold, dismal weather; one case only, two cancelled. Looked at book sent to me called *Strong Medicine*, on obesity and heart disease; an irritating medical potboiler.

Jan 11   The coldest night for 82 years. Judy has been

offered a place at Nottingham, gratifying for us in the midst of our anxieties, but what pains or pleasures can we expect from it? Kindled light as a memorial to my dear father of blessed memory. Thence, to Anti-coagulant clinic, not hard pressed; Ward 12 (full round), and Follow-up clinic. Lunch at 'The Organ'; the proprietress informs me that her life is in danger from a man who has been molesting her for four years! Advised her to see a lawyer. Medical out-patients finished late; brought Dr. D. and Dr. G. [*Indian house-physician*] home to dinner. Played Greek and Indian gramophone records for them, and then took them to catch bus; altercation with bus-driver, who had begun to move off though he could see them approaching.

Jan 12 [*Saturday*]   The seventeenth day of deep freeze in the British Isles. Remained at home all day, chiefly at rest. Studied Vol 59 of the *Book Auction Records*, and read Carlton on Timothie Brighte (1550–1615), Bart's physician, an inventor of shorthand and author of *A Treatise on Melancholie* (1586). 'That Was the Week That Was' very good tonight, but blasphemous effort by David Frost on comparative religion.

Jan 13   Very drowsy; temperature minus 8°C in Manchester, astonishing frost pattern on the trees in the garden. Read interesting articles in *Sunday Times*, including on the gulf between parents and their adolescent children, and a review by Cyril Connolly of a new book on Von Humboldt, the scientist and explorer who inspired Charles Darwin. Had to look up 'obreptitious' in Shorter Oxford Dictionary = 'containing a false statement for the sake of obtaining something'.

Jan 14   At lunch, Mrs. F. [*gynaecologist*] rude and verbose. Her tongue runs away with her in a neurotic sort of way. Home at 5.30 p.m. Judy expresses her hatred of Judaism, and declares her agnosticism. Am pained at her declaration, and M. depressed thereby. 'Panorama': Sir Edward Boyle interviewed on education, old school buildings and shortage of teachers; Lord Gladwyn and William Pickles, L.S.E., for and against Common Market. De Gaulle has made a speech today against British entry into the Common Market, and rejected Kennedy's offer of Polaris.

Jan 15   Disturbed night. Slight thaw, but still bitterly cold. M.'s birthday today, a somewhat conjectural date, but God bless her in any case. Card from David, somewhat formal. Arrived at Anti-coagulant clinic at its completion, Dr. F. having taken over. My Prothrombin time 12 secs = 100%; blood urea, by finger-prick method, 43 mgm%. Ward Rounds 7, 12 and 15. Talk to Matron, anxious about her 3 stones' loss in weight. Attended Medical Advisory Committee meeting to discuss power cuts. Snow crisp on the ground.

Jan 16   Wards 11 and 15; talked to Dr. F. about his wife's irresponsible verbosity. St. John St., one case. Home early, and further altercation with Judy about a forthcoming interview. She is intensely rude to me; I will put it down to her being edgy and apprehensive, but I am in serious doubt whether she merits further education at my expense (cf. David). Hugh Gaitskell seriously ill, in mortal danger. Virus infection, we are told.

Jan 17   Disturbed night, depressed and suffering from insomnia; had not taken Methyldopa, which usually acts as a soporific. No intention of going to hospital today. Left house at 11.0 a.m.; bitterly cold, Arctic conditions, biting wind, appalling. To St. John St., for letters; found that Miss James had failed, as usual, to give me messages before Xmas. Thence to tailors for fitting, and Sherratt and Hughes. Purchased Marie Renault's *The King Must Die*, about Crete and Knossos, and a signed copy of Lawrence Durrell's *Alexandria Quartet*, number 130 of 500 signed copies. Compton Mackenzie is 80 today, and declares that the secret of longevity is to sit instead of standing, to ride instead of walking, and to avoid physical exercise, especially golf. I am inclined to agree. Artificial kidney to be used on Mr. Gaitskell, who is deteriorating rapidly.

Jan 18   Encountered E.E., who talked about his work as a magistrate. Told him that I have observed in the last year or two, from their names, that many of the local juvenile delinquents have parents who were once my patients when I first came to the district. Thence to domiciliary visits: coronary thrombosis (aet 58, Stalybridge, ECG taken, admitted); cardiac asthma and congestive heart failure (aet 64, Denton, admitted). In Stalybridge, saw H.J. [*former patient*]; he has aged, but I was glad to see him. Ward round, 15, in full and Medical out-patients until 6.0 p.m. Watched BBC film on Abu Simbel. Afterwards, while 9.15 p.m. news was being read by Robert Dougall, an announcement was made of the sad death of Hugh Gaitskell; a lamentable end to a promising career, and the probable next Prime Minister.

Jan 19 [*Saturday*]   Arctic conditions. Made breakfast for M. and spent restful day reading Levine, *Cardiac Disease and Trauma*, my diary of recent visit to Rhodes and Crete, and obituaries of poor Gaitskell in the *Guardian*. The freeze-up ever worse, extreme cold and snow, with roads blocked and gross disorganization of all forms of transport; the sea frozen for 5 miles out of Dunkirk, M.1 blocked, etc. etc. Have decided to cut out Tuesdays in St. John St. in future. Will notify Miss James on Monday [*Jan 21*], and will begin to take things easier. It is essential to live a bit longer and see the world with my dear wife, whilst we are still together. The children have disappointed us after all our efforts to educate them. Besides giving up Tuesdays, I may also give up Thursdays and domiciliary visits later on. We shall see. On TV, broadcast by Prime Minister of tribute to Gaitskell; Bernard Levin excellent on the subject in 'That Was the Week That Was'; George Brown and Wilson have made statements wrapped in sinister hypocrisy.

Jan 20   Visited S.P. [*dentist*]. He is depressed with his dental work, and hates it: hard work, and little return for his efforts. Six guests to tea, including Prof. Lipson, F.R.S.; showed my library to him. Watched 'Monitor': poems read by Yevtushenko, the Russian poet, 'Babi Yar' and others.

Jan 21   M. left for London with Judy, for her interview with Professor Cobban at King's College. Roads icy and full of snow; called at garage and gave cigars to foreman. Ward rounds, 14 and 15, in full; Mrs. C. [*private patient*] has slight relapse. St. John St., one case; have cancelled Tuesdays for the next few weeks [*cf Jan 19 1962*]. Home by 4 p.m., in heavy snow, with drifts, and no let up. House very silent. Today, 3 Methyldopas and one Saluric taken. Intended to have a quiet evening sitting peacefully, but Hans S. [*friend and patient*] came for a check-up. Thereafter, numerous phone-calls; Dr. F. telephoned for good measure. Took another Saluric, 0.5 gms, and 10 mgm Guanethidine. M. phoned on arrival in London at midnight, after eight-hour train journey. Went to sleep, reassured they were safe.

Jan 22   Rose at 8.0 a.m. and read the *Guardian*, after making myself some dilute coffee. The house very lonely without my dear M. and Judy. Left at 10.30, having decided not to do the Anti-coagulant clinic; there were only 19 cases I was told later. To domiciliary visit: congestive heart failure, in cold icy room (aet 67, Hyde, admitted). Bright sunshine, roads slippery, but slightly warmer. Ward 12, full round; a woman with multiple sclerosis has been found to have a bronchogenic carcinoma also. Home by 4.0 p.m., to calls of domestic interest. David phoned; I feel deeply sorry for him. He told me about a fellow called Booth at Hay-on-Wye, who has an antiquarian book collection worth inspecting. After six o'clock news, left for Lodge meeting. Departed early, after Worshipful Master's speech, and was pleasantly surprised to find M. and Judy back from London.

Jan 23   Made breakfast for M., and proceeded to domiciliary visit: arthropathy and rash (aet, 22, Hyde, admitted, case for diagnosis). Thereafter, to hospital; my BP, 155/95. After lunch, to St. John St., 3 cases.

3:0 p.m. [*Male, aged 22, joiner*] He was a healthy young man, of short stature, who told me that he plays rugger and does weight-lifting. Three months ago the back of his bicycle was struck by a lorry; he 'woke up on the side of the road' and has no recollection of the impact, but thought he had been knocked out for '2 or 3 minutes'. Two stitches were inserted in a small laceration over his right eyebrow, he was not detained in hospital, and no X-rays were taken. Thereafter, however, he was off work for 4 weeks and 2 days, getting weekly certificates from his doctor because, he explained, his 'back was aching' and he 'couldn't move in bed'. When I asked the young man what his GP had done during these weekly visits to the surgery, he replied that the doctor had put a stethoscope to his chest, asked him if he had headaches, issued a certificate, and gave him no treatment. (None was needed). I regard the absence from work for over a month of an active and fit rugger-playing weight-lifter of 22, after a trivial accident in which he was knocked out for a couple of minutes, as excessive. It should not have upset him for more than three or four days at the most. The case disturbs me.

Home by 5.0 p.m. Colder and colder, −18°C. Sea frozen, the Mersey frozen, ice floes, fog and chaos. Cuts in power: gas and electricity. Hugh Gaitskell's funeral today, cremated.

Jan 24   Domiciliary visit: congestive heart failure (aet 61, Denton, admitted). To hospital; discussed ward cases with Dr. F., and reprimanded Sister G. for not walking round with me. One of Dr. V.'s cases, a woman of 34 on steroids for asthma, and who had a hip operation a few days ago for an alleged abscess in the joint, has died. Thereafter, to domiciliary: angina of effort (aet 54, Ashton). No cases at St. John St., home early. Tonight's news: 814,000 unemployed.

Jan 25   Forty patients in Anti-coagulant clinic; my blood urea 40 mgm%, had to be done twice due to error in tube solutions. Medical out-patients, and thence to domiciliary in Hadfield, Derbyshire; myxoedematous coma (aet 67, admitted). The village was isolated and the patient's street steep, with huge banks of snow on either side of it, but a thaw is slowly setting in.

Jan 26 [*Saturday*]   Restful day. Began to prepare

collection of Restoration Plays for disposal to Michael Papantoniou. It is a wrench to part with them, but it is better for me to dispose of them whilst I am alive than that they should be frittered away, lost, damaged, or stolen. M. would not appreciate or understand their value, and would be imposed upon easily by unscrupulous booksellers. Men like Kenneth Maggs and Percy Dobell [*London antiquarian booksellers*] are with us no more, alas. They were pillars of integrity.

Jan 27   Read the papers, and made further attempt to tidy up the library and improve on chaotic situation. Many wonderful books unearthed, which will keep me happy for quite a time. M. phoned David; his loyalty to his wife is a point worthy of note. She is alleged to be writing to me. Thaw has continued, temperatures rising; the floodwaters also.

Jan 28   Could not sleep; Saluric caused nocturia, three times. To Mrs. K., Dukinfield; ring removed, gave her Xmas present and had coffee. Ward round 12 (females), in full, and thereafter to four domiciliaries. St. John Street, 2 cases. Miss Miller [*secretary*] came for filing, and much rubbish, including some old reports, was discarded. Home by 6.0 p.m., but called out urgently to private case in Ashton of another broncho-pneumonia, right base chiefly, paid 12 guineas, admitted. Returned home exhausted, and entered this Journal; cannot delay it.

Jan 29   Rather lame letter from Hazel this morning, with effort at apology for past ill-humour, but intend to ignore it. Electricity account astronomic, £20.15s.4d. To Mrs. K., Dukinfield, ring reintroduced, £1.11s.6d., and anti-coagulant clinic. Thereafter, to casualty dept., where Miss Miller's father has been brought in with a broken humerus. Ward rounds, 14 and 15; saw R.H. [*private patient*], a neurotic with angina. Dr. D. gave me a picture of his parents taken with us in Crete, with small note from his mother. Talk to Mr. C. [*consultant surgeon*] about David and our grief. Home by 4.0 p.m.; wonderful not to have afternoon at St. John Street. Maurice G.'s [*friend*] sister-in-law commits suicide, a young woman.

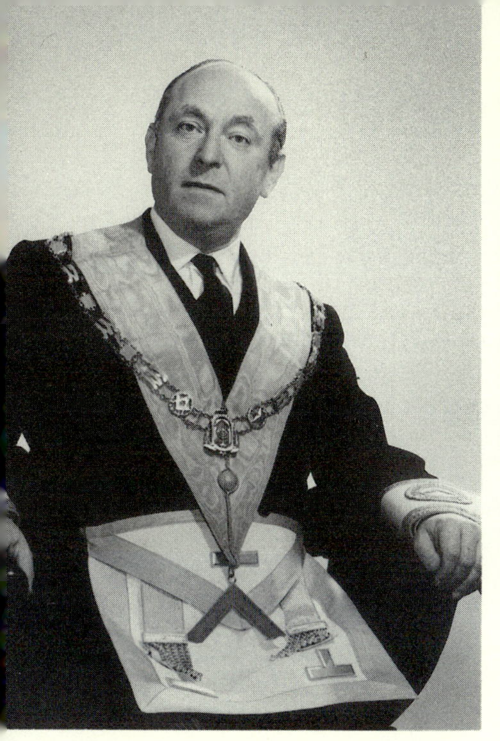

Worshipful Master of his
Masonic Lodge

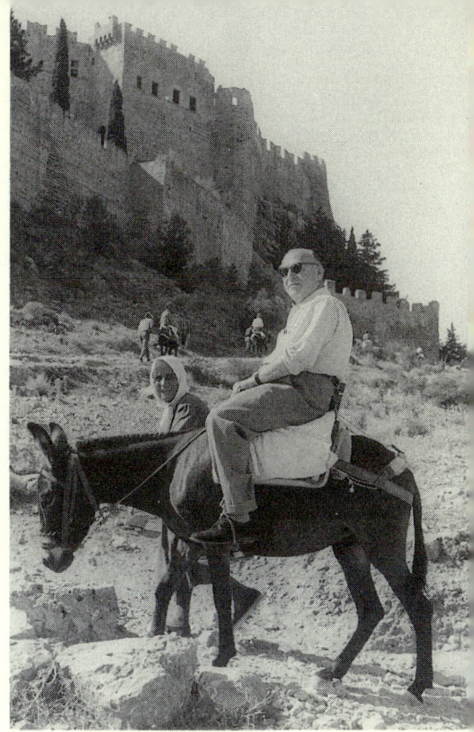

In Lindos, Rhodes,
October 1962

Dining with 'M.' in Manchester

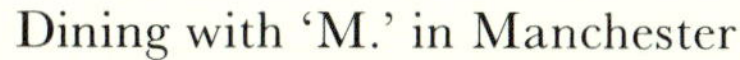

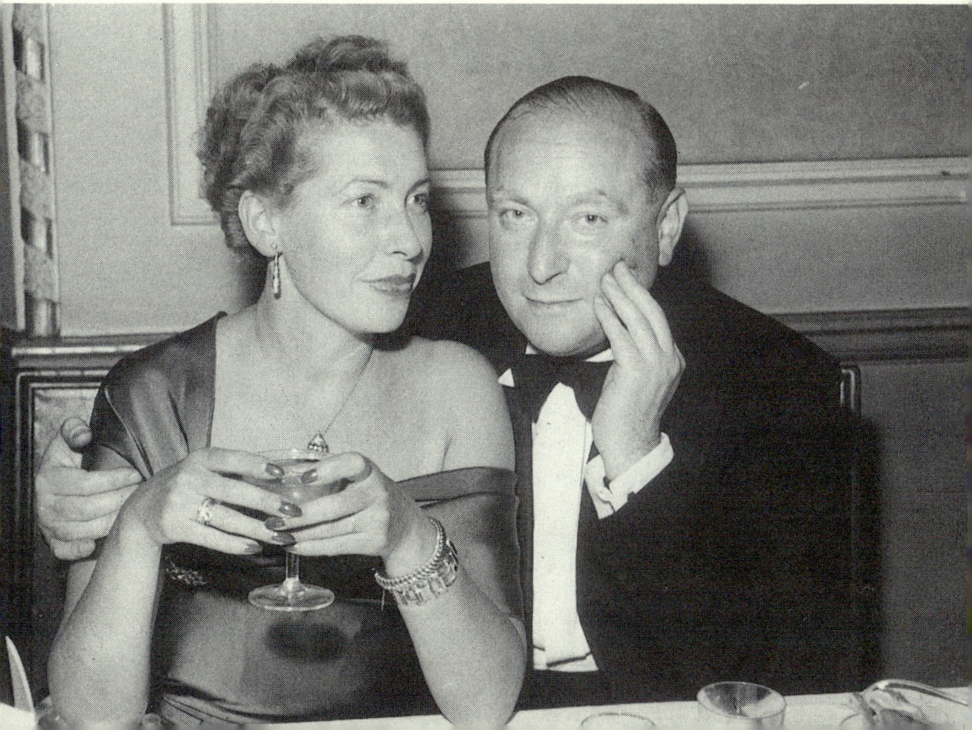

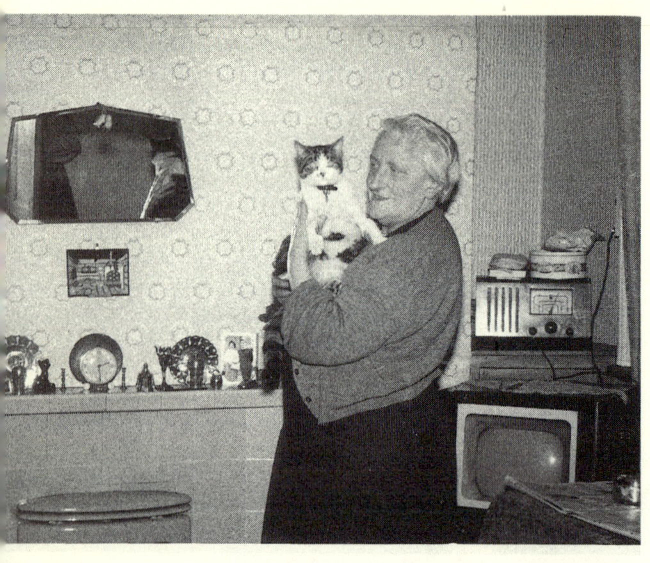
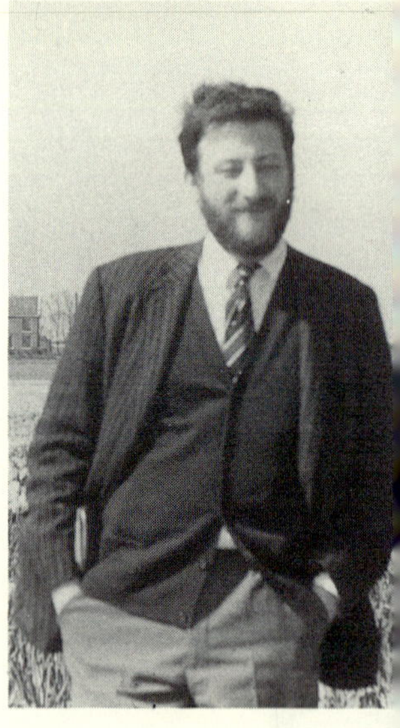

Above Miss James, receptionist and factotum at St John's Street, Manchester, 1962 and, *right*, David Selbourne, early 1964

Uncertain relations: Judy, 'M.' and Hazel in 1964

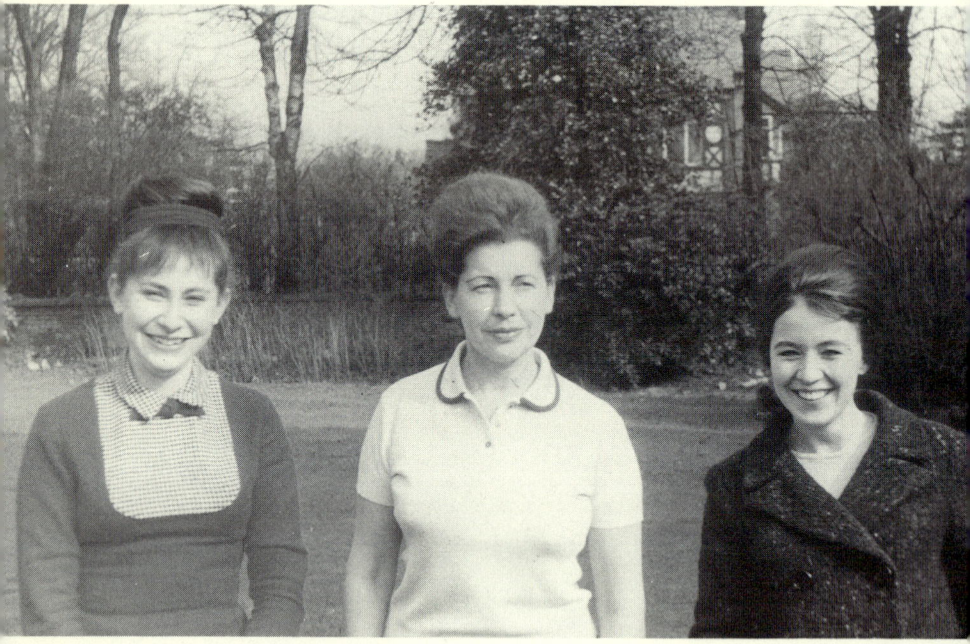

Jan 30   Out of the Common Market for the time being; De Gaulle does not want Britain in. St. John Street, 2 cases.

3:30 p.m. [*Male, aged 42, electrician's mate*] He was on the night-shift at about 2.30 a.m., eight months ago, when he was struck on the forehead by the balance-weight of an overhead crane. He says that he was 'knocked dizzy', saw a 'lot of spots' before the eyes and fell to the ground, but was not unconscious. He was then 'picked off the ground', with his right forehead bleeding, taken to the First Aid room where a dressing was applied and from there to hospital, where three stitches were inserted in the laceration. Next morning his skull was X-rayed, but this revealed no fracture. He was off work for a month with headaches, but has 'kept up' since. Today, he told me that he still has 'sickly headaches' over the right forehead, which 'come on at any time'. 'I have no idea what brings them on', he told me, 'the cold weather could do it'. These headaches, in his account, last 'about 20 minutes', they do not radiate, and they are 'not improving'; 'I've got one now', he added for good measure. He was a well-built man, depressed in appearance and somewhat humourless, who had an almost invisible ½" scar close to the hair margin over the right forehead. There was no tremor of his hands, his pulse, blood pressure and reflexes were normal and co-ordination tests, optic discs and cranial nerves were also normal. I could find nothing much the matter with him. His headaches are essentially subjective. He was a miserable looking fellow.

When I rang the uncouth solicitor in this case, he did not talk to me but put his secretary on to take the message. Real ethics!

Jan 31   Judy gets into King's College, London. God bless her. Regional Hospital Board pay slip, gross £519.14s.1d.; basic salary £273.17s.9d., plus £210 for domiciliaries and £23.4s.4d. travel allowance, less deductions including £148.18s.3d. income tax = £370.15s.10d. Watched fine programme, 'This Week' (ITV), on 'The Common Market Failure'; interview with Lord Home, Foreign Secretary, and talk by A.J.P. Taylor, the acid Oxford historian.

Feb 1   Heavy snow. To domiciliary: coronary thrombosis, congestive heart failure (aet 58, Denton, admitted). Thereafter, in very bad weather, to Anti-coagulant clinic. Full ward round, 12; paper round, Ward 15. After lunch (3/6), to further domiciliary: pneumonia (aet 38, Ashton, to be admitted if worse). Thence, back to hospital for Medical out-patients, including an incoherent and lachrymose Yugoslav, who complained of '18' erections daily.

Feb 3 [*Sunday*]   Read *Observer* and *Sunday Times* before lunch. Ruth gave me a knitted waistcoat she had made for me herself. Getting books ready for Michael Papantoniou. Selling the Restoration plays is like tearing out my vitals, but what alternatives have I? To keep them for my worthless son, my grasping son-in-law, or my impudent young daughter who is so rude to me at the slightest provocation?

Feb 4   To St. John St., and sorted out large mail. Thereafter, proceeded via John Dalton Street to Shaw's Bookshop, and then to Sherratt and Hughes; Mr. N. [*see March 22 1962*], a strange type, is quite unpopular in the shop. Lunch at Masonic, 14/6d; paid for 8 coffees. St. John St., 4 cases, including A.Y., a nice fellow, who called about his wife in Ward 12 (multiple sclerosis and bronchogenic carcinoma). To M., 4 weeks' pay in advance, £60. Arranged cartons of books for Michael Papantoniou, including Massinger, Wycherley, Otway, Shirley, Suckling, Chapman, Waller, Beaumont and Fletcher, George Herbert's *The Temple*, Farquhar, Habington, Colley Cibber and Milton's *Paradise Lost*.

Feb 5   Cold weather has not yet abated. Domiciliary visit: bronchial asthma, hypertension, anaemia (aet 43, Audenshaw Vicarage, admitted). Here, I was attacked by a large and lanky dog belonging to the Vicar, which made my coat and hands dirty. A stupid dog; very much winded thereby. Did not do Anti-coagulant clinic. Ward rounds, 14 and 15; 27 male medical cases. After lunch, to tailors', to try suits. One of them botched up and ruined; the dinner suit,

£18.18s.od. paid, a very slapdash job also. Will discontinue my patronage. Did not go to Consecration of new Lodge in Oldham; am getting tired of these effete and aimless performances, in which megalomaniacs saunter about with a deluded sense of their own grandeur.

Feb 6   Death of sister of Dr. Ellis [*his St. John St. landlord*] and Lord Samuel, aet 92. Ward round 12, in full; two private patients still present. No cases at St. John St. this afternoon; deliberate. To Sherratt and Hughes on foot, and thereafter to Lodge meeting. Today, noticed bullying attitude of the Police towards the public. Home by 11.15 p.m.; cant stay up late these days.

Feb 7   St. John St., 5 cases, including bookmaker for investigations, and G.H., aet 65, Miss James's friend [*see Nov 28 1962*], seen gratis.

3:0 p.m. [*Male, aged 34, engineering inspector*] He was on holiday in Italy on a motor-cycle, with his wife (a sewing machinist) sitting pillion, when a private car ran into them near the small township of Santhia, on the road from Turin to Milan. The most serious injury he suffered, together with multiple abrasions, was a burn on the outer side of the lower calf of his right leg, which came into contact with the hot exhaust pipe of his motor cycle. His wife sustained friction abrasions, a fractured bone in her right foot, lacerations to the right ankle and over the right eyebrow, and was concussed. He was deeply shocked, and she was 'flat out'; her first clear recollection was of waking up in an Italian hospital. ('I saw nuns looking at me', she said.)

While they were in hospital – as in-patients for 17 days – he developed a large ulcerated area at the site of the burn, which made an arc around the back and sides of his right leg. They returned home together by train; a skin graft was recommended to him, but he decided against it, and the leg gradually healed with regular Acriflavine dressings. Two months after the accident he returned to work; but 10 weeks later he developed an eczematous rash over the lower end of both legs, and over the area where the ulcer had been. He was readmitted to hospital and was an in-patient for 6 weeks, until three weeks ago, receiving hydrocortisone treatment. He has not returned to work. (His wife returned to work a week after getting back from Italy, but she said that for some time she had kept having the same nightmares of not being able to get help to find a train home, 'because of the language problem'). On examination, he was a healthy young man, of good type, who had a horizontal band of scar tissue, 5″ long and 2½″ broad, affecting the lower third of the right leg. It was not ulcerated, and not painful, but was covered with a bandage. It is possible that some chemical irritant produced the bout of eczema; but it is also not uncommon for a 'traumatic' dermatitis to develop after a shock or an accident, in a predisposed individual. He is fit to resume work immediately. There was no evidence of neurosis in his wife.

Feb 8   G.H., 'ovarian cyst', to be readmitted to Ward 11; informed Miss James of it.

Feb 9 [*Saturday*]   Michael Papantoniou purchased 42 choice items, including George Chapman's *Revenge of Bussy d'Ambois* (1613, first edition), which once belonged to Swinburne, Massinger's *Great Duke of Florence* (1636), Chapman and Shirley's *Tragedy of Chabot*, Goffe's *Tragedy of Orestes* (1633) bound by Rivière, Edmund Waller's *Pompey the Great* (1664), Wm. Abington's *Queene of Aragon* (1640), John Fletcher's *Monsieur Thomas* (1639), and Milton's *Paradise Lost* (1669, first edition). He paid me £1,800. An interesting day spent with him, and to bed very late.

Feb 12   Arose at 4.40 a.m. and read article on Indo-Pakistan relations until 5.20 a.m. Talked to F. [*travel agent*] on phone about sailings for West Indies; dopey about arrangements, but all travel agents are lousy.

Feb 14   Woke at 4.5 a.m., went down to make tea for myself and read yesterday's *Guardian*. Later, received Stilton cheese from Fortnum and Mason, sent by Michael Papantoniou, a nice gesture. M.'s charwoman failed to arrive; she has been insufficiently mollycoddled. Home by 6.30 p.m., and opened Stilton. Received two Valentines today.

Feb 15   Slept well. Cold grey morning with frost; Judy's 18th anniversary, God bless her. Harold Wilson elected leader of the Labour Party. To Anti-coagulant clinic; dealt with many problems. Medical out-patients very heavy indeed, but able to deal with cases with celerity and few interruptions. Lost my way going home. This evening watched excellent Russian film of 'Lady With the Dog', from story by Chekhov.

Feb 16 [*Saturday*]   Gave Judy finely bound 6-volume Clarendon Press Shakespeare, in leather box, no date, as a birthday gift. Stayed in bed for greater part of the day, reading and preparing talk to University students next Tuesday [*Feb 19*], on Thirty-Five Years of Medical Practice. Dressed in the evening and went to the Josephs [*friends*] for dinner, and to discuss forthcoming cruise with them to the West Indies.

Feb 17   Gave Geoffrey *Thesaurus of Hebrew*, Plantin Press, Antwerp, 1578, extremely rare. Jonathan very noisy and unpleasant; needs firm training. Promised them £500, to assist them when they move to a new house. Watched ITV play 'Paradise Suite', with Sam Wanamaker and Carroll Baker ('Baby Doll'); cf. the end of Marilyn Monroe.

Feb 18   Insomnia again; up at 2.30 a.m., to 4.0 a.m., intrinsically sad about David's silence, and his treatment of his mother. Paid telephone account, £12.10s.11d. for quarter. To hospital at 10 a.m., for examination of 13 trainee nurses. Two of them, young ones, had lost their husbands, one aged 23 in a car accident, and the other from a subarachnoid haemorrhage; a third, an Indian girl from Ghana, aet 30, lost her only child, aet 1, of polio. A fourth, called R., wants to nurse, but has a psychopathic history and has been in umpteen hospitals. Saw Matron about them, and their circumstances.

Feb 19   Anti-coagulant clinic, and full Ward rounds, 12 and 15. After lunch, called to private patient: aet 54, Ashton, coronary thrombosis, urgently admitted. When I phoned the hospital from a neighbour's house to get him admitted, the charitable good Samaritans asked me for 3d! Thence, to St. John St.; rested in Miss James's kitchen, in front of the fire. No cases, and at 5 p.m. to University of Manchester Union, to talk to students on my 35 years as a doctor.

I spoke about the relative ease of becoming a medical student in London in the 1920s. At St. George's Hospital, for example, there were only 9 candidates for 11 scholarships. If one had matriculated in 1922 or before [*he matriculated in 1922, at the age of 16½*], it took 5 years to qualify as a doctor. I qualified in 4 years and nine months [*in fact, he qualified to practise as a doctor in January 1928, at the age of 21 years and 11 months*], and all my teachers, such as Lord Horder, are now dead.

I told them how, as a young doctor, I saw patients dumped into wards with what were then incurable diseases: diabetes before insulin, TB without antibiotics, pernicious anaemia (for which 1lb of raw liver, or hogs' stomach, would still be prescribed in those days), myxoedema, and S.B.E. [*sub-acute bacterial endocarditis, causing inflammation of the lining of the heart*] which was deadly before penicillin. On the other hand, although cigarettes were so cheap, cancer of the lung was rare.

Before taking up my first hospital appointments and studying for my M.D. [*which he obtained in 1931, aged 25*], I went in 1928–29, as a young assistant of 22, to a general practice in Dowlais near Merthyr Tydfil, at a salary of £18. 10s. 0d. a month. I saw people in Merthyr buying spectacles for themselves for 1/- on the market stalls; and so many people suffered from pneumonia in winter, their beds standing on damp stone floors. In one case I vividly remember, a man in Dowlais with a First War VC lay in a sodden bed, with rain dripping on it through the ceiling.

I described how I returned to London in 1929, took my final M.B., B.S. with Distinction in Medicine in June of that year, and became a House Physician at St. Bart's Hospital in Rochester. In those days hospitals were essentially voluntary and were often sustained by well-buttressed fat ladies who felt great pride, with the rest of the community, in the hospital as a local institution.

All this has gone now. There were 200 beds at St. Bart's in Rochester, and three resident doctors who did everything; now Parkinson's Law is in operation, with more medical staff, more administrators, more expenditure, more delays and much less efficiency [*see July 6 1962*]. Worst of all, £92 million a year is spent on Prescriptions, 64% of it on proprietary medicines, while the frustration of doctors is growing.

Finally, I told them two truths: that 'human nature is weak, my own included, and will not resist temptation' and that, 'in general, hard workers live longer than lazy ones'. Dr. F. had come to my talk to listen, and seemed pleased with it. Thereafter, to poor fish meal in the cafeteria. Home by 8.30 p.m.

Feb 20 To bank: am advised to convert 5% Registered Debentures into Bearer Shares. God knows what it means; some new form of thievery thought up by somebody. Phoned Sam Barr [*accountant*] from hospital, re loss of income since accident [*see Sept 11 1960*]. Ward round, 7; Dr. F. warns me against Dr. X., house physician, whom he says is a deceitful gambling fellow, and disloyal. I agree.

Feb 21 No hospital today. Proceeded instead to Manchester, to second trial of suit at tailors'; appalling. I will leave them after this. Thence to Royal Mail Lines, to organize trip to Amazon for next year. Thereafter, to Shaw's Bookshop (nothing doing, and what he has is too dear), and lunch at Masonic Temple, 7/-. To St. John Street, 2 cases; one failed to turn up, the fourth this week, growing discourtesy of patients. At 6.0 p.m. to tea in Central Library and boring talk on 'Highlights of Victoriana' by City Treasurer. Have walked much today in the city. Angina.

Feb 22 A long letter to M. and I, from David. Marvellous prose, but not true, and self-revealing. To Anticoagulant clinic, and Follow-up session; a most unsatisfactory arrangement in having two clinics simultaneously. After, to domiciliary visit: cerebral haemorrhage, moribund (aet 56, Dukinfield, unfit to move).

Feb 23 [*Saturday*]   Persistent praecordial pain, and mid-sternal, whilst in bed this morning. Caused me considerable uneasiness. Trinitrini tablets taken, and rested quietly until discomfort passed. Too busy and worrying a day yesterday, and sadness after reading David's letter. Took 500 mgm Methyldopa, 6 mgm of Marcoumar, 5 mgm Bendrothiazide. Slept until 5.45 p.m., after another 250 mgm Methyldopa.

Feb 24   Ruth, Geoffrey and Jonathan to lunch. M. depressed and lachrymose. Good articles in the Sunday papers: Malcolm Muggeridge on The Fabians and the ridiculous capers they have always cut, reviews of the *Kama Sutra*, the political situation in Burma, and the art of enjoying retirement at 60. Good leader against the independent nuclear deterrent in the *Observer*. Also views on the British by foreigners, and an excellent 'Colour Supplement' in the *Sunday Times*. Watched Paul Getty interviewed by Alan Whicker, a magnificent programme.

Feb 25   Took 250 mgm Methyldopa, Guanethidine and Esidrex-K. Thence to post office: telegram to Dr. F. for New Year's Day (Moslem). St. John St., 5 cases. Home to find that Micky, the bird, died this afternoon. Would have been twelve in April; saddened by its death and Judy tearful. Watched 'Panorama' on earthquake in Libya; recruitment in the Forces, with interview of Profumo; and flight of British scientists to the USA.

Feb 27   My application for new life insurance cover rejected. Ward 15, and entered yesterday's Journal entries. Lunch, 3/-, owe 6d. After lunch, full ward rounds in 12 and 14. No cases at St. John St. 7.0 p.m. to Halle, the first time conducted by a woman (Nadia Boulanger): Mozart's Concerto No. 22 in E Flat, played by a Turkish pianist Idil Biret, and Faure's *Requiem*. Splendid.

Feb 28   My 57th Anniversary. Many cards, also letter

from Hazel. Proceeded to domiciliary visit: congestive heart failure, cor pulmonale, *in extremis* (aet 45, Ashton, admitted). Lunch, 4/-; extra 6d from yesterday. My BP at 2.10 p.m. 160/80, very good; albumen, a trace. St. John St., 4 cases.

3:30 p.m. [*Female, aged 77, spinster*] She was a fragile, tiny woman, with markedly round shoulders, who lives with her sister, aet 81, who accompanied her. Four months ago, she went out alone at 4.0 p.m. for a loaf of bread, and was knocked down on a pedestrian crossing. She was struck violently by a car on the right side of her body, suffering generalized bruises and abrasions, especially to the right leg and hip; she also struck the left side of her face on the ground, but no bones were broken. An ambulance came to take her 'away', but she refused to go; 'my sister would not have known where I had got to', she told me.

The police therefore took her home, and her sister said that she sent for the doctor. By then her knee had become swollen, she was unable to walk, her face too was swollen, and she had a black left eye. (They provided this description together.) She remained at home for three days, when her doctor insisted that she go to hospital. There, under examination, 'a doctor' found a 'lump' in her right breast, and a mastectomy was performed; she remained in hospital for 13 weeks thereafter.

Today, she said she 'cannot walk much'; and that she stays at home, reading the papers and listening to the radio. (The sisters have no television). 'The hip is all right now', she added, 'but I haven't been out much'. On examination, there was osteo-arthritis of both knees, but the right knee was worse than the left, swollen and painful, and looked partly disorganized because of the arthritic condition, which had been exacerbated by trauma. She also had a deep and nasty pressure sore on the right heel, which was exceedingly painful, penetrating, and had a dressing over it. Her feet were cold, and the pulses were not felt very easily; the circulation in the right foot was particularly bad.

She was a frail old lady, lucid and rational, but with generalized arteriosclerosis, in whom the normal processes of ageing and disintegration have been appreciably accelerated by the accident on the pedestrian crossing. Her pulse at the wrist was weak, and at times so thin as to be uncountable.

March 3 [*Sunday*]   Spoke to V.N. on the phone about the psychological and social changes wrought in her daughter by having her nose 'lifted' by plastic surgery. Afternoon spoilt by overwhelming naughtiness of Jonathan [*grandson*]; when he left, M. and I were thoroughly exhausted, limp and palpitating. Gave M. Soneryl gr.1½, and she went to bed at 8 p.m.

March 4   Rose at 7.0 a.m.; made M.'s breakfast and took Judy to school. Letter to Professor Umezawa of Tokyo; prodding preliminaries re contemplated visit next year. Visited Miss A. [*private patient*], Dukinfield, for injection and dressings applied to ulcerated legs. Ward round, 7. After lunch, St. John St., 6 cases, including a man from Abbey Hey who had asked his G.P. if he could see a 'private specialist' but thought that he was being seen free.

4:30 p.m. [*Male, aged 59, fireman-stoker*] He had washed his face at work and was drying it with a towel, nineteen months ago, when a metal staple, which had been left attached to the towel by the laundry, cut the side of his face at the corner of his left eye. The cut was only ¼″ long, but bled rather profusely, and he put a dressing of pink lint and adhesive plaster on it in the Ambulance Room. He said that he 'did not bother with it at all' for three or four days, during which time the dressing remained where it was; when he removed it, the cut had not healed. For the next ten months it did not heal either, during which time he kept up with a sort of careless supervision of it, intermittently dabbing it with boracic lotion. Eventually he went to the Works Doctor, who referred him to the Skin Hospital: as soon as it was seen, a local anaesthetic was given, and the ulcer which he had at the site was excised, together with the surrounding area. After it had healed, radium was applied to the site and he was discharged.

Today, he said of the scarred area that he had 'irritation with it', that his eye 'keeps flicking', but that he sleeps and eats well. However, he has only worked ten days this year, has been 'on and off with rheumatism' and 'collapsed' at work recently. He was a man of slender build and poor colour, who did not look very robust, had a regular pulse, no tremor of his hands, and a very good blood pressure (150/90). There was a triangular scar – its base about 1″, its perpendicular height ⅞″ – at the outer corner of the left eye, which was soundly healed but had the tissue-paper appearance of all radium scars. It faded gradually into the surrounding skin and was not noticeable. There was also some evidence of rheumatoid changes in his fingers and wrists; around the right wrist he had tied some red flannel.

What has happened to him is that a small cut on his face did not heal, and continued on to ulceration and malignant change. That is, he had a rodent ulcer, though it is not at all common in my experience for cuts to turn malignant. (If he had got an epithelioma of the skin, for example, it would have been much more malignant, and been accompanied by glandular enlargement in the neck with widespread extension into the system.) It was a cancerous change which flowed directly from the accident of cutting his face. Recurrence is not very likely.

Many phone-calls this afternoon in the Rooms. It is almost like the old days, when I was very busy upstairs, but there is no point.

March 5   Dr. H. tells me about relationship between Dr. X. and Sister in Ward 12. To Mrs. F.N. [*patient and friend*], Dukinfield; she is to undergo hysterectomy. Hope she goes through operation all right. Gave some books to her daughter, Susan. Home by 4 p.m., and siesta. Narrowly escaped electrocution thereafter, when pulling burned-out plug from socket. M. in bad mood; David's silence is sapping her stamina.

March 6   Letter from J.W. [*husband of former patient*] refusing to pay fee for my visit to his wife, and informing me of her death on Monday last [*Feb 25*]. A stupid woman, penny foolish. Reading W.H. Davies, *Autobiography of a Super-Tramp*.

March 7   Visited Mr. F.N. [*see March 5*] to explain his wife's admission for hysterectomy, and Miss A. [*private patient, see March 4*], unguent given, legs much better. Lunch, 3/6; my BP, 165/85. Summoned to Casualty Dept; case of cardio-respiratory failure in obese female, aet 47, weighing over 30 stones. Home at 6.30 p.m. M. in better mood after talking to Maurice G. [*rabbi*], but Judy studying too hard. Gave her some books from the Top Library, to cheer up her spirits.

March 8   Pouring rain. Received letters from solicitors re accident case: great opposition to be encountered from the defendant and a hostile witness, as anticipated [*see Sept 11 1960*]. Made appointment to see Dr. W.F. [*his heart physician*] on return from West Indies. Ward 15, full round, discharged 5 cases; indecent haste exhibited by Mr. C. [*consultant surgeon*] to get his private patients in. Fruit purchased at Rayner's, £1.10s.0d., before starting drudgery of Medical out-patients; but not too heavy. Noted that Dr. V. had a glazed look again. Dr. L. called with medical books I had loaned him, now battered; some personality types are incorrigible about treating books badly.

March 9 [*Saturday*]   With M. to town to buy shirts at Moss Bros; she contributed £3.15s.0d. towards it by cheque. Collected letters at St. John St., and collided with small van on way home. My fault, I think. Phoned garage on return to organize repair on Monday; will make no claim. Felt depressed at noon: combination of forthcoming litigation re accident of Sept. 1960, today's accident, effects of Methyldopa, David's affair and M. tuning up for a row. David arrived at 2.30 p.m. He looked well and gave sound advice about the litigation, but has tendency to be intermittently morose. Gave him an envelope with £5 in it for Hazel. M. had a go at him about Hazel's conversion, which she refuses. Ran him to the railway station and thence, with M., to dinner at the hospital, but very tired and left early. Watched 'That Was The Week That Was': rubbish.

March 10   Rose early and made breakfast for M.

Read David's play in part, and snatches from the papers. No patience, anxious to get away. Tidied up Library; heartache at the sale of my Restoration Plays, but I am used to suffering and depression, and life appears fairly aimless. Would like to circle the globe. I can afford it, but the tyranny of the children and other anxieties keep me back from one bold stroke. Had a good sleep this afternoon, and resumed reading the papers. Play in West Germany against Pius XII [*Hochhuth's The Representative*], who did not pronounce against Jewish persecution, has aroused an outcry by R.C.'s and neo-fascist organizations. Pro-Nasser Syrian revolt consolidating; Jordan next, possibly. At 8.0 p.m., to the Josephs [*friends, who would go to the West Indies*]; Albert is working much too hard. He looks pale and grey, worse than me.

March 11   Awoke at 3.30 a.m., made some tea, and prepared today's work. Returned to bed at 4.40 a.m. At 9.0 a.m. telephone engineer came to the house to instal new phones; given 2 cigars, 2 books for his children and 5/- cash. Then to police to inform them of our departure. Ward 15; D.R. [*private patient*] gave me Masonic handshake. To Moss Bros, to purchase white braces for evening wear and bow-tie. To Miss James, 10/-; to Judy £21 (£1, plus £20 for house-keeping charges during our absence for 4 weeks). God keep her in good health. Phoned Maurice G. to bid him farewell. Exhausting day; always so before going abroad.

March 12   Day of Departure. Thank God we have reached it. Received letter and book from David. Hazel wishes me a pleasant journey and omits to mention M., who is naturally annoyed. Have smoothed matters over as best I can. Sotheby price-list of Sale of Scientific and Medical Books received. Newton's *Principia* – which I could have had for £100 ten years ago – fetched £2,300, but I have the 2nd and 3rd editions in reasonable state. Will be leaving my Library for a month; will make selection for Sotheby's on my return. Dr. F. telephoned from Anti-coagulant clinic to wish me 'Bon voyage'. Final instructions given to Judy; feel tensed up and sad for M., Judy and David. He is fully preoccupied with his marital state, scribliomania, self-pity and illusory happiness, which I have seldom found. The beauty of the world around me has been my chief source of consolation. Boat train from Waterloo to Southampton, and boarded 'Antilles' (French Line) for West Indies and Venezuela at about 8.15 p.m.; cabin 413 cramped and unsatisfactory. Sailed at 10 p.m.; cold, with moderate sea. Poor seats in dining room, but excellent dinner. Complained; alternative accommodation being arranged.

March 13   Storm, rough sea, many sea-sick, including M.; Mrs. Joseph sick and confined to cabin. Very cold and windy. Watching events carefully.

*

[The Journal breaks off here, but it is very probable that a diary was kept in a separate note-book. It has not survived.]

*

April 11   Arrived home at 3.0 a.m., weary in mind and body. Never again will I travel from the North to Southampton, or vice-versa. Went through some of the Mail, and then to bed until 10 a.m. Ruth called with Jonathan. He is a loveable little boy. Phoned Dr. F.; Mrs. F.N. [*see March 5 1963*] had successful operation. Miss James phoned; her friend Miss G.H. has cancer of the ovaries. Slowly breaking the back of my correspondence. I now have a bad memory for names; Easter holiday a Godsend. 14% increase in Doctors' Salaries, announced during our absence.

April 12   Woke at 8.30 a.m.; first bath since 12th March. Went directly to Miss Miller [*secretary*] for St. John St. letters, which she had carefully tabulated and arranged. To hospital: gave Dr. F. mirror and comb for Mrs. F., purchased in Curacao. Thereafter to Albert J., mourning the death of his father, aet 102. Sat with him for a while, and home by 3.30 p.m. Sorting out letters is a tedious business.

April 13 [*Saturday*]   No official work commenced as yet. Rate demand received for £131.5s.0d; will appeal. Took

Judy to Piccadilly station for train to Birmingham on visit to David: 1st class single, £1.10s.9d. Gave her a letter to take to him. Restful day. Read back-numbers of papers to keep abreast of the News. House very deserted; thank God M. and I are together. We are back where we started 27 years ago. Very drowsy with Methyldopa. Impossible to cope with volume of work ahead, if present dosage maintained. Watched 'TWTWTW': Bernard Levin, an arrogant type and Jewish anti-semite, was not in programme this week.

April 14 [*Easter Day*]   Made breakfast for M., and gave her £15 shopping money. Read Alec Waugh on Haiti, in *Black Republic* [*1929*]; he viewed the country through rose-coloured spectacles. Very good *Sunday Times* 'Colour Supplement' on Cuba. Also read how the New Rating System is assessed; an In Memoriam on the 20th Anniversary of the Warsaw Ghetto uprising, with touching extracts from diary of a survivor; and an article on travel in Communist countries. In the evening, TV discussion by 4 Church Ministers on Life after Death; gibberish.

April 15 [*Bank Holiday*]   Purchased 2 gallons of petrol, 9/6d, and ½ lb of Butter, 1/9d. To Mrs Faulkner [*secretary*]; gave her a present from Haiti. Thence to domiciliary with Dr. J.: lymphadenoma (aet 51, Ashton, readmitted). Whilst I was out, Judy had been deposited at the house by David who drove up with her from Birmingham; he came and left at once, at 12.30 p.m., saying to Judy that my letter to him [*see April 13*] was insulting. It had been nothing of the kind, and only conciliatory. Watched Laurel and Hardy film, *A Chump at Oxford*, partially amusing, and 'Panorama': the Aldermaston Marchers with Canon Collins, and British plays on Broadway with Peter Ustinov and Kenneth Tynan.

April 17   After lunch, to St. John St., 5 cases, including M.E., who brought me a large tin of Benson's Toffees, and D.G., who is a mildly hypertensive neurotic on Librium. The latter, who has gone bankrupt, took up nearly two hours of my time. Watched TV film on Dead Sea Scrolls and recent explorations by John Allegro in Jordan.

April 18   Received box of Flor de Lancha cigars from J.F. [*friend and private patient*]. To hospital and Ward rounds, 12 and 15. Thence, after lunch, to St. John St.; 2 cases, 2 failed to attend. One week today since return from Cruise; have dived in at the deep end.

April 20 [*Saturday*]   To St. John St. for letters, and thereafter to Manchester and Salford Council of Social Service; discussed charitable donation. Returned *Violins of St. Jacques* and Aspinall's *Guide to West Indies* to Central Library. From there to domiciliary visit: bronchial asthma (aet 52, Ashton, admitted), and proceeded to Ward 12 round. Watched Red Army Singers and Dancers on TV, and 'That Was The Week That Was'; Bernard Levin assaulted.

April 21   Execution in Spain of Grimau, Communist, causes world reaction. Much ado also in 'Royal' circles at forthcoming marriage of Alexandra to Ogilvy. Effete and decadent princelings of an outdated aristocracy are foregathering en masse. They have high-sounding titles, such as 'Archduchess of Austria' (aged 6) and so forth. What bull! But the working classes will swallow all this rubbish with wild acclaim, and thus perpetuate the travesty.

April 22   Called on Dr. W.F. [*heart physician*], to discuss medico-legal problems arising out of my accident claim. He was helpful; left him 2 bottles of Hock. Appointments flowing in rapidly. Dead tree in garden inspected, with large glutinous toad-stool and Robin's nest. Not to be disturbed.

April 24   To domiciliary: congestive heart failure, *in extremis* (aet 72, Ashton, for admission.) Waited at house for arrival of Dr. R. [*geriatrician*], who came with the Almoner in the ambulance. Then saw T. [*friend*] in street; he seems to be going off his head, marked paranoidal attitude. Ward Rounds, 12, 15. Presented by Dr. F. with Jar of Indian pickles.

April 26   Anti-coagulant clinic almost completed on arrival: signed reports, and phoned travel agents about short

Baltic cruise in June. Have half a mind to go, but do not want to leave M. [*Judy was to do her exams, and M. would have to stay*]. Will await developments. Rested after lunch, and started Medical out-patients sharply at 2.0 a.m. Home by 6.0 p.m. Gaitskell left £80,000 gross, £75,000 net. Spoke to Geoffrey about obese woman seen in today's out-patients, 21 stone. Walk with M., discussing our constant heart-ache.

April 27 [*Saturday*] M. had breakfast in bed, which I brought up for her. Discarding old *BMJs* and *Lancets*. Skimmed through them, with their Honours Lists, Obituaries, Promotions etc.; room for reflection on the ever-changing pattern of Medicine, and on Mice and Men. Watched tennis match on TV from Bournemouth (hard court): Ann Haydon (Mrs. Jones) won against an Argentine girl, aet 20. To the Horwichs [*friends*] this evening. Met Stanley G. [*friend*], who is taking a cruise in June. My own enthusiasm for going away without M. is rapidly declining. There are worthier things to do, such as go to London and organize sale of books at Sotheby's.

April 29 To Follow-up clinic, 10 a.m.; 14 cases, mostly interesting. To St. John St., 4 cases, the 5th failed to attend. The discourtesy of the public towards their doctors is growing. Have never experienced anything like it; no wonder doctors are emigrating.

April 30 Received letter from Professor Umezawa of the Tokyo Institute, setting out an interesting schedule for our visit. Regional Hospital Board statement: gross pay £529.0s.3d. (basic £273.17s.9d., domiciliaries £222.12s.0d., ECGs £12.12s.0d., travel £19.18s.6d.); net £371.4s.8d. (income tax £124.19s.0d., superannuation £29.15s.9d., national insurance £3.0s.10d.) Spoke to F.B. [*ENT surgeon*] about X. [*prominent Tory on Manchester City Council*], an ambitious and uncouth mountebank. Lunch, 3/6d; next to me Dr. Y., an arrogant and disagreeable fellow. Domiciliary visit: congestive heart failure (aet 74, Denton, unfit to move). Thereafter, to St. John St., 3 cases.

3:45 p.m. [*Male, aged 55, labourer*] He was formerly a senior officer in the Polish army, a man of good build and type, who was struck on the top of his scalp above the right forehead twenty-two months ago, when a 'loose iron bar' fell from an overhead crane. He said that he 'fell to the ground unconscious'; he came to as he was being lifted on to an ambulance stretcher, which he claimed was 'half an hour later, the minimum'. At the hospital, where he was detained overnight, a cut on his scalp was dressed, and he was found to have suffered three chipped teeth on the left side of his upper jaw, as the result of the impact; but an X-ray of his skull revealed no fractures. He was off work thereafter for 8 weeks, with 'very much pain in the head'. When he resumed work, he was put on to light labouring duties, checking cables. Six months ago, he began to 'lose his memory', his headaches worsened – they were sometimes so severe that he 'fainted', and on one occasion when he was on night duty, he 'had to take a taxi home' because of his headaches. At this point, he was referred by his GP to a consultant psychiatrist, and was given electric convulsion therapy. He told me that he received six shocks, and thereafter 'felt better'. I also elicited that he had had previous accidents to his head; for example, when he was in the Polish Army in 1939 he was accidentally struck on the head during military manoeuvres, but his helmet saved him. On that occasion also his skull was X-rayed, and he was told that 'the joints were separated between the bones of his skull'. Today, he said that he has headaches 'every day'; that these headaches are what he called 'striking', and that they go 'right through' his head and across his forehead.

At this stage, I called his wife in, with whom I conversed in German. She said that since being struck on the head by the iron bar he had 'changed altogether', that he was depressed by being a labourer after having been an army officer – she told me that he was a survivor of a group of Polish officers who were murdered by the Russians – and that he was difficult to live with. (They have no children.) She added that he was constantly complaining of his headaches, and was 'not interested in anything'; this she said in English. On examination, there was a featureless 1″ scar on the top of his scalp over the upper aspect of the parietal area, and a small scar of ½″ on the opposite (left) side of his scalp, due to his accident when in the Polish Army. His pulse was rapid but regular, there was a tremor of his outstretched hands, his blood pressure (140/90) was normal, his central nervous system was normal, his urine contained no abnormal constituents, and his other symptoms were normal. He has developed a severe post-concussional neurosis, to the point of psycho-neurotic illness, which has already required psychiatric intervention. There are two relevant factors: one is that such psycho-neurotic symptoms often follow head injuries, and the other is that a psycho-neurotic personality such as his is not unusual in Central Europeans. His headaches are psychogenic, but the disability they have created is permanent; he is unlikely to improve beyond his present state, but I thought him fit to continue working.

May 1   M. woke me up at 3.0 a.m., unable to sleep; gave her a Nembutal, which was ineffective. She was fretting over the renegade David and his spouse. She also fainted badly in the morning; arranged for Golda S. [*neighbour*] to keep an eye on her. Thereafter, to domiciliary visit: anxiety state, drunken husband (aet 39, Ashton, to arrange convalescence). Lunch at hospital, phoned M., and to St. John St., 5 cases.

3:25 p.m. [*Female, aged 55, widow, housewife*] She was crossing the road in Salford, 20 months ago, in order to get to a waiting taxi, when she was knocked down violently by a car and suffered a severely fractured pelvis, a dislocated right shoulder and contusions to a previously osteo-arthritic spine. She spent eight weeks in hospital thereafter. In the third week of her stay she was found to have sugar in her urine. She was started on insulin treatment but this was replaced with 'diabetic pills', which she is still taking. Shortly after leaving hospital, when she was beginning to 'get about', she developed a pain 'all over her chest'. At its first onset, this 'pain' made her cry, lasted 'ten to fifteen minutes', and was relieved by brandy; she has had further attacks of the pain, which also 'comes on' when she is in bed, but claims that she has had no treatment from her doctor for it. Today, she told me that she is 'always thirsty' and 'always tired'; that she 'cant bend' to put her stockings on; that, she is short of breath and her feet swell, so that she has 'had to take a size bigger'; that she gets up at night to pass urine and has insomnia. (Despite all this, she said that she feels 'much better' than she did, and has had no chest pain for the past two months.)

She was a thick set, sallow woman, accompanied by her daughter; she said that she had 'three girls at home' who do 'the washing and cleaning', while she does 'the shopping and cooking'. On examination, she had a conspicuous scar on her forehead from a laceration sustained in the accident; clear heart sounds; and no evidence of swelling of the ankles or any other signs of heart failure. Her blood pressure (140/80) and pulses were normal; and her urine contained neither sugar nor albumin. It is also noteworthy that she is not on a diet. (The orthopaedic aspects were outside my province).

This is a complex situation. As to her 'diabetes', there was no sign of sugar in her urine, even though she is not on insulin, nor on any special diet. This evidence suggests, despite her symptom of thirst, that her 'diabetic condition' cannot really be considered a grave matter. As to her chest pain, it is certainly not unusual for angina of effort, as well as diabetes, to be triggered by a serious accident such as she had, and even less unusual for a stout or obese person to develop angina on getting out of bed after a long period of immobilization. But I am not convinced that she suffers from (untreated) angina of effort. The reasons are, first, that she said she had the pain even when she was in bed, and that it was relieved by brandy, which is not a feature of angina. Second, because she said the discomfort lasted ten to fifteen minutes and made her cry. This too is against another typical feature of angina: people usually remain very silent and still, and are afraid to move.

However, the fact that there were no detectable abnormalities in the heart itself on examination does not disprove her angina: angina can occur without such abnormalities. Indeed, some of the worst diseases of the heart, even those of an acute nature, can occur in apparently healthy hearts without anything being apparent on clinical examination. Nevertheless, I found the evidence of her angina, on balance, to be clinically unconvincing.

Heavy traffic on way home, getting worse daily. Found M. more cheerful. F. [*travel agent*] came round, offering me a place for £120 on a Black Sea Cruise in three weeks' time; very tempting.

May 2   Bought a transistor radio set for M. on approval. Thence to two domiciliary visits: pernicious anaemia (aet 64, Droylsden, to be admitted tomorrow); and old cerebral thrombosis, with severe hemiplegia, who happened to fall downstairs (aet 65, Ashton), a case which wasted my time and which the G.P. should have dealt with. After finishing St. John St. had half-hour nap to avoid traffic; came home in 20 minutes instead of 40. M. purchased machine for washing-up dishes, £78.15s.0d.

May 3   Made breakfast for M. Collected passport photos; frightful. Thereafter, Anti-coagulant clinic and Ward round, 14; Ward 12, paper round. Everest climbed by the Americans for the first time. Spoke to Albert J. [*who accompanied him to West Indies*]; a threat of him coming on the Black Sea Cruise with me. Dreadful to contemplate.

May 4 [*Saturday*]   Restful day, but Albert J. still seems to want to come with me.

May 5   Grey skies. Read newspapers, including Colin Legum on South Africa in *Observer*: very serious oppression of the coloured population, negation of elementary rights. The whites are doomed. Fidel Castro in Moscow; Kozlov has a stroke. Good article by John Strachey on 'Pasternak's Children'; description of present-day Warsaw by Patrick O'Donovan; and analysis of Papal policy and Pius XII's silence during the war, by George Steiner (*Sunday Times*). Watched Sammy Davis Jr. on TV; I fail to see his talent.

May 6   Made breakfast for M. To hospital, and ran into holiday snag, solved by applying for 'compassionate' leave at the instigation of P. [*hospital administrator*]. St. John St., 3 cases.

4:30 p.m. [*Male, aged 61, machine-hand*] He was bending down, stacking some bricks at 9.45 a.m., when a section of steel bolt, 3″ x 6″ and weighing about 10 lbs, fell about 3 feet and struck him on the left forehead. He said he was wearing his cap at the time; 'it saved me', he added. There was a laceration, but no stitches were needed. He was then off work for a fortnight.

Today, two months later, he said that he has headaches 'if there is too much noise', has a 'pricking feeling' over the left temple, but that if he rubs his forehead 'that seems to ease it'. He also claimed to 'feel the pricking' when he turns round 'sharply'. On examination, he was healthy and looked at least ten years younger than his age. He has consulted solicitors, claiming continuing disability of one kind and another, but when I asked him whether in all honesty there was anything wrong, he said there wasn't.

Summons to Assizes tomorrow morning.

May 7   Letter from L.F. [*solicitors*] re my car accident [*see March 8 1963*]. Made breakfast for M., and thence to Assizes, with George Carmel Q.C. before Mr. Justice Fenton Atkinson, but no medical evidence called on our side. St. John St., 3 cases, including woman with BP of 220/110.

3:30 p.m. [*Male, aged 54, boilerman*] He was banking up a boiler with sawdust when there was a blow-back. He received extensive burns to the hands and arms, chest, shoulder and back, to the waist; he was also burned on the right side of his face and on the right knee. He was intensely shocked on admission to hospital, where he was detained three months; three weeks after admission, and to add to his troubles, his left lung collapsed and he had to do breathing exercises six times a day for some weeks. He also had pneumonia, which was treated with antibiotics. He had blood tranfusions, and underwent skin grafting operations; he has had five in all so far, the last 12 months ago when some skin under his left armpit had to be divided, because contractures had developed and he was unable to raise his left arm over his head. He is on the waiting-list for a further skin graft, due to contractures which have developed over the shoulder and because of the unsightliness of some of his scars. (When he first came out of hospital he had open wounds for about six months, which had to be dressed with impregnated gauze dressings.) He went back to work 14 months after the accident and is now 'stamping cartons', for the 'same money' as he was earning as a boilerman.

Today, he told me that he can't sleep without sleeping tablets; that the right side of his face was 'sore' when he shaved; that he had a fortnight's holiday last summer at Prestatyn; that his skin itches a great deal and is 'ugly'; that he sweats a lot when he walks, but not from the burnt areas; that he has no energy, and that the accident has 'weakened' him. He was a pale, unhealthy looking man, tall and thin – he lost 3 stones after the accident, but is 'picking up a little now' – whose face was discoloured and blanched on the right side; there was a similar blanched area right round his neck, which looked like a grey collar.

On examination, much of his trunk, arms and under both armpits was scarred over, with thickened and heaped up keloid formation in strands, and there was gross discolouration of the skin, apart from the alteration of its texture. Some areas were brown, such as the back of the arms, and others were paler in colour. He himself said that his scars were 'going softer'; movement of the elbows and joints was satisfactory. His pulse was slow (42) and his blood pressure 120/70. I thought his pulse rate was of some pathological significance; it needs further investigation and watching carefully. None of his scarring is likely to improve much, and the contractures may cause further trouble in future. The remote possibility also exists – I have seen two or three cases in my 37 years of practice – of the development in the scars of epithelioma, a malignant condition of the skin. His own estimate was that he was 'about 60% to 70% recovered', but he was being too generous. Indeed, he made no attempt to exaggerate his disabilities, which are grievous.

May 9   Went with M. to vote in council elections; both of us for Liberal candidate. Purchased petrol and oil from Cheetham garage, 17/0½d, objectionable type of Jewish proprietor. Made donation [*see April 20 1963*] of £116.17s.6d.

to Manchester and Salford Council of Social Service. Phoned P. [*hospital administrator*], re leave of absence. He said that the false excuse of 'compassionate' leave is not necessary, and that I can deduct the time from next year's holiday allowance; very gratifying.

May 10   Sweeping victories by Labour throughout the country in Council Elections; gain of 550 seats, heavy losses by the Tories. To Anti-coagulant clinic: my Prothrombin time 17 seconds, 37% activity. Is Methyldopa causing toxic changes? Ward rounds 12, 14 and 15. After lunch, excellent today, to Dr. G.W. [*heart physician*] for medical examination [*re his accident case*].

[*Extract from Report on Dr. Hugh Selbourne, dated 10th May 1963*] '. . . He made a reasonable recovery from his 1953 coronary thrombosis but it left him with a liability to angina of effort. Nevertheless, he was able to live a normal life and carry out his duties as Consultant Physician, and his condition remained static until 1960. On 11th September 1960 he was driving his car along the main road near his home, when another car, emerging from a side road, collided with him. He was thrown against the steering wheel, and sustained shock and bruising to the abdominal wall, right leg and iliac crests. That same evening he had a severe attack of anginal pain coming on at rest, and lasting for ten minutes [*but see Sept 11 1960*]. After the accident, his angina was more easily provoked and more troublesome. On 21st December 1960 he had a further severe attack of angina coming on at rest and lasting for over an hour. I admitted him to the Royal Infirmary with a diagnosis of acute coronary insufficiency. On admission, his BP was 140/90 and there was electrocardiographic evidence of myocardial ischaemia. He was put on to anti-coagulants, settled down reasonably well and was discharged on the 11th January 1961. I have seen him at regular intervals since. In the main, his condition has not changed very much, but towards the middle of 1962 his blood pressure began to rise, is currently about 190 or 200/110, and he is being treated with anti-coagulants and hypotensive drugs.

Road traffic lighter this evening. Looking forward to my trip through the Black Sea [*see May 1*].

May 11 [*Saturday*]   Wynne, the spy, gets 8 years; the Russian involved gets death sentence. To Middleton, to see case for National Union of Mineworkers.

9:30 a.m. [*Male, aged 68, retired miner*] He was a very sick man, dysphasic and incoherent from his left sided stroke 5 years ago, and with long standing severe bronchitis with emphysema. Fourteen months ago he developed a gangrenous patch over the left heel – his wife said he had been having 'terrible pain in his leg' – and was re-admitted to hospital, where his BP was found to be 130/100 and the gangrene diagnosed as due to arteriosclerosis. To save his life, his left leg was amputated above the knee, and an artificial limb fitted. (There is a note in the surgeon's handwriting which says 'I do not think this man will ever do anything to help himself to walk, and that further treatment would be a waste of time'.) I found him in bed this morning. Through his wife, who was very vague about the details of his condition, I learned that he is regularly visited by his doctor but is not on any treatment, that he sleeps reasonably well, and that he is 'putting on weight'; in fact he used to be 14 stones, but is 8 stones today. On examination, his left arm was stiff and almost functionless, the stump of his leg was healthy, he had wheezing respirations, and his movements were slow and painful. The artificial leg was not being worn, and he hobbled on one leg for me to examine him. (He could not tell me, when I asked him, why he had originally had his leg off.) I found his blood pressure to be normal, 140/80, but this is likely to be because his general health is failing; a consistently high blood pressure which suddenly falls, as his has done, shows an extremely gross condition. He and his wife have had 9 children, seven of whom are living, all married.

Thereafter, to St. John St., to collect my letters. Siesta, after lunch. Bitterly cold, like a November day. At 8.30 p.m. visited Ringway with the Josephs to inspect new airport building; a remarkable transformation from its original drab condition. Compares favourably with continental airports. Interesting day, on the whole, and better than the dawdling about I have done in the recent past.

May 12   Read further article by Colin Legum [*see May 5 1963*] on South Africa and its problems, and comments on Labour successes, all over the British islands, at local Council elections. Also, on the attitude of the Public to illegitimate births and the mothers; cruel and unforgiveable. Visited by Geoffrey, Ruth and Jonathan for tea. Told Geoffrey a few home-truths. His reluctance about my foreign travel suggests a desire on his part that I should spend as little, and leave as much, as possible.

May 13   Talked to Dr. Y. at lunch on exfoliative cytology. St. John St., 3 cases, including dress machinist, aet 50, a very thin-chested greying woman who carried her head a little to the side, and has been off work for ten weeks. She was knocked down by a car and suffered cuts and bruises, including to her knees and elbows. When I asked her when she would go back to work, she looked as if she had been struck by a thunderbolt. 'My leg will have to be all right,' she said with asperity, 'before I go back on that treadle.' Watched 'Panorama' on the USA: Robin Day in Birmingham, Alabama, Rev. Martin Luther King and Robert Kennedy interviewed, negro vs. white problem discussed.

May 14   M. again without daily help. Did Anti-coagulant clinic; loaned Dr. Y. article on exfoliative cytology. P. [*hospital administrator*] signed leave of absence forms; promised to take him out to lunch next week. Ward Rounds 12, 14 and 15. Thence, to Medical Advisory Committee luncheon meeting; the customary balderdash, with Dr. M. [*consultant*] winning useless administrative argument on points. Home by 5.0 p.m. Winston Churchill visited the House of Commons today. Warm reception given him; maybe his last visit. Watched 'This is Your Life' for the first time, and impressed by a remarkable woman: Gladys Aylward, missionary in China.

May 15   At lunch, Mr. D. [*consultant surgeon*] said he was going to Australia, to explore possibilities for himself; I dont blame him. St. John St., 3 cases, including life examination of consultant radiologist at Manchester Royal Infirmary. Met M., and to cinema to see Peter O'Toole in *Lawrence of Arabia*, at the Gaumont. Announced on news that American astronaut has been 9 hours in orbit.

May 16   Fine day. Left for Liverpool at 9.45 a.m. Arrived at 11.15 a.m., and looked round Liverpool Cathedral; talked to verger, aet 74. Thence to Rodney Street, and medical examination by Mr. L.T., thoracic surgeon, on behalf of defendants in my accident case. He seemed reasonable, but it was a cursory examination.

May 18 [*Saturday*]   To St. John St., to collect my letters. Son David came at 12 noon, and stayed for lunch and tea. General conversation. He is still on his guard, still bearded; very beatnik-like, or am I wrong? His writing shows promise, and is being encouraged by Coghill in Oxford. Asked him about his wife, etc., and ran him to the station. To the Livingstones for dinner.

May 19   Interesting article on China Today in the *Observer* and customary book reviews. Putting on weight, unfortunately: ½ stone in past 6 weeks. Must definitely lose it. Sorry to be going away without M.; can't be helped this time, however.

May 20   Dictated testimonial for Dr. C. [*house physician*]. After lunch, St. John St., 4 cases, including W.A., accompanied by French wife; a hypertensive, aet 57, member of Dukinfield Lodge; and a Yugoslav antisemite, who fought for King Peter. Watched Panorama on Ethiopia with James Mossman; interview with Haile Selassie.

May 21   Took Judy to school, and then to bank; withdrew travellers' cheques from my account, £50.10s.0d. Bespoke bed for yesterday's hypertensive, to be admitted on my return. Farewell to P. [*hospital administrator*]; called at Dispensary to order necessary substances for travel in Middle East and Black Sea. St. John St., 2 cases. Very exhausted today.

May 22   To Arnfields, and thence to Dispensary for medical supplies for voyage. Gave attache case and keys to Miss Miller, plus postages and fares for collecting my letters from St. John St., £3.0.0. Ward round, 12, and thereafter to Mrs. F.N.; tabs. for her hot flushes delivered. After lunch, called on Dr. K. [*see Dec 12 1962*]; he appears to be always in the doldrums. Gave him advice and £1, but he is a sad case. Thence to Manchester for travel insurance: Medical cover £100, luggage £100, wrist watch £100. To M. for 2 weeks, £30.0.0. John H. [*friend*] called round this evening, wanting advice about changing his GP, whom he said had 'gone mental'. Geoffrey and Ruth came to wish me a happy journey.

*

Next morning he flew to Venice, where he boarded ship for a two week voyage to the Black Sea, calling, among other places, at Piraeus, Haifa, and Odessa. There are only a few notes extant of this journey, including references to 'organized chaos' and to meeting a 'talkative Roumanian doctor, who told me his tale of torture in Bucharest'.

*

June 10   Pleasant flight back to London, rotten food, arrived 2.0 p.m. Phoned M., and took plane for Manchester, flying time 40 minutes. Met by M. and Judy; Ruth, Geoffrey and Jonathan called at the house later. Gave out gifts, unpacked, and dawdled about. Profumo affair the rage.

June 12   Claims lodged re torn suitcase and damaged blouse, bought at alleged duty-free shop on liner, and wrote final warning letter to C.D. [*private patient*] re account. To domiciliary visit: thrombo-phlebitis of leg (aet 70, Audenshaw). Lunch at hospital, 3/6d.; talked to Dr. V. St. John St., 5 cases.

3:0 p.m. [*Female, aged 27, single, clerk*] She was a slender girl, of good appearance, with extensive multiple sclerosis. At the beginning of 1962, when I first saw her as a hospital in-patient, her life was despaired of, as she was suffering from an acute and fulminating disseminated encephalomyelitis. She recovered, and after discharge was on a fairly even keel, attending my out-patients and follow-up clinics, at 2 or 3-monthly intervals. She also began to receive physiotherapy and attend a Rehabilitation Centre; and was looking exceedingly well when I again saw her two days before her accident.

However, on Feb 10th this year, when on an outing to the Pennines with her young man, a car struck their Ford Zephyr in the rear, and in the impact her neck was 'jutted' backwards, her left shoulder and back were 'twisted', and she struck her left knee against the dashboard. Her left knee thereupon went into a spasm, and she cried very much and was frightened. She got out of the car, and the people at the nearby road-house, the 'Hare and Hounds', took her in and gave her a drink of tea. She said that her head was 'jerking', and her leg was in a clonic spasm, easily explained as a feature of multiple sclerosis. For about 10 days she had great difficulty in walking, but she was greatly helped by the physiotherapist at the Rehabilitation Centre, completed her course, and resumed her work as a clerk.

Today, she told me that since the accident she has developed a foot drop, cannot dorsiflex her left foot, limps when she walks, is unable to kneel down and tires more easily. She also said that she gets cramps in her right foot if she crosses her legs, and of late her right hand has become weaker. Her tearfulness, a consequence of her multiple sclerosis, has increased, and she has lost half a stone since the accident; she now weighs 6st. 13lbs. The accident has clearly aggravated her condition, but it is too soon to say whether the deterioration will continue. I told her that I would like to see her in six months time. She is a seriously sick girl, and well informed as to her condition; though I minimized her disabilities to her, she has read about her disease and discussed it fully with other sufferers, so that her own apprehension is justifiable.

Milk at St. John St., 9d. Timothy Birdsall, the TW3

cartoonist, has died of a blood disease. Tragic indeed; he was only 27.

June 13   Acted as Chairman at Hospital Appointments Committee; new senior House Officer and Indian House Physician appointed. Ward 15, round. After lunch, to St. John St., 6 cases. Watched extraordinary interview of Lord Hailsham by Robert Mackenzie, on Profumo affair.

June 14   Domiciliary visit: virus encephalitis (aet 48, Dukinfield, admitted). Home by 6.30 p.m., much traffic. Michael Papantoniou arrived about 8.30 p.m. Sat up with him until 2.0 a.m. Sold him 21 items for £400, including Wycherley's *Gentleman Dancing-Master* (£55), Suckling's *Discontented Colonell* (£75), Davenant's *Cruell Brother* (£75), Cartwright's *Royal Slave* (£55), and a presentation copy of Humphrey Ward's *Robert Ellesmere* (£17). Am quite satisfied.

June 15   Michael Papantoniou is ruthless as a book-buyer, but likeable somehow. Breakfasted at 8.30 a.m., and took him to Gibb's bookshop; nil there. Thereafter, to Bob Walmsley's, where I purchased De la Rivière, *Le Miroir des Urines* (1763); John Ball M.D., *Modern Practice of Physic*, 2 vols. (1760); and Antoine Baumé, *Chymie Experimentale et Raisonnée*, 3 vols (1773). Total cost, £18.

June 16   Tidied up books in Library disarranged by Papantoniou. Woman astronaut in space sent up by Russians; man and woman now separately in orbit. Ben Gurion resigns, for personal reasons. Listened to Romanes Lecture given at Oxford by Lady Violet Bonham-Carter, on 'Personality and Politics'; the first time the lecture has been given by a woman.

June 17   Profumo debate in Parliament today. Government majority of 69, with 34 abstentions; Macmillan will probably resign in the Summer. Gross incompetence.

June 19   Ward 12; case of acute encephalitis [*see June 14 1963*] worse, spoke to relatives. Lunch and proceeded to

St. John St., 3 cases. Russian astronauts have come down. Held evening party, eleven guests; gave Edward K. [*friend*] Porny's book on heraldry. A fairly tiresome, dull evening.

June 20 Case of acute encephalitis dying. At lunch, argument between Dr. X. [*physician*] and Mr. Y. [*surgeon*]; the former put his foot in it re sepsis in the operating theatre, and the latter lost his temper. To St. John St., 5 cases, including hiatus hernia or aortic stenosis, to be admitted for investigations, paid 6 guineas.

June 21 Acute encephalitis case in Ward 12 still dying; a dreadful pity. A new Pope elected, Paul VIth: Cardinal Montini, Archbishop of Milan, a progressive.

June 22 [*Saturday*] Read *Manchester Guardian* in bed, bathed and shaved. David came for lunch, and to collect some of his books from his old study. I hope to go to see him in a fortnight, and call at the small town of Hay [*see Jan 22 1963*]. Spoke to his wife on the phone; I am trying hard for a rapprochement between M. and Hazel, the contending parties.

June 25 M. wakes at 3.0 a.m. with nausea; she settled down afterwards. Made her tea in the morning. Preliminary inquiry to F. [*travel agent*] re visit to China or world tour on the 'Willem Ruys'. Sent off £62.12s.0d., for Judy's holiday in Salzburg, including festival tickets. Thereafter, to hospital and Ward round, 7. Dictated letter to the Misses S. and B., my fellow travellers on Black Sea Cruise.

[*Excerpt from letter to Miss S. and Miss B., London NW2, dated 25th June 1963*] . . . 'I thought I would write and ask you how you were getting on, after the serenity of the cruise, since we all seem to have dispersed into thin air. I have now been home for a fortnight, and often think of the very happy days we spent, together with our friend Mr. K. When I got home I found everybody looking forward to my return with some anxiety . . . Would you ever go to Russia again? If you did, I am sure you would wish me to come with you, so that you could peel my oranges and apples. I trust that you will both call upon us whenever you are in Manchester, and I will certainly do my best to visit you if I ever come to London, which these days is a rare event . . .'

Dr. F. [*leaving hospital to go into local general practice*] wants to purchase surplus hospital blankets; saw Matron and P. [*administrator*] on his behalf. Refused; parsimonious. Listened to President Kennedy in West Germany, making his speech to bolster the Atlantic Alliance as a counterblast to Gaullist nationalism; I hope it will work. Also, heard Geraint Evans in Cimarosa's *Il Maestro de Cappella* on BBC TV.

June 26   To domiciliary visits: pregnancy and alleged murmur, could not hear it (aet 18, Audenshaw), and secondary anaemia due to intestinal carcinoma (aet 66, Denton, admitted). Thereafter, to Arnfields; E.G.T. [*managing director*] gave me a bottle of John Haig whisky. After lunch, visited Dr. A. [*local GP*] at home; he is leaving his practice tomorrow and going into public health. He looked rather thin and dejected, and his wife disconcerted. St. John St., 4 cases. Spoke on phone with incompetent insurance company employee about one of today's life cases; the rot is setting in with clerical staff, increasingly lazy and discourteous. Excellent party political broadcast by Mr. Harold Wilson, Leader of the Opposition.

June 27   Heavy rain, cloudy and overcast. Dr. D. phoned to cancel today's domiciliary visit, as the patient had died. Thereafter, to Woods Hospital with Dr. F. to get bedding for him from Miss E., then to inspect his house in Ashton. No lunch today: feel better as a result. St. John St., 3 cases, and home by 5.30 p.m.

June 28   Mr. B., insurance agent, called at 9.0 a.m. re damage to suitcase; reprimanded him for veiled threat to discontinue cover because of my claim. He will repair the broken glass in the Hall and a broken window. Thereafter, to two domiciliary visits: cor pulmonale, emotional disturbance with wife, divorce etc. (aet 57, Audenshaw, admitted), and acute asthma (aet 24, Ashton, admitted). Gave cheque for £2.2s.od.

to Miss Miller [*secretary*] for her birthday, aet 38, and further farewell to Dr. A. [*see June 26*]; he looks sad and washed out. (Mortality high: Dr. P., Dr. G., Dr. T. [*recently deceased local doctors*]). This evening, discourteous phone conversation with David. He does not wish M. to light candles at his home if we call next week; we are much distressed and unhappy. M. and I go for a walk afterwards, as we always do when worried about David.

June 29 [*Saturday*]   In bed most of the day, pharyngitis with severe weakness. Unable to swallow, but improvement as the day progressed, sorting out papers. Reading Fosco Maraini, *Meeting With Japan* and Bertrand Russell, *What I Believe*, written in 1925; in 1940 there were proceedings against him in the New York Court as a result. ('The good life is one inspired by love and guided by knowledge'.) Dr. F. visited me, gave me throat lozenges, and stayed for tea. M. gave him a dreadful illuminated fish, purchased in Jamaica, some table-cloths and a table for his new house.

June 30   Article by James Baldwin, *The Fire Next Time* in *Sunday Times*. [*This was a pre-publication excerpt from Baldwin's book, which came out two weeks later.*] Dr. F. phoned to inquire about my health. Solution of hydrocortisone prepared by Geoffrey for spraying my throat. At 2.30 p.m. my BP 170/110; had taken no Methyldopa this morning, therefore took 500 mgm straight away; felt better for it.

July 2   [*The entry has attached to it an article by David Holbrook, from the Manchester Guardian of July 2, on 'The Image Woman', about the continuing Profumo affair. In it Holbrook asks, of the current 'moral indignation' about Christine Keeler and the other participants, 'Where do the strong feelings originate?' and answers that 'Since we spend a great deal of our inward energy sitting on our own libidinal urges . . . we are enraged when we see someone apparently enjoying the release of these controls without remorse – and even without ill consequences. So we feel envy and hate'. He also calls this release the 'happy, reckless life of abandoned sex which we would all dearly like to live.' Holbrook argues further that the fact that the image of Christine Keeler (whose name he nowhere mentions) is*

*'splashed on every popular newspaper's front page . . . has a profound
cultural significance: she suggests an ideal'. His own position is that
'her behaviour suggests that the whole impulse behind her career is a
compulsive need to prove to herself that she is feminine' – which 'should
engage our deepest compassion' – while 'for a man the image-woman
engages with his unconscious anxiety about his own potency, and his
own worry about his capacity to form good relationships. I daresay this
anxiety is one which compels a man to take a mistress or prostitute . . .
In middle age, when anxiety about potency increases, a man is more
likely to go in for his potency over again, and thus allay fear – for
a time. So the lapses of public men in this way evoke our strongest
responses . . .']*

Made breakfast for M. Thereafter, to Chatsworth (car
park, 2/-; entrance to fascinating gardens, 4/6d). Enjoyable
trip; will go again with M. on a future Tuesday and have a
mid-week break. On return, watched TV about a day in the
life of an intern at Bellevue Hospital, New York. The first
realistic film of hospital life I have seen, in marked contrast
to the 'Dr. Kildare' and 'Emergency Ward 10' poppycock.
Row in Commons over the Philby affair, the '3rd man' with
Burgess and Maclean. Always suspect to me, but of course
protected by his Conservative Establishment friends, and
actually recommended to the *Observer* by the Foreign Office
after his dismissal.

July 3   Letter from the Misses S. and B. in London.
After lunch, to St. John St., 5 cases, including road transport manager with undescended testicle and varicose veins,
and case of dyspepsia with C_2H_5OH problem and excessive
smoking.

July 5   To hospital, and Anti-coagulant clinic; my
two private patients seen in Wards 11 and 15. Thereafter, domiciliary: broncho-pneumonia, alcoholic (aet 68,
Ashton, admitted). Dr. T. [*the GP who called him*] looks
old and groggy; has just been to Llandudno for a two
week holiday, appalling. Home for lunch with M., short
rest and packed for Birmingham. M. took me to the station,
and arrived Birmingham (New Street) at 7.30 p.m. Met by

David and taken to his flat in Edgbaston. Depressed by it, the long estrangement, and the conditions under which my beloved son is living. It must be nearly 30 years since I was last in Birmingham. I dont mind missing the place for another 30.

July 6 [*Saturday*]   Breakfast, and off with David and Hazel to Hay-on-Wye, via Hagley, Leominster, Tenbury and toll-bridge. Weather fairly bad; run lasted just over 2 hours. Lunch at Crown Hotel, Hay for three, including beer, £2.10s.0d. Poor service and boorish manners of proprietor. They never make anyone welcome; no wonder people increasingly go abroad for their holidays. Interesting day. Purchased books from R.G. Booth, owner of book-and-furniture shop, for £13.0.0. These included Johnson's *Lives of the Poets*, 2 vols, fine vellum binding by J. Rees of Bristol, 1821; Henry Dana Jr., *To Cuba and Back*, 1859; Barbey d'Aurevilly, *What Never Dies*, translated for private circulation, Paris, 1902; S.P. Laplace, *Exposition du Système du Monde*, 2nd edition, 1799 (10/-); Newton's *Principia*, 3 vols, 1803, uncut and in original boards, the first complete translation of *Principia* into English and the first translation of 'De Mundi Systemata', which Newton originally intended as the 3rd Book of the *Principia*; Ada Lawrence and Stuart Gelder, *The Early Life of D. H. Lawrence*, 1932; P.J. Barthez, *Nouveaux Éléments de la Science de l'Homme*, 2nd Edition, 2 vols, 1806; Wm. Whewell, *History of the Inductive Sciences*, 2nd Edition, 3 vols, 1847; Jethro Tull, *Horse–Hoeing Husbandry*, original boards and uncut, with introduction by Wm. Cobbett, 1829, and others. Good value; Booth also included a fair-sized bottle of Leather Polish.

July 7   Arose at 7.30 a.m.; better weather after yesterday's rain. Wimbledon singles Finals had to be abandoned yesterday because of torrential downpour; the Test Match at Edgbaston was also abandoned. After breakfast, had run around in car with Hazel and David to the centre of Birmingham; great developments, but it appears from what I am told that Birmingham is a conservative stronghold, with much aggressive ill-humour towards coloured people. (That is, shits and fascists.) Took 10.20 a.m. to Manchester, but because of customary ineptitude of B.R. employees, misinformed of time of arrival at 1.25 p.m. Met by M. who had been waiting for more than an hour; handed her a letter from Hazel which appears to have reestablished normal relations. Read First Act of David's play, *The Old Man*, approved by Professor Coghill of Oxford. To bed early, throat not too good.

July 8   To Follow-up clinic, and thereafter domiciliary visit: thyrotoxicosis (aet 67, M/c 11, admitted). Went home for lunch with M. Took her to Ringway for her journey to Marseille [*to visit her sister*] and waited until the plane left; God speed her safely there and back. Thence to St. John St., 4 cases, including case of 'battered baby'. Talked to Miss James, on leaving. Watched 'Panorama' interview with King and Queen of Greece; they have outlived their usefulness, if they ever had any.

July 9   To Anti-coagulant clinic, and Ward Rounds, 12, 14 and 15. Home by 4.30 p.m. Phoned David and Hazel this evening, long conversation and congratulated him on his play *The Old Man*. Riots in Trafalgar Square today, over the state visit of the King and Queen of Greece to England.

July 11   To St. John St., 4 cases; including conference with solicitors about 'battered baby' case.

3:15 p.m. [*Male, aged 44, textile merchant*] He was wearing dark glasses when he entered the room and said that five weeks ago he had driven down to London, with his wife and four children, in order to see the new Hilton Hotel and to have tea there. However, in attempting to enter the building he walked into a glass door which he took to be open, bumping the right side of his forehead and temple. (He said that he felt 'so sick and dizzy' – though no bump came out on his forehead, despite the gravity of the collision – that he was unable to drive home to Manchester that day, and had to get rooms at the Cumberland for the night.) The next day his wife drove them home, and the day after that he visited his doctor, asking him to examine his right eye; the doctor, he asserted, 'thought there was a haemorrhage in it'. At this point he 'went off' work, and has not been back to work since. Instead, he has seen an eye specialist, whom he claims 'was not sure whether there would be permanent damage', but who felt that the bang on his head had precipitated astigmatic changes in his right eye, and that he needed glasses.

Today, he said that he has 'rotten' headaches, his right eye is blurred, he has to wear dark glasses, he has to 'squint when reading the newspaper', and he has not been able to attend to his business. I told him to remove his dark glasses, which he was still wearing, so that I could examine his eyes, and found that he had a widely dilated right pupil from the drops, probably Atropine, which the specialist had inserted in it. (No wonder that he cant see properly!) On examination of his fundi, there was neither haemorrhage nor other damage to the eye, and no evidence to suggest that he was suffering from migraine or any other post-traumatic phenomenon of a neurological nature.

The situation thus seems to be as follows. First, if, when he collided with the door of the Hilton Hotel, he had received a blow sufficient to interfere with his vision, one would have expected at least some bruising of the forehead. Second, if he needs glasses, it is only to be expected at his age; I do not for one moment believe that the bang on his head has accelerated the need for them. Third, I am sure that he is attending to some part of his business. Fourth, the blurred vision in his right eye could easily be improved by instilling some Eserine drops in it in order to contract the widely dilated right pupil. If this were done he would not have to walk about in dark glasses, which I am sure he takes off at home.

Anti-Greek demonstrations against Frederika and Paul of Greece during State visit. Disgraceful hooliganism.

July 13 [*Saturday*]   Letter from M., posted in Marseille on Wednesday. Left at 10.30 a.m. for Southport with Judy to see medico-legal case of fractured femur. (I advised the solicitors that I was not an orthopaedic surgeon, but they nevertheless wanted me to go). Reading *Cuba There and Back* by Henry Dana.

July 14   Restful day, tidying up my Library a little; Judy kept me company browsing around. To keep the place in order is an insoluble problem. Wonderful rediscoveries of books, purchased wisely in the past and almost unobtainable now. Watched extraordinary BBC TV broadcast on Sex, with Dr. Alex Comfort and Prof. Carstairs. Excellent and enlightened views expressed.

July 15   Heavy and incessant rain. Test-ban talks to begin today; hostile exchanges between Russia and China. St. John St., 4 cases.

4:35 p.m. [*Female, aged 55, 'assistant greengrocer to her husband'*] She was a woman of slender build with a red face, nicotine-stained fingers, and a marked tremor of her outstretched hands. Four months ago she was out in their travelling grocery van; they were stationary on a hill outside a customer's house – she 'standing up inside the van' and 'handing provisions' to her husband – when a car, which 'came up from below', ran into the back of them. (She told me that in the mêlée that followed the driver claimed that the sun had 'blinded' him). She was 'knocked over' by the impact, falling and striking her left hand against a box of groceries; and, as she fell inside the van, her husband 'fell off into the street'. 'The car did not actually touch us', she added. She was then taken briefly to hospital where her hand was 'looked at', no X-ray was taken, and although she claimed that she had 'pulled all the muscles' in her left hand, she was sent home.

The next day, however, she 'felt the shock', and called on her doctor, who gave her some 'quietening pills'. She was off work thereafter for three months; whenever she went to the shop during this period it was 'only to talk to the customers', and she has not been out in the grocery van since the mishap. Today, she said that she was 'still under the doctor', who continues to give her 'quietening pills' since she 'keeps trembling', though she is 'not as bad' as she was.

On examination there was nothing abnormal in the left hand, but her blood pressure was considerably raised (220/140), and her fundi showed changes compatible with a severe degree of hypertension. Her accident was a minimal matter, compared with the serious constitutional disorder from which she suffers, and of which she was completely unaware. She smokes '25 to 30' cigarettes a day. 'Sometimes I'm smashing, and sometimes I go off', she told me.

Watched 'Panorama' on the Rachman case, British Guiana and the beating up of suspects by Sheffield police. Interruptions, as usual, by telephone calls.

July 16 Rose at 6.0 a.m. after good night's sleep. To domiciliary visit: hypertension, diabetes and polyneuritis (aet 60, Ashton, advice given); Dr. Z. [*the Polish general practitioner who called him*] was a prisoner in Russia during the war. Thereafter, to Assizes and preliminary discussion with Derek Hodgson Q.C., followed by lengthy harangues in Court over piffling medico-legal case before Mr. Justice Fenton Atkinson. Case adjourned; to resume tomorrow with further waste of time. David rang this evening. He is moving to Stratford-on-Avon.

July 17 Judy's last attendance at school this morning, and the last day I took her to school as a pupil; an end of an era for me. To Assizes, 10.30 a.m.: evidence given, Hodgson on sticky wicket. Thereafter, to Bob Walmsley and purchased Wm. Stokes, *The Use of the Stethoscope* (1825); Wm. Heberden, *Commentaries on the History and Cure of Diseases* (1802); Thos. Willis, *Pharmaceutice Rationalis*, Oxford, 1674, six folding plates, fine copy.

July 18 Advised by solicitor to charge 60 guineas for yesterday's Court appearance and Tuesday's [*July 16*] attendance. Two letters from M.; she is very miserable indeed. Proceeded to Arnfields; better relations, and even Miss Griffiths [*secretary*] seemed to smile. Thence, to domiciliary visits: coronary thrombosis (aet 50, Ashton, admitted), and sub-arachnoid haemorrhage, *in extremis* (aet 74, Ashton).

On leaving met R.M. [*former patient*] in the street. He is a commercial traveller now, and told me that his boss 'treats his staff well always' and is 'very charitable', but is dying of cancer. Ward rounds 7, 12, and 15; my BP 160/100, with some angina due to rushing about.

July 20 [*Saturday*]   Earth tremors in the South of France. Eclipse of the Sun visible today in N. America. Partial nuclear test-ban treaty between Russia, USA and Britain appears imminent. Read significant account by Lord Altrincham in *Manchester Guardian* of his recent visit to Russia. [*In the article, which is attached to today's entry, Lord Altrincham takes issue with Mr Macmillan who, a week earlier in an interview with the Daily Express, had said that Russia had become a 'much more modern society . . . a much more bourgeois society'. Altrincham expresses himself to be 'amazed that anybody can use such language' about a country 'more mysterious than ever', lacking in personal freedoms – 'especially the freedom to own property' – and 'reactionary' despite its material progress. 'Obviously', he writes, 'Mr. Khruschev has quarrelled with the Chinese. But does this mean that he is any less of a dedicated Communist, any less interested in conquering the world for communism than Mao Tse-Tung?'*] Thereafter, to domiciliary visit: probably coronary thrombosis, blood pressure nil, *in extremis* (Mrs. N.T., aet 59, Denton, admitted). Returned home to continue reading. At 8.0 p.m. to the Opera House with Judy to see *The Ides of March*, based on the novel by Thornton Wilder, with Marie Lohr, Irene Worth, and John Gielgud as Julius Caesar; excellent.

July 21   Awoke at 2.0 a.m., and again at 4.0 a.m. Read a little and then slept to 10 a.m. After lunch, tidied shelves in library, and read Dr. Antommarchi's report on the post-mortem which he conducted [*in 1821*] on Napoleon. Watched Sir Fitzroy Maclean talking about Moscow, and heard Bach Harpsichord Concerto in C from Zurich. Some praecordial pain today.

July 22   Full Ward Rounds, 12 and 15; poor Mrs. N.T. [*see July 20*] died of a massive infarction. After lunch, to St. John St., 3 cases. Home at 6.0 p.m.; gave Judy private press edition (1929) of the *Poems of Catullus*, discovered yesterday while dusting and rearranging books. Dr. O'C. rang; the Irish in general practice are a queer lot.

July 23   Two letters from M. She is coming home on Thursday (July 25); thank God. To Anti-coagulant clinic and Ward Round, 7. Sent telegram from hospital to Dr. Mc. [*local general practitioner*], another bloody Irishman, reminding him again about my domiciliary forms, overdue since the 15th inst. Bought chocolates, 5/6d, and straight home thereafter at 4.0 p.m.; many zombies on the road, driving selfishly.

July 25   10.30 a.m., attendance at Crown Court No.5 before Mr. Justice Gorman; medical evidence given in Witness Box. St. John St., 3 cases, including inspector of AGIP petrol stations, 15st. 10lbs; during afternoon, M. phoned from London on arrival. Home at 6.0 p.m; M. looks well. Partial test-ban treaty between Russia, USA and Britain ready for signature.

July 28 [*Sunday*]   Fine sunny weather today. Report on Skopje earthquake in Yugoslavia; vast exodus of holiday makers to the coast and Continent. But nothing of sterling note in Sunday papers; many comments on Nuclear Test-Ban agreement, a boring subject by now.

July 29   After lunch, to St. John St., 3 cases.

4:15 p.m. [*Female, aged 20, Inland Revenue clerk and housewife*] She was a healthy looking young lady who fell off a motor cycle on Whit Sunday a year ago, while riding pillion with her fiancé, whom she has since married. (She said that the motor cycle fell on top of her). She suffered bruises and abrasions to the right arm, right thigh and right calf, and was shocked. She did not knock her head, and was wearing a helmet. She said there were 'very few people about', but a woman in an adjoining shop phoned for the police; she made a statement to them and then went home by bus. She was off work for three days, but two weeks after the accident, she told me, boils 'came out' on her 'stomach'. She complained that she had had no boils on this part of her anatomy before, but has also had none there since. (She also displayed the back of her right calf to me, intimating that I might see a scar or other disfigurement on closer observation; there was nothing to be seen whatever.) The suggestion that falling off a motor cycle could provoke boils on the stomach is beyond the remotest stretch of the imagination.

Watched 'Panorama': De Gaulle wants his own H-Bomb.

July 30   Very fine day; temperature in the 80s. To Anti-coagulant clinic; fairly hectic, my BP 160/90. Ward Rounds, 7 and 15. Opera House, 7 p.m., for premiere of 'Six of One', with Dora Bryan and Richard Wattis. Full house, sweltering heat, appalling show; one of the most ghastly I have ever seen.

July 31   Twenty-two domiciliary visits this month. Quite a good record for a July. St. John St., 4 cases, including little man with bow-tie examined twice previously, and case of myocardial ischaemia, admitted; paid 6 guineas. Stephen Ward, found guilty of living off immoral earnings, attempts suicide. Leaves 12 letters; unconscious in Hospital at present.

Aug 1   Very hot and sunny day. Ward rounds, 12 and 15; James S. [*friend*] has had a posterior infarct. Gave him 10/- I owed him. After lunch, proceeded to St. John St. One case failed to attend, leaving one case only: old publican with amputated left leg. Macmillan interview on Associated Rediffusion, evasive about his resignation. Bad news about Stephen Ward in St. Stephen's Hospital, just alive.

Aug 2   To Anti-coagulant clinic; including American, attending for (free) anti-coagulant supervision for himself, who tried to cadge a (free) consultation for his wife. He started to say she had a headache, etc. and I gave him an appropriate reply. Thence, to domiciliary visits: simple-minded spinster, undernourished and unable to look after herself (Miss N.D., aet 54, Denton, spoke to Almoner re arrangements for protection); folic acid deficiency anaemia, post-partum (aet 23, Hyde, admitted); and diabetes insipidus (aet 82, Ashton, to be admitted). Ward 15; Sister M. is emigrating to Australia at the end of the year, where her wages will be £18.0.0. per week.

Aug 3 [*Saturday*] Atrocious electricity bill for £31.11s.2d; will query it as a routine procedure. My basic salary raised to £312.3s.2d. per month = £3,745.18s.0d. p.a. Visited S.F. [*travel agent*] with M. in afternoon, to discuss next trip abroad; India and Ceylon being mooted. Returned home in pouring rain. Watched Zizi Jeanmaire dancing on television. Death of Stephen Ward announced.

Aug 4 Taking it easy; continued cataloguing my books in Main Library. Heavy rain, cold and gloomy, roads flooded. No one at the seasides. Further treasures unearthed in the 'Lumber Room', including excellent early travel books on Australia, *The Surgical Works of John Abernethy* [*1816*], and D. H. Lawrence's *Collected Short Stories*, 1140 pages, published at 8/6d in 1934 by Secker, beautifully printed. Ruth, Geoffrey and Jonathan called for tea and supper. Jonathan does not improve. He is mischievous, disobeys, strikes his father, hurls his glasses across the room, and climbs on the furniture with his boots on. So nice and quiet after they have gone. Nothing much in the papers: Stephen Ward obituaries mainly, and China's anger with Moscow over Test-Ban agreement.

Aug 5 [*Bank Holiday*] Heavy rain, one of the worst Bank Holidays in living memory. Was thinking of a pleasant, restful day with M. – just the two of us – but, alas, the phone went at 9.30 a.m. while I was reading in bed. Called to Prestbury to see B.A. [*daughter of friend*], aet 27, complaining of abdominal pain. Diagnosis: dysmenorrhea and depression, lachrymose. Heard of very sad goings on, between her and married man, from her mother, who is herself unhappy and frustrated. Came home with her father, and discussed case on phone with M.C. [*psychiatrist*]; found 25 tabs of Librium which I gave him for her, 10 mgm to be taken three times a day. Felt very drowsy after lunch; siesta with M. Further pleasant cataloguing thereafter: John Hunter on *Human Teeth*

(1771) and Wm. Harvey's *Anatomical Excercitations* (1653).
Watched Alan Whicker in Texas, and 'Panorama': signing
of Test-Ban Treaty in Moscow (direct vision). Sat up until
1.30 a.m. reading book reviews, including of Yevtushenko's
Autobiography, unjustly slated by Toynbee in the *Observer*.

Aug 7   To Arnfields, and domiciliary visit: cerebral
vascular lesion, hypertension, congestive heart failure (aet
50, Dukinfield, admitted). Thence to hospital; felt rather low
and depressed, my BP 160/95. Thereafter, to St. John St.
in pouring rain, 3 cases. David and Hazel came for tea and
dinner. Gave David £25.0.0. for a 3-piece suite, as promised.
M. took the visit very well, and the atmosphere was quite
pleasant. I am happy that it went off so well. Listened to
Brahms' Fourth Symphony on radio.

Aug 8   Went reluctantly to hospital; no wards today.
To St. John St. for siesta, to 2.50 p.m.; thereafter, 2 cases. I
like the leisurely pace of my work at present. Any faster tempo
would be unwelcome. Home at 6.0 p.m. Pleasant supper
with M., but chaos thereafter; chicken-man [*who delivered the
weekend chicken*], electrician, radio-repairman, Ruth on phone,
etc. etc. Watched TV broadcast of 'Aida' from Verona,
with 25,000 audience in Roman amphitheatre; disturbed
by visitors. Unearthed more books, including Ibarra edition
of *Don Quixote* [*1803*], Claude Bernard on *Diabetes* [*1877*] and
Florence Nightingale's *Report* to the 1858 Royal Commission
on the Sanitary State of the Army. Announcement of terrific
mail-bag robbery of £1,000,000 from London to Glasgow
Mail train, at 3.0 a.m. this morning. [*A later correction says
'£2,600,000'.*]

Aug 9   Ward Rounds, 12 and 15. Phoned M., and
Ruth on her 24th Anniversary. Feel low and tired, very
short of breath, BP 150/90. Talked to Dr. V. during
luncheon interval; heard that Sister H. might be getting
married. Wonderful news, the only way to be rid of her.

Aug 10 [*Saturday*]   Restful morning; made breakfast
for M. and did some more exploring of interesting items.

Found nice boxes for the 2 copies of Lind's *Treatise of the Scurvy* [*1753*] and for Woodall's *Surgeon's Mate* [*1639*]. Discovered Sydenham's *Schedula Monitoria De Novae Febris Ingressu* (1686), which contains the first description of 'Sydenham's Chorea'. Collected letters at St. John St., before walking up to Palace Theatre with M. to see Bolshoi Ballet. Maya Plisetskaya, leading ballerina, superb as the Dying Swan.

Aug 11   For supper to Ruth's at 6.30 p.m. She made a good meal. Well-built greenhouse, with cucumbers and tomatoes. Worried about her; she feels sick and looks drawn. Her BP 90 mm. systolic, 4 months pregnant.

Aug 12   Bad night, nocturia 4 times. St. John St. 3 cases. More travel literature arrived by the second post. Hard to make one's mind up. Also, a letter from Judy in Germany, among the butchers of Europe.

Aug 13   Rose late; my wrist-watch had stopped. Also forgot my Methyldopa today. To Anti-coagulant clinic; a Prothrombin estimation carried out on Mrs. Y. [*private patient*] was '16 per cent', but repeated a few moments later it was reported as '90 per cent' = ineptitude of the highest possible order. Full Ward round, 15, accompanied by Drs. F., C., and D., with Sister G. After lousy hospital lunch, purchased chocolates, razor blades and 2 pieces of Imperial Leather (£1), and proceeded to domiciliary visit: ulcerative stomatitis and gingivitis (aet 24, Denton, admitted). To St. John St., to collect letters. While there, Dr. B. rang about Miss N.D. of Denton [*see Aug 2*], making unsubtle threats of the Coroner in the event of her death, if she is not admitted. Gave him the polite works, with shafts of venom. Monotonous evening, nothing constructive. The *Guardian* lost, either thrown out or destroyed. Irritating.

Aug 14   To Arnfields; nothing doing, Wakes. Ward Rounds, 12 and 14. At lunch, talked to Dr. H. about barbiturate poisoning. Thereafter, to St. John St., 6 cases.

3:0 p.m. [*Male, aged 51, grinder*] He said that four months ago he and some of his mates were 'overcome' by fumes which contained carbon monoxide, and which were wafted from an adjoining department at work. When he went outside, helped by a mate, he was 'shaking like a leaf'; he found 'about half a dozen other people' standing there, complaining of the fumes. He was thereupon taken by ambulance to hospital, where he was given an injection, admitted for 26 hours and then discharged home.

He was off work for one week, returned for a day and a half, when 'everything began going round' and he felt 'mazy', and was off work for a further six weeks under the care of his doctor, during which time he was referred to a psychiatrist. He returned for a month, but has been off work since, attending the psychiatric unit of his local hospital. He has also consulted solicitors, who have issued a writ on his behalf.

Today he told me that his legs were 'peculiar' – he has to sit down if he attempts anything manual – that he has a 'dull head' and 'yawning spasms', and that he dreams 'silly dreams'. (In one, which he said had made him 'frightened to death', he dreamt that he had committed a murder at the Town Hall, where he once worked as a porter.) However, he also said that he was 'getting better', had 'never had any previous nerve trouble', and that he had been to Bispham in July for a week's holiday. 'When are you going back to work?', I asked him. 'I'm in the hands of Dr. W. [*psychiatrist*]', he answered.

On examination, he was a healthy looking man, with regular pulse and excellent blood pressure (140/80), all of whose systems were normal. He would feel much better if he went back to work, as I told him. Instead, he was very careful how he worded his sentences, and insisted that I wrote down everything as he had said it, without altering a single word or inflexion.

Further attempts to create order in my Library. Listened in to Brahms Concert on radio.

Aug 16   Letter from Judy sent from Vienna; her adventures with boys. To domiciliary visit: congestive heart failure, cor pulmonale (aet 63, Droylsden, admitted). Thence, to Anti-coagulant clinic; American [*see Aug 2 1963*] came to nag me about his wife's giddiness, but her problem essentially is that she 'wants to go home'. Ward Round, 12. This morning, dawdled about mostly; very slack, Wakes week, Residents away, Dr. C. [*consultant physician*] off, few domiciliary visits, but talked to Dr. L. about thyrotoxicosis. Quiet evening. Train-robbers captured, remarkable achievement.

Aug 17 [*Saturday*]　　Return of Judy from Vienna; went to meet her at Central Station at 2.30 p.m., calling at St. John St. on the way. Sad news of the death of George Weldon [*associate conductor of Hallé*], in Cape Town on tour. Died in his sleep, single, aet 55. Very upset.

Aug 19　　Judy gets her 3 A-levels, 'A' in English and History. Anniversary of my Mother's Death 13 years ago; may her dear soul rest in peace (light kindled).

Aug 20　　Ward Rounds, 12 and 15. After lunch, to Manchester University Medical Library: chat to Wilson [*librarian*]. Things may be moving nearer an exchange of volumes. Home for siesta. Later, watched fascinating TV programme on Abraham Lincoln's promise, 100 years ago, to the Negroes, not kept by his successors. Interviews with prominent U.S. negro leaders, Dr. Stephen Clark, James Baldwin, Reverend Luther King and others. Also Malcolm X of the Muslim Brotherhood preaching Negro superiority, militant and aggressive.

Aug 21　　Purchased Mrs. Robert Moss King, *The Diary of a Civilian's Wife in India, 1877–1882*, 2 vols, with numerous illustrations, London, 1884; original brown cloth, octavo, mint condition, £1.5s.0d.; a bargain, I think. Lunch at Masonic and to St. John St., 5 cases, including intelligent boy of 12 with headaches ('like a thumping all over'), and a myocardial ischaemia with angina of effort; an unpleasant smart alec trying to get things on the cheap.

Aug 22　　Full ward rounds today, 7, 12, 14, and 15.

After lunch, phoned M. Thence to Medical Library; saw Wilson, hopeless fool. He is about the laziest loon I ever saw, books generally in poor condition, situation worse than ever.

Aug 24 [*Saturday*]   Further clearing in play-room: found interesting prints, catalogues, books, letters etc. Much rubbish. Made tea for TV repair-man, and watched Test-Match, M. at synagogue. Further afternoon session of clearing. Walk with M. to local bookshop; the owner a shifty sort of fellow.

Aug 25   My Wedding Anniversary, the 27th. God bless M., the children and grandchild, and the yet unborn one. Ruth phoned; the only telegram was received from them. Israeli and Syrian border-clashes. To wedding reception for Felix C.'s daughter, and thereafter to further party at the Lindemanns [*friends*]. Feel unrested today. Gave lifts left, right and centre, to and from parties, including to Carlebach's cousin from Belfast, and his two daughters doing Classics, with few thank-yous. Rabbis are particularly ill-mannered.

Aug 27   Arose early, suffering from infected insect-bite at bridge of nose; antibiotics (Tetracycline, 1 gm) taken today, with much relief. Took M. and Judy to Central Station for 9.25 a.m. train to London, fixing up 'digs' for Judy. To St. John St., for mail; asked M.F. [*consultant surgeon who had rooms in same building*] about my 'conk'. He advocated broad-spectrum antibiotics. Back home exhausted.

Aug 28   Awoke at 2.0 a.m. to read an article on Spain by James Morris in yesterday's *Manchester Guardian*. [*Entitled 'Spain's shrunken autocracy' the article has been attached to the day's entry. In it Morris says that contemporary Spain, 'urged on by the momentum of the world outside', is 'unmistakably on the move'. Morris notes the 'immense new gusto and magnetism of Europe' and the 'growing prosperity of the people, the queues of foreign cars along the Costa del Sol and the television sets in the shop windows' while 'there in the middle the dictator sits, an ageing veteran of the blackshirt era'. Morris describes him as a 'plump and unprepossessing figure', whose 'Cause' is being negated by 'almost everything that is lively, promising* *and reassuring about the New Spain'.*] Judy has been fixed up in Hampstead at £7 a week, with 8 guineas retainer. Freedom March in USA by Negroes; mass rally in Washington. Nose improving on antibiotics.

Aug 29   To St. John St., 2 cases.

3:45 p.m. [*Female, aged 41, housewife*] She said she was of 'intellectual background', and Hungarian Jewish by birth. At the age of 22, in April 1944, she was sent to Auschwitz, where her parents and other members of her family died; 'they have taken all my family', she stated. She was in Auschwitz until January 1945, and was then transferred to Belsen, until April 1945. In these camps she suffered scarlet fever, typhus and frostbite from exposure, tattooing of the left arm, beatings and starvation. During this time, she said that her monthly periods ceased. She also spoke about the forced labour, 'regulating the soil at the edge of the river in winter', and described to me the cold showers at 2.0 a.m. 'in a small room with broken windows' at Auschwitz, 'where there were no towels'.

Today, she complained of 'nightmares', in which she feels as if someone is 'chasing' her and she 'cant get away'; backache, 'especially between the shoulder blades', radiating to the small of the back which sometimes 'locks' her in a position so that she 'cannot move'; 'swollen eyes'; and 'very bad nerves'. She also said that she could not concentrate on anything 'for more than half an hour'. 'All these complaints have come since my starvation and ill-treatment', she added.

On examination, her blood pressure was normal, there was no evidence of thyrotoxicosis, or of any serious organic disability, though she had treatment for 'kidney trouble' in 1947, and her rheumatic pain is undoubted. She also had an intermittently aggressive and unsympathetic demeanour ('to qualify for any compensation, at least 25 per cent disablement is necessary', she said to me), but she has endured atrocious sufferings at the hands of an evil race of persecutors. She has recently been examined by Dr. X.Y., who showed her, she says, no sympathy for what she has experienced. (If so, he is a bastard). 'I was in excellent health before I went into the camps,' she said to me; 'now I have permanent nightmares'. A dreadful case.

Home for supper alone; opened a tin of salmon, and listened to Bach and Purcell on the Third Programme.

Aug 31 [*Saturday*]   31 domiciliary visits so far this quarter, 13 for August. 'Spring cleaning' in main Library; pamphlets and early medicine etc. sorted out, and some Maggs and Quaritch catalogues cleaned and backed [*wrapped in paper*]. The dust ruins them. Gave Judy a copy of Drucker on Renoir, very comprehensive, a quarto volume of his reproductions, text in French. It cost me 4 guineas. Called at Ruth and Geoffrey's house [*they were away*]; inspected hot-house, and took some tomatoes.

Sept 2   Chat to Judy, in her Youth and Happiness.

Sept 3   At lunch, discussed steroid withdrawal case [*see Sept 4*] with Dr. V.; a report to be sent tomorrow. To St. John St., one case only. In the evening, watched excellent TV film on Guatemala, with commentary by Alan Whicker.

Sept 4   Woke up late, at 8.30 a.m.; no nocturia. To Arnfield's; examination of 7 apprentices. Dictated report re A.R. (deceased), the steroid withdrawal case. [*In this case, he had been asked for advice by a firm of solicitors about the accidental sudden reduction, as the result of a misunderstanding between a General Practitioner and a Chemist, of a patient's steroid treatment; the man suffered from asthma and rheumatoid arthritis, and had a heart attack two days after the reduction (to one third) of the dosage, and died shortly thereafter. He wrote that* 'the reduction may have contributed to his death, but it is well to know that sudden death can occur in asthmatics on steroids whether the drug is withdrawn or not. In fact, asthmatics who are on steroids are arguably more prone to sudden death than those who are not. Nevertheless, a sudden reduction might easily have "rocked the boat" and precipitated his disintegration . . . But there is much to be clarified before rushing headlong into a case of this sort; accusations of incompetence cannot be made without careful appraisal. For example, if this patient's death is alleged to be due to acute adrenal insufficiency, promoted by a sudden diminution of steroids, it is necessary to know what features of it, if any, appeared during the last few days of his life. Thus, was there salt deficiency in the blood? Were there other disturbances in the blood chemistry, the signs of which are lassitude, fatigue, listlessness and a fall in blood pressure, followed by rapid deterioration? It is important, to begin with, to know the mode of death; that is, how he died . . .' *Nearly four months later, on Dec 30 1963, 'with the major part of my questions unanswered', and with 'only vague information given to me', he wrote that 'no useful purpose will be served in proceeding with this case.'*]

Sept 5   Eating too much again. Dreadful air disaster yesterday; 80 dead near Zurich, Swissair Caravelle, crashed 5 minutes after take-off on way to Rome. A mystery. Purchased chicken for Miss James's 65th Birthday. To lunch at Masonic; chat with Dick H. [*stockbroker*], no season for investments at present. St. John St., 6 cases, too many to deal with, including a potato-merchant.

Sept 6   Ward Rounds, 14 and 15, including case of thrombocytopenic purpura; shown to Mr. C. [*surgeon*] for splenectomy. After lunch, medical out-patients; also saw Mrs. F. [*gynaecologist*], with painful 'rheumatic' left elbow; treatment arranged for her. Thereafter, to St. John St., for letters; noted that yesterday's potato merchant had not kept his promise about the potatoes, which he said he would deliver at St. John St. People are very glib with their promises; cf. the man who promised samples of soap. Still waiting.

Sept 7 [*Saturday*]   Some further 'spring cleaning'. Death of J.G. Wilson reported, aged 87, late of Bumpus [*the old-established Oxford Street, London, booksellers of which Wilson, a Scot and friend of Shaw, Edward Garnett, Forster, Walter de la Mare and many other writers, had been managing director*]. Happy memories of him, of his courtesy and hospitality, and of snack lunches with him. Purchased Woodall's *Surgeon's Mate* [*see Aug 10 1963*] from him.

[Attached to today's entry, without explanation – though it may have been found during the day's 'spring-cleaning' – is an article by Sir Hugh Walpole, 'Things that Remain', from the Listener *of July 25th 1940. In it, Walpole tells how on a 'lovely June evening' that year, at his home in the Lake District – with its 'rose garden, rock garden, bees and a library with fifteen thousand books' – he had heard 'terrible' news of the war on his radio. 'I looked out on my acre of ground', Walpole writes, 'and knew that it was all in this world, beside work, friends and health that I wanted . . . At that exact moment, I saw my acre taken from me, the concentration camp, the loss of my freedom.' He then describes how his 'panic' is allayed by the sound of a broadcast of a Beethoven Trio, by a 'picture above my mantelpiece by Utrillo', and by reading one of his favourite passages from* David Copperfield. *'Like every other man', Walpole concludes, 'I have known great disappointments – in myself, my ambitions, my friends, world events – from time to time. But books have never disappointed me, pictures have radiantly encouraged me, music has carried me forward . . . These are the things in which we may always trust.']*

Sept 10   Early domiciliary visit: J.H., broncho-pneumonia, C_2H_5OH (aet 50, Stalybridge, admitted); a schoolmaster who recently killed 2 people when drunk-in-charge, and spent 6 months in prison. Ward Round, 15. After lunch, visited Wilson at the Medical Library. His dilatory manner exasperated me. I told him that I had ceased to be interested in his piffling scientific pamphlets, and would have nothing to do with him unless he contacted me first. I think I have now done with him; his books are in a frightful state, and unworthy to be in my Library. Thereafter, to St. John St.; no letters. Home at 5.30 p.m. Wrote letter to Woodall [*local builder and repairer*] about his recent rudeness to M., when he came round like an infuriated bull, after I had complained of his unsatisfactory work.

Sept 11   *Manchester Guardian* did not arrive at usual ᵗime. Visited P.W. [*private patient with 'grossly severe hypertension'*] ᵃrd 15; discovered that the imbeciles had not yet started Methyldopa, although I had asked for it 3 days ago. ᵒ him personally. He said he felt better 3½ minutes later! Obviously a neurotic also. Heard today that L. of Glossop [*a Jewish 'brush manufacturer'*] had died of aplastic leukaemia. He was cremated at Dukinfield Cemetery and his ashes were scattered in Glossop Churchyard; no religious service was held. Depressed at home this evening; Judy's conduct the cause.

Sept 12   Admissions slack at hospital. Visited Wards 14 and 15; discharged 4 males. After poor lunch proceeded to St. John St.; two cases.

3:0 p.m. [*Male, aged 37, labourer*] He was a miserable-looking fellow with 7 children, aged from 2 to 11. While pushing a barrow of sand under a low girder (at 11.10 on a Saturday morning) 9 months ago, he said that he 'straightened up too quickly', and struck the lower part of his spine on the girder.

He claimed that he was in bed for the first two or three days, during which time his doctor gave him a 'rubbing liniment', and tablets to 'ease the pain'. Thereafter, apart from consulting solicitors and making a claim for damages, he 'started having blackouts' and began to lose the 'use' of his 'legs and arms'; during these 'blackouts' – his wife told him, and he told me – he was 'crying'. His doctor, who has found nothing organically wrong with him, referred him to a psychiatrist, who has since been treating him with 'blue' tablets and 'thick' medicine. 'Coming out of the post office' eight weeks ago, he continued, 'everything went dizzy', and he felt as if he was 'spinning round'; he said that he 'fell against the wall', but 'got home all right'. (Note how these types never fall in front of buses.)

Today, nine months after bumping his back, he said that if he walks any distance his back 'starts aching' ('it aches now', he added); that he feels tired; that he keeps having headaches 'like pains' at the back of his head; that his appetite is poor and that he takes 'sleeping capsules'. 'I want to go back [*to work*] but I dont know when I shall be able', he said to me; 'but I am not as bad as I were', he added.

On examination, he had normal blood pressure (120/70), a very rapid pulse (120, nervous tachycardia) and nothing wrong with his back, though he jumped whenever he was touched. This is a case of a trivial injury which has fallen on poor soil, and produced a gross neurosis; his rapid heart-beat, his only real symptom, is due to this neurosis. Types like him usually profess an anxiety to 'go back to work', but they never do until everything is settled to their satisfaction. I told him that there was no reason why he should not try to do something to rehabilitate himself; but I know he will not try, and that even if he did he would start flopping all over the place at the outset. [*A supplementary note reads: 'Good case for presentation to MRCP Class'.*]

Visited G.H., Miss James's friend, at her flat. Cancer of ovaries, tragic state of affairs. She knows not her fate. Further tidying in upstairs room; found Christopher Sympson on *Music* (1727), a pleasant little book, and a good Mormon Collection, of intrinsic value. Terrible air crash of Viking near Perpignan; charter-plane, British tourists on way to Costa Brava. No survivors, 36 passengers and 4 crew, many young couples. French radar inadequate it appears, or non-existent.

Sept 14 [*Saturday*]   Home by 1.0 p.m. After siesta, did further tidying up. Much rubbish eliminated. Gave Judy some Owenite and anti-Owenite Tracts, 1830. To the Josephs after dinner, for champagne celebration of the birth of their grandchild. Pleasant evening; home by 11.30 p.m., and so to bed. Made myself tea at 1.45 a.m. and entered this journal after reading a few *Listeners* of 1957 vintage. Poem on 'Death' attached hereto, rather striking. [*By K.W. Gransden, it appeared in the* Listener *of April 11th 1957. 'And our turn will come, our turn will come,' writes the poet; 'not a newspaper death, an undifferentiated death / At which you can shrug your shoulders and turn to another page – / But a death for you to deal with.'*]

Sept 15   Disturbed and restless night. Decided to take Japan trip with British Scandinavian Study Group [*on Oct 13, for one month*]. Fine and sunny day, 80°F. No siesta.

Sept 17   Talked to Dr. V. [*consultant physician*], a queer fellow, I must say. Also saw E.E.; he seemed to imply that my Masonic promotion is nigh. Dr. N. [*friend*] telephoned, distressed in General Practice. He said he loathes it.

Sept 18   Eve of New Year, went to synagogue. I miss David to complete the circle. Fair amount of general depression.

Sept 19   Many New Year cards. To synagogue at 10.30 a.m.: good sermon, well phrased, but service frightfully uninteresting. Home by 1.0 p.m. David and Hazel arrive from Stratford-upon-Avon. Began to sort out the books David wants to take from his study. To St. John St., 2 cases; young girls (aet 18 and 21) who are next-door neighbours, involved in an accident together. Home, to continue disposal of books with David, which he stuffed in the boot of his car. Judy 'rude' (??) to M. at tea, in front of Hazel and David; M. very sensitive in front of the visitors, but Judy non-apologetic. All this adds to my depression, and occasional anxiety about continuing this harassing type of existence.

Sept 21 [*Saturday*]   M. nags me, Judy is rude to me. I left home in a hurry, on verge of collapse. Cumulative exploitation of my resources by parasitic children; no paranoia about it. To St. John St.; tidied shelves in bookcase. Proceeded to Walmsley's bookshop. Conclusions: he is an ass who knows nothing about his books, charges too much and is parsimonious. Will not call for some time now. Had a mind to prolong my absence, but home by 1.45 p.m. Broke down and wept. Survey of my wasted life, bringing up useless children. Very depressed and despondent. Am seriously considering stopping financial assistance for Judy's education. Read *Bart's Hospital Journal* and *Guardian*, thoroughly. Did more shelf-arranging. Soothes me.

Sept 22   Slept in Guest-Room and felt rested. My Library as chaotic as ever. Read the *Observer*, which has reprinted part of one act of a play [*Hochhuth's The Representative*] attacking Pius XII, justifiably, for his silence during the murders of millions of Jews. First injection against cholera for M. and I, passport photos signed, etc. Everything almost ready [*for visit to Japan*]. Mist and fog appearing.

Sept 23   Watched 'Panorama' on a) Destalinization of Czechoslovakia; b) Conservative MPs on the Next Election and Leadership of Party; c) Interviews with Governor Wallace and Fascist Youths in Birmingham, Alabama. Funeral of Negro children after Bomb explosion in Church.

Sept 24   Heavy rain. Am much better after cholera injection. Two domiciliary visits: multiple sclerosis (aet 44, Denton, needs electrically-controlled wheelchair), and mongol, deteriorating (aet 41, Denton, arranged out-patient investigation). To Lodge meeting at 5.30 p.m.; a very good ceremony indeed by Sam F. [*Worshipful Master*], his last. Home by 10.0 p.m. Listened to David Oistrakh playing Brahms' Violin Concerto; went to sleep in the middle of it.

Sept 25   Arose at 7.0 a.m. and entered this logbook for yesterday. Made breakfast for M., God bless her. Proceeded to domiciliary visits: congestive heart failure (aet 59, Hr. Openshaw, to be admitted tomorrow); and coronary thrombosis (aet 60, Ashton, admitted). St John St., 3 cases.

4:20 p.m. [*Female, aged 40, housewife*] She was an intelligent and attractive woman, pale in appearance, who, when she came into the room, seemed depressed and anxious. She told me that she has 'always had her hair bleached once a month', and 'washed and set' twice a week, procedures which she has had regularly carried out for the last fifteen months at a local hairdressers', the Maison D. (When I asked her about this activity she admitted that she had always been preoccupied about her hair; 'it used to be very beautiful', she said.) Two months ago, she was prevailed on by an agent of X. Products to try a 'guaranteed Perm' at the Maison D. One week thereafter, last July, her hair started to come out on the right side of her head; she screamed when she saw the hair on her towel. Her doctor told her it was 'nerves', but she was subsequently unable to 'eat or sleep', and still cannot do so. Today, she said she has a feeling as if 'something is crawling' across her head, is sleepless, never wants to go out, smokes 20 cigarettes a day, and has 'sick headaches'.

She lost her first husband; they had two small sons, whom she brought up alone. Eight years ago she married again; two years ago she had a child who died a few days after birth. This incident of her hair loss has now supervened, and the distress it has induced seems to have led to the cooling of her second husband's affections. 'He has not been coming home', she said; 'it has definitely caused a break', she added. When I asked her what she meant, she said that she used to have sexual intercourse 'two or three times a week', but 'had only had it once in the last 6 weeks'. (At this point, she repeated that 'he sometimes comes in at 2 or 3 o'clock in the morning, without kissing me like he used to').

On examination, she had had her hair cut short; its colour was not uniformly blonde since she has been unable fully to attend to the bleaching of it in the recent period. Her blood pressure was normal, but her pulse was rapid and irregular; and there were three scabs on the right side of her head. This poor woman is simultaneously preoccupied with her hair and with her marital relations. (In fact, she seemed to consider the affection of her husband and the condition of her hair to be of equal importance.) But considering all the shocks to her nervous system she has suffered in the past, the loss of her hair has come as a severe blow; it easily explains her own attitude to it, her depression, sleeplessness etc. However, there is no likelihood whatever of permanent damage to her hair, as I told her. Rather, it is her nervous state, aggravated by her concern for her appearance, which is probably retarding the hair growth. What she has to do now, I said, is to leave her hair to grow back again without fiddling with it, or scratching her head. I told her I would see her again in three months' time. [*An additional Ms. note reads: 'Tragic life'.*]

Sept 27   Did no Anti-coagulants today. Dr. V., a queer bird, looks stormy. Ward Rounds, 12 and 15; told by Mr. J.H., schoolmaster [*see Sept 10*], that I am 'a character'. Fruit purchased, 19/-. After lunch, Medical out-patients, short session. Home early, before the 'Black Fast' begins [*for the Day of Atonement*]. M. depressed; David silent so far. Reading *Meeting With Japan* by Fosco Maraini; nicely got-up book, but hard going in parts. To eve of Day of Atonement Service, dull as usual; got soaked in the rain walking home afterwards.

Sept 28   Day of Atonement. David telephoned first thing this morning; in M. a faint glint of joy as a result. She does not look well; the holiday will do her good. Read Neville Cardus on John Barbirolli's 20 years' service to the Hallé; he is receiving a gold medal at tomorrow's Hallé concert, seats sold out, Artur Rubinstein playing. Proceeded to synagogue; returned home with Judy for lunch at 2.15 p.m. She leaves tomorrow for London, and then M. and I will be alone. Back to the synagogue at 5.45 p.m., and home in time to see *That Was The Week That Was*; splendid satire, with Sir Cyril Osborne and Bernard Levin, and including a song on Pius XII. M. flattened out by useless Fast.

Sept 29   Poor night, disturbed at 2.0 a.m. by loud bang: aircraft breaking sound-barrier, picture falling down, or burglar jumping in through window? Went down to make tea for M. and self. Wakened by Judy at 7.45 a.m. We got ready, and M. and I (and her friend Susan S.) took her to Central Station to get the 10 a.m. for London; she then left us for University. Have stood up to a great deal of rudeness from her in the past years; can hardly claim to have gained their [*his children's*] respect and love. If I have, there has been a signal absence of practical, demonstrative behaviour to warrant such an assumption. David's silence for three years and his contemptible treatment of his parents, Judy's rudeness, and Ruth's blatantly mercenary attitudes and indifference have made me cynical, and glad to be free of them. Thank God M. is here, to share my remaining years. Later phoned Judy at her new abode; no reply. Phoned David; Hazel answered. He is in bed with a chill; cycling excursion on Day of Atonement!

Oct 2   Woke up at 5.0 a.m., and collated Robert Boyle's *Medicinal Experiments, or a Collection of Choice and Safe Remedies*, 3rd Edition, 1696. Lacks frontispiece portrait and twenty terminal pages. Also collated 4th edition, 1703, complete as in Fulton [*bibliography of Boyle's works*]. To Dr. J., for second cholera injection. He nearly murdered me; gave me painful arm with discomfort, a rotten injection. St. John St., 3 cases, including Her Majesty's Coroner for City of Manchester; 400 Inquests and 2,500 post-mortems per annum.

Oct 3   Not going to hospital today. To St. John St. for letters, and proceeded thereafter to Masonic Temple; saw H.W. [*Masonic official*] re overpayment of donations to Benevolent Fund. I have paid double throughout in error, thanks to X.'s objectionable touting. St. John St., 3 cases. Home by 6.20 p.m., to find letter from Judy, with her first impressions. She does not like her digs, but appears overwhelmed with college life and its activities; long may it last.

Oct 4   To Anti-coagulant clinic; E.E. [*freemason and patient*] attends. Talk re Masonic promotions; quite on the cards that I have been promoted. Proceeded to Ward rounds, 12, 14 and 15. Thereafter, talked to Dr. S. in the Cancer and Radium Clinic, who said there had been no real progress in the last 10 years for the bulk of Mammary Cancers. Total cost of Japanese trip so far £1,104.8s.7d., with passports and visas yet to arrive. After poor lunch, Medical out-patients; energetic today, feel well, thank God.

Oct 5 [*Saturday*]   At home all day, reading and tidying. Generally depressed. Read *Guardian*, and Maraini on Japan. Phoned Miss James [*receptionist*] and asked her to lunch. She could not come; there is something horribly impudent in her demeanour. Distressed to hear from Judy today that she is unhappy at her digs; her landlady, it seems, is a prying woman of low intelligence, who is charging 7 guineas per week for very little comfort.

Oct 6   Did some 'spring cleaning', and found a volume of works by Fabrizzi [*Hieronymus Fabricius*] of Padua, pupil and successor of Fallopius, and one of the greatest of all teachers of Anatomy, who taught Wm. Harvey. My copy contains writings On the Formation of the Foetus in the human and in a calf; on the Development of the Chick; On The Structure of the Pharynx; and On The Openings of the Veins. To bed early to read *Sunday Times* and *Observer*: criticism of method of choice of Tory leader as 'undemocratic', oppression of the Jews in Russia, and trouble in South Vietnam. My usual apprehension building up prior to plane flight. God will be with us.

Oct 8   To domiciliary visit: anxiety state and depression, old case of electro-convulsion therapy 15 years ago (aet 73, Denton, not admitted). Harold Macmillan admitted to Hospital for prostatic obstruction, on the eve of the Conservative conference; great excitement in the Establishment Camp.

Oct 10   Dreadful disaster in N. Italy: bursting of dam which flooded valley in the night. 3,000 dead, bodies washed down for 6 miles. Cancelled newspapers, magazines for one month. Ward Rounds, 12, 14, 15; am glad to be getting away from the evil R. [*consultant surgeon*]. St. John St., 5 cases.

3:20 p.m. [*Male, aged 55, widower, 'steam-raiser, lights railway-engine fires'*] He was thin and emaciated, and had a hoarse voice which was hardly audible. He told me he had had bronchitis in the winter-time 'for years' – 'about twelve to fourteen years' – but that this year it had become 'worse than ever'. He also said that he has been losing weight, 'over a stone since last February', has a 'hard' cough, occasionally expectorates blood, is short of breath, and has lost his voice 'since August'. He sleeps well, but has a poor appetite. He told me, too, that he had smoked 20 cigarettes a day 'since leaving school'; he still smokes '10 a day', despite his condition, and has an 'occasional Guinness'. On examination, I noted that he was markedly short of breath on dressing and undressing, that there was an impaired percussion note at the right apex of his lungs and posteriorly, with diminished breath sounds, his chest expansion was 1½" (35" to 36½") and that his blood pressure was low (110/80). His cough was unproductive; the sort of cough which occurs in malignant growths of the throat or lungs, pressing upon the nerve supply to the vocal cords.

The poor man is suffering either from cancer of the lung or a carcinoma of the bronchus, and it is probably inoperable. He, of course, is unaware of all this. He said to me towards the end of our conversation that he thought he was going to get better. I doubt it very much.

Home by 6.30 p.m. Harold Macmillan has had his prostatectomy today, and promises to resign before the next election; Lord Hailsham has announced his wish to give up his peerage and stand for parliament, if a constituency will accept him.

Oct 12 [*Saturday*]   To hospital. Signed all reports and letters up to date, gave key to St. John St. to Miss Miller, and paid her up to date, plus fares and postage, £2.10s.0d. Saw Mrs. A. [*private patient*] in Ward 11, improving. Also visited case of surgical emphysema in Ward 1 for Mr. H. [*consultant surgeon*]; very extensive, felt as low down as the wrists, patient gravely ill. Home at 4.0 p.m., to find that a beautiful book had arrived: Norma Russell's *Bibliography of Wm. Cowper to 1837*, Oxford Bibliographical Society (1963).

*

There are no further journal entries until Nov 13, nor any other record of his visit to the Far East. A page of notes on Japan, however – with the words 'to avoid sensationalism' pencilled in the margin – sets out, perhaps for the purposes of a talk, details of Japanese geography ('get map'), population statistics ('625 inhabitants per square mile'), economy, religion, language ('Japan has the lowest illiteracy rate in the world, 0.3%, and three of the largest circulating newspapers on earth, with 35 million copies sold every day of each one'), and ceremonial customs. On the last, he writes that 'the Japanese are a courteous people, and their traditional politeness dictates the form and manner in which everything is done . . . For reasons of class, age, sex, seniority in the family, no Japanese is considered another's equal: one of the two must show deference to the other.' Another matter which is noted is that 'the Japanese belong to several religions and may practice more than one religion at a time'.

*

Nov 13   Arrived late in London, at 11.0 a.m.; transferred by BEA to charter company for flight to Speke Airport. Poor plane, but smooth landing, and driven home by taxi; 5/- tip to driver. Opened part of my mail: many catalogues (heaven knows when I will get cracking on perusing them). To bed by 8.0 p.m., dead beat. David telephoned from Stratford-upon-Avon. He is broke; frightening thought. Am depressed by his beatnik existence.

Nov 14   Went down at 4.20 a.m., and completed going through my Mail until 6.40 a.m. Had tea with M., and then returned to bed until 8. Proceeded to hospital. Saw Dr. F., who looked harassed; Dr. V. as mad as a hatter, he stated. Lunch at hospital; residents a lousy bunch, and poor types as doctors. Home in heavy rain and gloom.

Nov 16 [*Saturday*]   Our grandson Jonathan's third Birthday Anniversary; God bless him and his parents. Watched 'Juke Box Jury' by mistake; astonishing rubbish.

Nov 17   Nil of note; an aimless day, nothing gained.

Nov 19   To Anti-coagulant clinic; found that telephone in my room had been removed by J. [*hospital administrator*], a stupid gesture. Reported it to P. [*senior administrator*]. Dictated reports to Miss Miller, who wept on being told off for errors. Ward 12, round. Lunch at hospital and long talk to Mr. C. [*consultant surgeon*]. He confirmed the rancour and jealousy of local GPs, and their lack of goodwill towards me.

Nov 20   To St. John St., 6 cases, including L.S. of Chorley [*see June 13 1962*], with coronary spasm.

3:30 p.m. [*Male, aged 60, furnace-keeper*] He was a man in fairly sound health, but with a marked tremor of his right leg, from the hip downwards. More than five years ago, he inhaled some carbon monoxide gas when he was rekindling the furnaces at the Iron Works where he had worked all his life; he was taken to hospital, detained overnight, and discharged without special treatment. He was then off work for

23 weeks. Today, he said that he was 'not getting any better', was still unable to 'get hold of' himself, 'can't sleep' and is 'always trembling'. When I asked him whether he trembled in his sleep, he said he was not sure and went out to ask his wife, who was in the waiting room. He returned to tell me that he did.

On examination, he was in sound general health, but his right leg trembled so much that it tapped upon the floor and made my desk vibrate while I was writing at it. The tremor varied with the amount of enthusiasm with which he described his symptoms; if there had been no money at the end of this, I feel sure they would never have arisen in the first place. So far, he has secured a disability allowance for life and a lump sum of £209 compensation, so he is not doing too badly out of a whiff of carbon monoxide. I told him he would live to a ripe old age, but it did not stop his leg trembling.

5:30 p.m. [*Male, aged 24, bus-conductor, former butcher's assistant*] He was a young man of short stature who came in an hour late, and I was half inclined to send him away. He did not appear to be very alert intellectually, and he was profusely apologetic: I felt obliged to see him. Six months ago he was a passenger in a car which turned over after a collision late on a Saturday night. He received a knock on the head – which rendered him unconscious – and he was kept in hospital overnight; no fractures were found, and three weeks later he resumed work as a butcher's assistant. However, he found that he 'could not lift the meat' as he had pains in his back, and though he carried on as best he could for 3 months, he eventually 'had to give up'. He started work as a bus conductor on Monday [*Nov 18*].

Today, he said that he still has pains in his back when he lifts anything, that he has lost weight since the accident, that he gets headaches (which sometimes make him sick), and that he does 'not feel like going out'. A full examination of his central nervous system revealed no organic disabilities: his cranial nerves, fundi, reflexes and sensation were all normal. But there was marked tenderness over the sacrum and the sacro-iliac joints, and stooping was limited by about 40% to 50%. He winced with pain when he had to bend down.

He would obviously benefit from some physiotherapy, though working as a bus conductor will not give him much time to attend for treatment. He also still has migrainous frontal headaches as the result of the concussion he suffered; they have not yet cleared up. I thought that I ought to re-examine him in due course, perhaps in three months or so, to see what progress he has made. [*My father did not discover until July 27 1964 that the day following this encounter, Nov 21, the patient gave up his job as a bus conductor, and tried to stab himself with a pen-knife.*]

Nov 22   President Kennedy Assassinated. [*The sentence is underlined three times in red.*] Frightful news of his death came through this evening; Ruth telephoned to tell me while I was dining. A Light has gone out in the World. A criminal called Oswald captured and charged with this monstrous crime. Policeman shot dead who was chasing him. President was aged 46, shot in Dallas, Texas. Lyndon Johnson now President. In the morning Ward Rounds, 12 and 15 and Medical out-patients, long session. Thereafter, to domiciliary visit: pleural effusion, probably bronchogenic carcinoma (aet 48, Dukinfield, admitted). On way home, purchased toffees, 7/3d. Watched TV about Kennedy's death; speeches by Sir Alec Douglas-Home, Harold Wilson and Joe Grimond.

Nov 23 [*Saturday*]   Read *Guardian* about dreadful murder of the American President, and listened most of the day to World comments on this heinous crime. In afternoon, went with M. to domiciliary visit: nephrotic syndrome, deep venous thrombosis (aet 63, Ashton, admitted). Proceeded with M. and her new hair-style to the Livingstones, for tea. Came home at 7.0 p.m., approximately, in time to see young man obviously loitering in the grounds with intent. Phoned the police, who were fairly prompt and arrived in car-loads. In the meantime, the loiterer had decamped. Listened to 'The Meistersingers' and watched TV (BBC) on the death of John F. Kennedy, with film of his murder and excerpts from his speeches. A great tragedy has befallen the World.

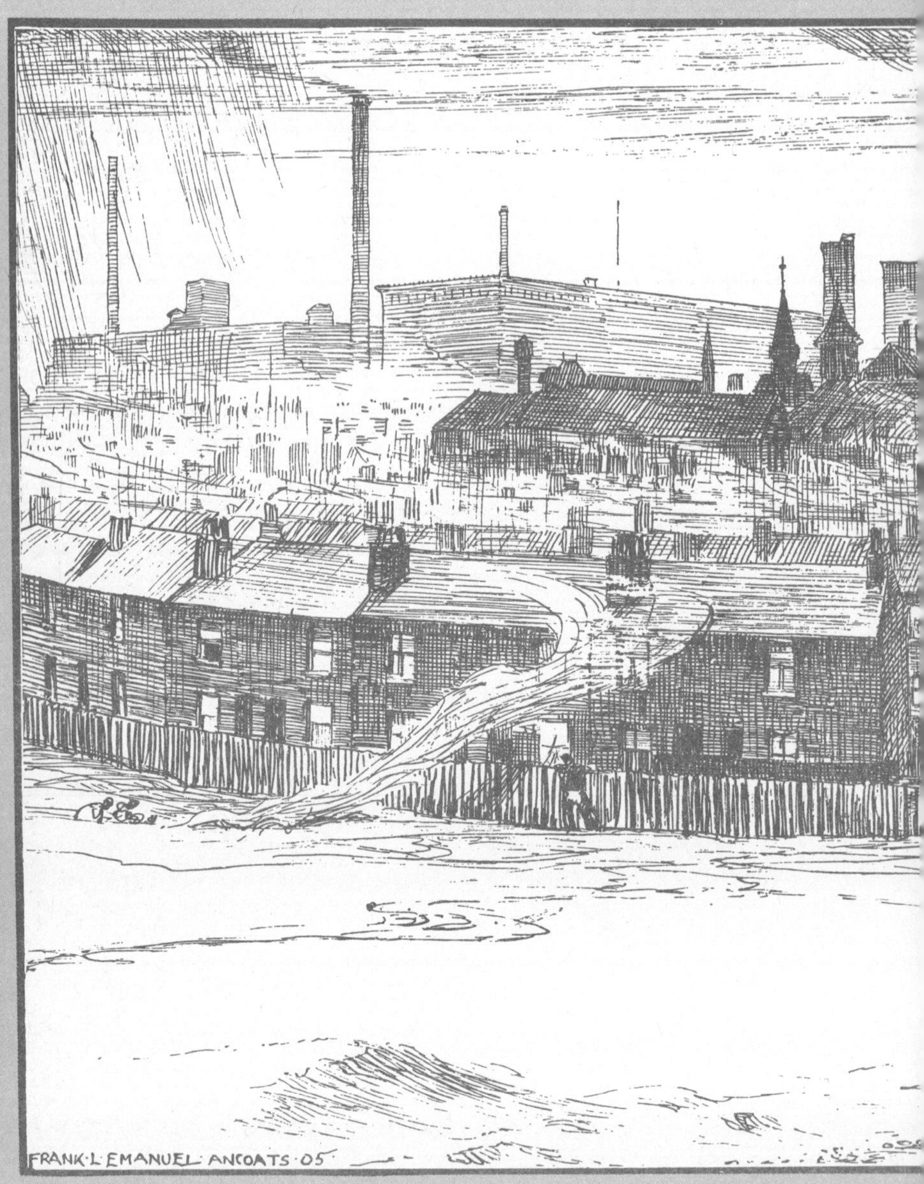

FRANK·L·EMANUEL·ANCOATS·05